Epidemic Encounters

Epidemic Encounters

Influenza, Society, and Culture in Canada, 1918-20

EDITED BY

MAGDA FAHRNI AND ESYLLT W. JONES

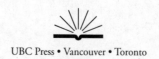

UBC Press • Vancouver • Toronto

20 19 18 17 16 15 14 13 12 11   5 4 3 2 1

Printed in Canada on FSC-certified ancient-forest-free paper
(100% post-consumer recycled) that is processed chlorine- and acid-free.

Library and Archives Canada Cataloguing in Publication

Epidemic encounters : influenza, society, and culture in Canada, 1918-20 /
edited by Magda Fahrni and Esyllt W. Jones.

Includes bibliographical references and index.
Issued also in electronic formats.
ISBN 978-0-7748-2212-1

1. Influenza Epidemic, 1918-1919 – Canada – History. 2. Influenza Epidemic,
1918-1919 – Social aspects – Canada. 3. World War, 1914-1918 – Health aspects –
Canada. 4. Medical care – Canada – History – 20th century. 5. Canada –
Historiography. I. Fahrni, Magdalena. II. Jones, Esyllt Wynne

RC150.55.C3E65 2012   614.5'18097109041   C2012-901036-7

Canada

UBC Press gratefully acknowledges the financial support for our publishing
program of the Government of Canada (through the Canada Book Fund), the
Canada Council for the Arts, and the British Columbia Arts Council.

This book has been published with the help of a grant from the Canadian Federation
for the Humanities and Social Sciences, through the Aid to Scholarly Publications
Program, using funds provided by the Social Sciences and Humanities Research
Council of Canada.

Cover illustration credit: "The Sœurs du Bon-Pasteur de Québec, like other female
religious communities, devoted themselves to the care of influenza victims during
the great pandemic." *Source:* "Des religieuses qui soignent les victimes de la grippe
espagnole," inconnu; Archives des Sœurs du Bon-Pasteur de Québec, Serge
Gaudreau, 2520.

UBC Press
The University of British Columbia
2029 West Mall
Vancouver, BC V6T 1Z2
www.ubcpress.ca

Contents

Figures and Tables

TABLES

Acknowledgments

Many people have helped to produce this collective work. We would like to thank the contributors to this volume for their unstinting efforts and their patience as this book made its way through the publication process. We also thank the two anonymous evaluators for their rigorous and detailed critiques. We are fortunate to have benefited from the financial support of the Aid to Scholarly Publications Program and from the enthusiasm and efficiency of everyone at UBC Press, especially Darcy Cullen, Jean Wilson, Megan Brand, and Valerie Nair. We thank Katy Hunt, of the University of Manitoba, for her administrative assistance, and Valérie Poirier, a doctoral student at the Université du Québec à Montréal, for her help with the bibliography. Our thanks, as well, to Mireille Bergeron and Céline Lacoursière, s.c.i.m., of the Archives des Sœurs du Bon-Pasteur de Québec, for kindly allowing us to reproduce a photo from their collection on the cover of our book. Finally, we are ever grateful for the encouragement and forbearance of our loved ones.

Epidemic Encounters

Introduction

MAGDA FAHRNI AND ESYLLT JONES

*It seems to me that everything that happens to us is a
disconcerting mix of choice and contingency.*

– Penelope Lively

INTERPRETING PANDEMIC INFLUENZA, 1918-20

The 1918-20 influenza pandemic, which crossed the globe and left
almost no society untouched, is perhaps the singular historical
contingency of the twentieth-century world: what should have
been a relatively innocuous disease developed a life of its own and affected
society in unanticipated ways. Although often difficult to interpret, and
poorly integrated into the major narratives of twentieth-century history,
it nonetheless increasingly commands the attention of historians and the
public. In the context of current anxieties and public discourses surrounding a global pandemic of H1N1 or another variant strain of influenza,
influenza's past is a topical subject of research. Indeed, the rise and fall of
its history throughout the twentieth and early twenty-first centuries closely
parallels patterns of broader public concern (or sanguinity) about a potential repeat of the 1918-20 pandemic. That all history is contemporary
history borders on cliché for an influenza scholar.

The pandemic has been the subject of a rather large recent outpouring
of popular works and has also been examined in a small number of English-
language scholarly monographs (two of them Canadian), two major collections, and a significant body of articles.[1] Much of the scholarship on
the pandemic is relatively new; a recent survey of the field concluded that
"the overwhelming majority" of works on the subject were published during the last thirty years.[2] The present collection is a specifically Canadian

examination of the pandemic, joining such international analyses as those edited by Howard Phillips and David Killingray; the European experience is addressed in a collection edited by Fred R. Van Hartesveldt.[3] Ours is a contribution to the history of medicine but also to Canadian social history more broadly. The authors gathered here are concerned with understanding the social structures and context in which the epidemic was rooted and experienced, and they look to social class, gender, ethnicity and race, age, and geographic location as key variables of analysis. Specific regions of Canada are studied here – British Columbia, the Prairies, Ontario, and Quebec – whereas a few authors (notably Mark Osborne Humphries and Linda Quiney) adopt a Canada-wide approach.

Like the field more generally, this collection is multidisciplinary, with contributors from a variety of fields including medical anthropology, geography, and history employing a diversity of methodological and interpretive approaches. It seeks to build on existing studies and introduces new work on the diffusion of the flu throughout Canada, taking us one step closer to a coast-to-coast picture of the pandemic's history. The contributors engage with current themes and debates in the global pandemic's historiography. Although some scholars have argued that influenza history is fragmented and lacks an overall synthesis or dominant "frame" of analysis (to use Charles Rosenberg's now classic formulation), thoughtful historiographical critiques in the field, such as those by Phillips and Killingray, Svenn-Erik Mamelund, or Guy Beiner, continue to push researchers in new directions.[4] Several themes have proven of particular interest to Canadian scholars and are reflected in this volume.

The first of these is the question of who contracted and died from influenza, and to what degree inequalities of race, ethnicity, and class led to differentials in mortality rates. In his 2006 article employing individual- and household-level data and mathematical analysis, Svenn-Erik Mamelund argues that there were socioeconomic differences in flu mortality in the city of Kristiania, Norway, challenging "the conservative view that Spanish influenza was an 'egalitarian' or classless disease."[5] Scholars in this collection, too, confront the notion that influenza was "democratic" in its effects. Their evidence reveals that race, social inequality, poverty, and pre-existing health crises all potentially played a critical role in shaping how individuals, families, and communities experienced the pandemic. Building on work by Mary-Ellen Kelm and Ann Herring on influenza in Aboriginal communities, where residents died at rates far in excess of non-Aboriginal Canadians, we explore here some of the reasons why this might have been the case.

Charles Rosenberg argued nearly twenty years ago that epidemics cut a "transverse section through society," laying bare its structure and revealing its fault lines.[6] Thus, a second area of interest is the social response to the pandemic, interactions between citizens themselves, and between citizens and state. Here, several of the essays shed new light on the experience of the epidemic "from below," as well as "from above," highlighting the role of non-state actors in attempts to address influenza and their interactions with government at various levels. These scholars reveal an active and engaged Canadian citizenry, commenting, often critically, on public health strategies or failures. Perhaps the most significant instance of civic engagement, in terms of coping with the millions of infected Canadians, was women's volunteer and professional nursing. Among the contributions made by this collection, then, is an analysis of influenza's history through the lens of gender.

Third, scholars in recent years have called for greater attention to the cultural history of influenza, particularly its long-term impact on memory, mourning, and modernity. This collection contributes to this debate through exploring individual and familial experiences of survival and grief, which challenge the public forgetting that has long surrounded the pandemic. In some ways, the crisis of 1918-20 might be seen as the last nineteenth-century epidemic: as these essays show, health professionals and political authorities were largely powerless to halt its spread and prevent its devastation. In laying bare the limits of modern medicine, the pandemic, like the Great War, demonstrated continuities with the previous century as much as it embodied twentieth-century modernity.[7] The high level of volunteerism and the critical role of informal networks of care from kin and community, as revealed by several authors here, bring into critical perspective the elite-driven process of pandemic preparation in Canada today.

Although historians are often wary of applying "lessons" from 1918-20 to twenty-first-century public health strategies, the reality is that we are often called on to do so and are occasionally offended if our expertise is ignored. Thus, it is appropriate that this collection concludes with reflections on past and present responses to epidemic disease, including Canada's experiences with SARS and the H1N1 influenza virus.

INFLUENZA IN CANADA

In September 1918, Canadian newspaper journalists anxiously followed the spread of an apparently serious influenza epidemic through cities on

the American eastern seaboard. Appearing virtually simultaneously in
Brest, Boston, and Freetown, South Africa, pandemic influenza killed
perhaps 50 million people between 1918 and 1920 – most of them during
the fall and winter months of 1918-19. Approximately fifty-five thousand
of these deaths occurred in Canada, where the disease entered virtually
every community across the country, no matter how remote from the
centres of contagion. Although the pandemic's less lethal spring 1918 wave
had been barely noted in the press, and despite wartime censorship,
Canadians were well aware of the extraordinary number of deaths that
were occurring south of the border and on the battlefields of Europe during the month of September. One of the cruelties of the disease was that
public health and medical personnel could do little to prevent its spread
or to treat its victims.

In 1918, much like today, influenza was a deceptive and difficult-to-
diagnose complaint, at times hard to distinguish from the common cold,
with a reputation as unpleasant but only rarely fatal. For reasons that remain
medically obscure, the variant of influenza that caused the pandemic was
not so benign. For those most severely affected, what began as chills and
aches could rapidly overtake the body, causing severe headaches, high fever,
nausea, and vomiting. Victims might turn blue from cyanosis as their lung
tissue deteriorated and their lungs filled with fluid, suffer from profuse
nosebleeds, and cough up blood. Eventually, they would asphyxiate or
suffer circulatory failure. Others were killed by secondary bacterial infections resulting in pneumonia, which was difficult to treat in this pre-
antibiotic era. Influenza appears to have affected the brain and nervous
system as well: sufferers exhibited psychosis and delirium, and some also
experienced paralysis. The 1918-20 pandemic had a very high morbidity
rate; perhaps as many as one-third of Canadians contracted it, although
statistics on morbidity are notoriously unreliable. The proportion of people
who died once infected was lower for influenza than for some other epidemic diseases such as cholera, for example. Yet, the flu pandemic was
deadly because such great numbers of people became ill and because of the
impact of secondary infections such as pneumonia.

Although the precise origins of the disease remain contested, most
scholars agree that it originated in the military camps of the US Midwest,
where it first appeared in March 1918.[8] Between the spring and the fall of
1918, it mutated into a dangerous virus. In a globalized world closely connected by military, commercial, and personal networks of travel, it spread
with all the speed of history's great contagions. Recently, scholars have

paid particularly close attention to how the prosecution of the Allied war effort affected its path: Carol Byerly in the United States and Mark Humphries in Canada have focused a critical gaze on the decisions made by military leadership in this history. From overcrowded military camps in North America and overseas in Britain and Europe, where soldiers received mostly inadequate medical care and lived in unhealthy conditions, influenza gained its foothold. Byerly and Humphries both argue that Canadian and US military authorities sacrificed the health of their troops, and of civilians, to the war effort. Caught between the demands of winning the war and the threat of pandemic, they mobilized soldiers without observing the quarantines that might have slowed the transmission of the disease during its second, deadly wave.[9] Canadian soldiers returning from Europe played a role in spreading the flu, which was reported among Ontario military camps by 19 September (see Chapter 9, this volume). It also spread from US to Canadian soldiers stationed in Eastern Canada, with cases appearing among troops in Nova Scotia and Quebec by 20 September 1918 (see Chapter 1, this volume).

In Canada, the first incidences of influenza outside of the military occurred during late September in eastern cities including Toronto and Montreal (where it arrived on 23 September 1918). However, as it spread rapidly across North America, civilians, too, carried it with them. In Winnipeg, the first civilian case occurred on 30 September, a woman who had recently returned from visiting family in Montreal. She died just one day after a school-aged girl in Toronto (see Chapter 9, this volume).

Canada's experience during the pandemic was, in a general sense, similar to that of other Western industrialized countries. Its overall mortality rate, at approximately 6.1 deaths for every 1,000 people, was comparable to that of the United States and slightly higher than that of England. The number of dead was nevertheless considerably lower than that of many African and Asian countries, which bore the brunt of the pandemic. It is more difficult to accurately assess the numbers of those infected, but probably one-quarter to one-third of the population contracted the disease. These aggregate figures, however, mask considerable differences in mortality and incidence as shaped by age, locale, social class, ethnicity, and race. For example, research in Canada by scholars including Maureen Lux, Mary-Ellen Kelm, and Ann Herring has demonstrated the disproportionate impact on Aboriginal people living on reserves and in remote communities.[10] Thus, it is impossible to speak of a universal pandemic experience, either globally or within Canada itself.

Unlike that of many European countries, Canada's public health infrastructure was rudimentary. There was no federal health department (this was established in 1919, partially in response to the pandemic); nor did every province have health departments (often, health was subsumed into other departments, such as immigration, public works, or agriculture). A synchronized national effort by the state to contain and respond to the flu was simply not possible given these fundamental structural limitations. However, health officials did communicate with one another, sharing ideas and frustrations individually and in medical and public health journals. Their transnational connections with US counterparts were critical. Toronto's medical officer of health, Charles Hastings, travelled to Boston, New York, and Washington to seek out information about the successes of US containment strategies. Winnipeg's William Boyd, city pathologist, went to the Mayo Clinic in Minnesota to obtain a vaccine for mass immunization.

Most of the human and financial resources that went into pandemic responses came from local governments across the country, with supervision from provincial boards of health. Despite the lack of national coordination, however, public health measures quickly took on a pattern during the pandemic, as communities throughout the country made similar efforts to control its spread. These included school and university closures, cancellation of church services, closures of public places of entertainment (such as theatres, movie houses, and billiard parlours), quarantine and placarding of infected households, and the compulsory wearing of masks in public. As the federal government had introduced a prohibition on the manufacture and importation of alcohol in March 1918, it was not necessary to close bars. Some cities also attempted vaccination campaigns. Although the aetiology of influenza was unknown in 1918 (the workings of the virus were not discovered until 1933), pathologists and bacteriologists developed vaccine serums that included what they believed to be the causative agents of the disease: these comprised bacteria such as streptococci, pneumococci, and Pfeiffer's bacillus, an organism isolated after the less severe but quite lethal 1889 influenza pandemic. It is difficult to assess the overall effectiveness of these measures, as we cannot know what might have happened in their absence. Any correlation between differing combinations of public health tactics and death rates across the country is as yet unclear.[11]

During an era that had witnessed significant medical advancements in bacteriology, epidemiology, and surgery, influenza caught medicine off-guard. There were no effective medical treatments for the disease, although all manner of interventions were tried. These ranged from venesection (bloodletting), to the use of intravenous saline and glucose, to oxygen to help patients breathe. Aspirin was given for fever, along with alcohol and stimulants such as atropine and strychnine. Pain and agitation were managed with cooling baths, chest poultices, or with opium derivatives such as codeine, morphine, heroin, and veronal. What was perhaps most helpful for patients fortunate enough to get it was bed rest, nourishment and hydration, and fever management, provided by nurses. Although influenza was a blow to the prestige of medicine and public health, it was a boon to the reputation and pride of nursing. In its aftermath, nursing leaders correctly pointed out the value of quality nursing care, which in the absence of effective medical intervention was especially important.

Yet, many flu victims, in both urban and rural settings, appear to have received little or no medical or nursing care. The high numbers of those infected with the disease generally overwhelmed hospitals, and they responded by finding temporary spaces (such as hotels or mission houses) where they opened emergency beds, which were exceedingly rudimentary and unsatisfactory for the provision of care. A significant proportion of Canada's medical and nursing personnel had volunteered for the war effort, leaving hospitals understaffed and lacking in experienced health care providers. Staffing the emergency hospital beds opened in communities throughout the country was thus a challenge. The disease posed a high risk for health care workers, and many doctors, nurses, and ambulance drivers themselves contracted it, further stretching the capacity to adequately respond to it. Many people remained in their homes, where they fought to recover from influenza with the help of family members. Whereas the better-off could afford private physicians or private duty nurses, many others did not have the resources to pay for a doctor, even should one be available. In this pre-Medicare period, the last vestiges of the Victorian sensibility of "less eligibility" also meant that hospitalization and medical care were not easily accessible to working people, who feared the expense of hospital bills and the interrogation of the means test often required to gain hospital admission. Many jurisdictions offered free hospital care during the pandemic, but this was not always made clear to the public.

By the spring of 1919, this variant of influenza had almost disappeared from Canadian communities, although another, much less prevalent, wave occurred during the following winter in some parts of Canada. This prompted an attempt by alarmed medical and public health officials to evaluate what had and had not worked in 1918-19, but their anxiety quickly

faded when the virus lost its strength. For many Canadians, however, the
flu had permanently altered their lives, having killed their parents, siblings,
and other family members, as well as friends and co-workers. Thousands
of Canadian families changed shape to care for orphans, and social welfare
institutions were forced to accommodate the needs of influenza widows,
widowers, and children. Although we know relatively little about its precise
implications for welfare state development, the memory of influenza is
embedded in such social institutions as state and family.

HISTORIOGRAPHY

Since the 1990s there has been an explosion in both popular and scholarly
interest in the 1918-20 influenza pandemic. It is no longer the "forgotten"
epidemic of the twentieth century, at least from the point of view of the
quantity of scholarship devoted to it: the field today numbers hundreds of
scholarly articles. Canadian scholars have long played an important role
in influenza historiography and are particularly well known outside the
country for their work on Aboriginal experiences. In the past decade, a
significant body of work has been produced in Canada, as elsewhere. There
is an emphasis on local or regional case studies, but scholars have benefited
from an increasing awareness of experiences globally, as the field grows and
matures. As the contributions to this volume attest, Canadian pandemic
scholars have always understood their research in a global context.

In a recent historiographic essay on the impact of influenza in Africa,
Matthew Heaton and Toyin Falola argue that the literature on the pandemic has developed along two parallel tracks that do not engage in genuine
debate with each other. One perspective emphasizes the universality of
the pandemic, regardless of place or social context, and is primarily concerned with tracing official health responses (similarly ineffective all over
the globe) and overall mortality rates (also generally similar). Heaton and
Falola suggest that many studies of the disease have glossed over important
variations in its impact, particularly those that attempt to track "diffusion,
demographics, and official response."[12] The other perspective, which can
be characterized as a social historical one, explores a series of diverse questions about the pandemic, such as how it affected religious faith, economic
development, gender, or race relations. However, Heaton and Falola assert,
the social history of the pandemic is fragmented, lacks a coherent analysis,
and avoids the thorny question of whether influenza's impact can best be
understood as global or as shaped by unique local conditions.

There is some truth to this schema within Canada; it is also true that scholars disagree in their interpretations of, for example, the significance of social relations. Differing methodologies, too, bring different questions to light: quantitative analyses of diffusion, for instance, generally do not speak directly to issues of memory. To some degree, Canadian scholarship has been unified by the exploration of questions about race, place, class, and gender that have been central to most studies of the pandemic written since the 1990s, and indeed, to social history more broadly. Although some of this work is based in local research, it addresses influenza's interconnection with social categories that are not explicitly local in nature. For instance, scholars such as Linda Quiney, Magda Fahrni, and Esyllt Jones have taken gender as a critical social relation within community responses to influenza in several Canadian cities and argue that gender roles shaped women's involvement in volunteer campaigns to provide care to flu victims. Nor is an interest in social difference necessarily disconnected from questions of epidemiology and public health. Scholars continue to improve our understanding of "diffusion, demographics, and official response" by seeking to know, for example, how diffusion affected the most vulnerable members of society, including Aboriginal people, workers, and rural residents. Integral to this work, which arguably takes a social historical approach in challenging a universalist thesis, is a sense that disease incidence and official responses remain an important component of any social history of influenza because they are still at issue and worth debating.

The meaning of the "local" in studies of influenza, as in the history of medicine more broadly, is one important path to resolving the "universal/ social" tension identified by Heaton and Falola. Place is often implicit in the historiography, but there remains some work to do in thinking through how and why place matters. Scholars such as Megan Davies have called for a more sustained attention to the local and regional, and a recent issue of the *Journal of Canadian Studies* edited by Peter Twohig was devoted to the theme of health and regionalism.[13] Certainly, no scholar of the influenza pandemic can ignore the local context, for in the absence of a federal health authority and infrastructure, almost all critical aspects of the public health response were locally developed and implemented. As this collection suggests, local studies remain important in the field. It is hoped that this volume will begin to facilitate a synthesis of the Canadian experience and will enable future discussion about the tension between universal and specific/local interpretations in the history of the pandemic.

Often, historians of the 1918-20 epidemic are frustrated by its continued marginalization in the history of the twentieth century. Its impact (great) seems out of line with the import (slight) assigned to it by historians. In Canada, many who have written most recently about influenza would not consider themselves primarily historians of medicine or disease: their interest in the pandemic has stemmed more from an effort to understand the social and cultural history of Canada and the place of disease in that history. They have attempted to integrate the history of the pandemic into their understanding of gender, class, and ethnicity as constitutive of social relations in early-twentieth-century Canada and have used those categories to enrich their analysis of the disease. Canadian social history was itself still in the process of development during the 1980s and 1990s as new work on influenza was emerging; as the practice of social history became more methodologically complex, researchers employed new tools and approaches that have proven well suited to the history of health and disease. To some extent, medical history has also shaped social-history practice – for instance, in its insistence on bodily experience as relevant to history. This exchange and dialogue have proven fruitful for our understanding of the influenza pandemic. One excellent example of this is the wide range of sources utilized by recent scholars, including the contributors to this collection. Sources such as newspapers or medical and health department documents often yield little insight into what living through this epidemic was like for ordinary people, or the longer-term impact of the disease. Supplemented by medical and social welfare case files, oral histories, diaries and letters, parish registers, and the records of civil society organizations such as volunteer groups, more meaningful insight into the pandemic is possible.

THE ESSAYS

Epidemics are of interest to scholars from various disciplines: most obviously, these include epidemiologists and medical researchers but also social scientists such as anthropologists, geographers, and sociologists, and those working in the humanities – historians and literary scholars, for instance. *Epidemic Encounters* embodies this wide-ranging interest in the influenza pandemic and is an implicit argument for the benefits of a multidisciplinary approach. Whereas the geographers and anthropologists represented in its pages are concerned above all with understanding who contracted influenza in 1918-20, who died, and why, the historians included here ask how medical authorities, health care workers, and various levels of the state managed the epidemic, and how individuals experienced and reacted to it. This diversity of approaches and objectives lends variety to the essays gathered here but, in the end, provides complementary perspectives.

Although tightly focused on a single event – the influenza pandemic of 1918-20, as played out and lived in Canada – this collection of essays exhibits a diversity of approach. A few common threads are nonetheless evident. To begin with, every chapter demonstrates that Canada, as much as any other country, was fully caught up in the pandemic and that much of what we know about it in other places – Britain, the United States, South Africa – holds true for Canada as well.[14] We thus find familiar elements of what has become the overarching global "flu narrative" in all the chapters. At the same time, all the authors would agree, we think, that there was no single experience of the epidemic. Locality and region mattered, as did race, gender, age, and social class. The chapters in this collection remind us of the geographical diversity of Canada: influenza played out quite differently in Fisher River and Norway House, in Montreal, in Winnipeg, in Hamilton, in Quebec's Arthabaska County, and among the First Nations communities of British Columbia.

Epidemic Encounters begins with essays exploring the ways in which various sectors of society – military and medical authorities, health care workers, and even ordinary individuals – responded to the pandemic as active citizens. In Chapter 1, Mark Osborne Humphries reminds us that, in Canada, the pandemic must be understood in the context of the war effort, and more particularly, the implementation and administration of the Military Service Act in the fall of 1918. The Canadian military, he argues, sacrificed individual and collective public health to perceived military needs. The transportation of Canadian recruits infected with influenza to Europe on troopships and, in the case of those intended to form part of the Siberian Expeditionary Force, to Western Canada on trains, contributed to the spread of the epidemic. So, too, did the vigorous enforcement of conscription, particularly in Quebec, during what Humphries calls "the pandemic period." Any hopes of wartime consensus were soon dashed: the Canadian public, he suggests, was prepared to make some sacrifices in the interest of military necessity but balked when military demands were clearly seen to be harming public health.

In Chapter 2, Linda Quiney focuses on the central question of the organization of the nursing labour force during the pandemic. Women – as family members, neighbours, volunteers, or trained nurses – were vital to the battle against the flu. In most circles, this was seen as only normal, given gendered assumptions regarding women's particular aptitude for caregiving, service, and self-sacrifice.[15] Arriving, as it did, in the throes of the Great War, the devastation of the pandemic exacerbated an already existing shortage of trained nurses. Volunteers thus stepped into the breach, and qualified nurses, many of whom had fought hard during the first two decades of the century to secure professional status, were "forced," Quiney writes, "to share their position and status at the bedside during the influenza crisis" (63). In this situation, differences between qualified nurses and dedicated volunteers were blurred; indeed, they were largely imperceptible to members of the public, including flu victims. Professionals and Voluntary Aid Detachment (VAD) nursing volunteers were united by their gender, often by their class background, occasionally by their uniform, and invariably by their appearance of sacrifice in the context of war and epidemic.

In Chapter 3, Magda Fahrni shifts attention from political authorities and health professionals to examine the ways in which ordinary citizens responded to the epidemic. Concentrating on Montreal, she discusses the phenomenon of "public letter writing" – letters from Montreal citizens to their local government and the press, proposing ways of managing the epidemic and reacting to policies adopted by the municipality, the military, and public health authorities. In some ways, her chapter provides an analysis from the bottom up, not because we hear from influenza victims per se, but because we are able to glimpse the responses of some Montreal citizens to state policy. Male, urban, and literate, most of these letter-writers were nonetheless considerably removed from the corridors of power. Some of them took the opportunity to share with local authorities their opinions on public health measures, both during the epidemic and more generally. Others – principally the owners of businesses small or large – were concerned with seemingly more mundane questions such as store opening hours during the epidemic and thus their own livelihood. These letters remind us of the flu's impact on bread-and-butter issues such as work and pay; Canadians just emerging from the context of "total war" found themselves plunged into one of "total epidemic," where everyday life was structured, to some degree, by the disease.

In Part 2 of the collection, the authors scrutinize the epidemiological data to arrive at a precise portrait of who fell ill, who died, and how the disease spread. In Chapter 4, Ann Herring and Ellen Korol undertake a detailed analysis of who, exactly, suffered from influenza. They focus on Hamilton, Ontario, employing death registers as their principal source, which they cross-reference with city directories to ascertain the residence – and by extension, the class position – of those who succumbed to the disease. The argument has often been made that, unlike tuberculosis or typhus, the influenza virus that proved so lethal in 1918-20 did not differentiate according to social class – although in most places, it did so by age, targeting young adults between twenty and forty, and in many parts of the world, it appears to have discriminated by sex, killing more men than women. Scholars who insist on the socially democratic nature of influenza point to the fact that it felled the wealthy as well as the poor, the socially prominent as well as the unknown, and that it swept through tree-lined residential enclaves as well as urban slums. There is some truth to this argument; as Esyllt Jones points out in Chapter 8, her essay on Winnipeg, "no sector of society was entirely immune to the disease" (197). Yet, though her contribution to this collection focuses on a particular middle-class family, she has shown elsewhere that Winnipeg's working-class and immigrant communities were especially hard hit by the epidemic.[16] In Chapter 4, Herring and Korol likewise demonstrate beyond a doubt that, although influenza could be found in all parts of Hamilton during the fall of 1918, the poorer north-end districts of this small industrial city suffered greater rates of mortality than their better-off counterparts in the south end. Contrary to what is frequently assumed, then, the pandemic was definitely not socially neutral.

In Chapter 5, Karen Slonim adopts what medical researchers and anthropologists call a "syndemics" approach, examining influenza's interaction with other co-existing factors and the ways in which this interface affected morbidity, mortality, and the management of the epidemic. She interrogates influenza's interaction, not just with other infectious diseases, but also with underlying social factors such as community structure, the nature of work, and the degree of access to informal networks of care. She looks at the social organization of two Manitoban Cree communities, Fisher River and Norway House, to understand how the epidemic could play out so differently in two such geographically proximate locales. She argues that better access to informal networks of care was a crucial variable that allowed residents of Fisher River to more easily survive the epidemic than their counterparts at Norway House. Factors such as the mixed economy of Fisher River (agriculture, fishing, and lumbering), the need for the Norway House Cree to trap further and further afield, and the key role played by the Hudson's Bay Company at Norway House may also have been determinant.

In Chapter 6, Francis Dubois, Jean-Pierre Thouez, and Denis Goulet combine an analysis of the data collected by Quebec's Superior Board of Health in 1918-20 with a close reading of the Montreal daily *Le Devoir* in order to examine morbidity and mortality on a Quebec-wide scale. Their statistical analyses are more detailed than any others that currently exist for Quebec. Among their conclusions is that, compared to the rest of the province, Montreal appears to have suffered from over-mortality. Such a deduction joins the international literature, then, in suggesting that population density was a significant factor for influenza mortality. It also infers the strong possibility that non-lethal incidents of the disease were under-reported. The authors also conclude, extrapolating from province-wide data, that, contrary to what the international literature indicates, sex does not appear to have determined who died in Quebec, as men and women were struck down in roughly equal numbers. A most useful aspect of their discussion is their focus on the 1920 "echo" wave of influenza, which is alluded to in Chapter 3 on Montreal but not seen everywhere in Canada. Although much less severe than the wave that hit Quebec during the autumn of 1918, it was nonetheless significant, lasting from February to April 1920 and killing almost two thousand Quebecers. Dubois, Thouez, and Goulet show that the Quebec regions worst hit by the fall 1918 wave appear to have been largely spared by that of winter 1920, and that the converse was also true. They also point out an intriguing factor noted by Quebec's medical community shortly after the 1920 wave – that it appears to have killed proportionally far more infants than its fall 1918 counterpart, which was (in Quebec as elsewhere) most devastating for young adults.

Part 3 of this book explores cultural understandings of, and responses to, the epidemic, as well as the ways in which its impact continued to be felt into the interwar years and beyond. If the pandemic was publicly forgotten for most of the twentieth century, it nonetheless lived on in the personal memories and family stories of individuals and communities. The two chapters in this section also suggest that the outbreak tested the limits of early-twentieth-century modernity.

In Chapter 7, Mary-Ellen Kelm analyzes a series of what she calls "flu stories" that were documented through various media in British Columbia during the epidemic and in subsequent decades. The official accounts of fatalities recorded in death certificates, the dramatic and occasionally boosterist articles published in the daily press, the oral histories conducted with elderly residents of Vancouver's Strathcona neighbourhood during the 1970s, and finally, oral and written narratives produced by First Nations people to detail their experience with influenza – these various sources attest to the different ways in which the disease affected diverse groups of British Columbians. Kelm sets her own family's flu story within the framework of the concept of modernity. Modernity, she argues, was marshalled in 1918-19 to explain both the spread of the pandemic, through "modern" lines of communication and "modern" worksites, and the means taken to deal with it – science and medicine. Yet, not all flu stories conformed to this narrative: in those told by First Nations people or by Strathcona residents, for instance, modernity was often absent altogether or incorporated into new hybrid forms. The universal influenza storyline was thus tempered by the peculiarities of local circumstance. Moreover, certain British Columbians – Aboriginals, people of Chinese, Japanese, or South Asian descent, religious minorities such as Mennonites and Doukhobors – were viewed by fellow citizens of Anglo-Saxon background as distinctly unmodern, and thus as potential "reservoirs" of disease.

In Chapter 8, through an examination of one Winnipeg family, the Hamiltons, Esyllt Jones explores the possibility that survivors of the epidemic, and particularly those who had lost loved ones to it, channelled their grief into spiritualism during the interwar years. Historians have frequently attributed the interwar revival of spiritualism to collective mourning in the wake of the Great War, but Jones argues that the even greater number of influenza deaths might well have played the same role. Like Mary-Ellen Kelm, she notes the ways in which the epidemic tested the limits of early-twentieth-century modernity; in a context where modern science and medicine had failed to provide significant solutions, it is possible that contemporaries sought answers in the realm of the spiritual. In exploring the links between the epidemic, death, grief, and spiritualism, Jones's contribution to this anthology is a pioneering cultural history of the influenza pandemic in the Canadian context.

In Part 4, *Epidemic Encounters* concludes by evaluating the usefulness of influenza's history in approaching contemporary struggles against epidemic disease. In Chapter 9, Heather MacDougall compares the efforts of Toronto's health department to manage the 1918 influenza epidemic with that body's responses to the SARS outbreak of 2003. Between 1918 and 2003, Toronto changed considerably, becoming a heavily populated, sprawling, multicultural metropolis. Yet, reactions to SARS by the media and the public in some ways resembled those manifested by Torontonians eighty-five years earlier. MacDougall concludes her analysis of the similarities and differences between these two health crises by arguing that local governments remain crucial in the battle against infectious disease. In 2003, however, the task of Toronto Public Health was complicated by jurisdictional disputes and recent cost-cutting measures implemented by the provincial government. In a postscript written five years after SARS and ninety years after pandemic influenza arrived in Canada, MacDougall reflects on the lessons that today's public health policy-makers might take from history, and from historians. In the case of SARS, she wonders, "What role did history play in persuading policy-makers, politicians, and the public that an immediate response to epidemic disease was necessary to protect citizens' health and to maintain the national economy?" (248). Indeed, she asks, is it even "the historian's responsibility to point out the 'lessons of the past'? If it is, to whom should her observations be addressed?" (247). These questions pertain equally to the Canadian experience with H1N1 in 2009-10. In their Conclusion, the editors of this volume reflect on the interactions between the 1918-20 pandemic and our recent confrontation with H1N1.

This volume does not exhaust the possible ways of exploring the 1918-20 influenza pandemic in Canada. As Guy Beiner has argued, much remains to be done in the area of cultural histories of the epidemic.[17] Furthermore, none of the authors gathered here tackles the epidemic from an environmental perspective. Pandemic influenza was a prime example of what Susan D. Jones calls the "nonhuman actors [that] have played important roles in 'making history,' influencing cultural practices and determining the shape of social institutions."[18] The potential for environmental histories of the flu is thus substantial.[19] Yet, the essays collected here offer a broad range of perspectives – demographic, political, social, and cultural – on Canadian experiences of illness and death during the waves of influenza that struck between 1918 and 1920. They thus provide significant insight into a pandemic that continues to exert a considerable hold over the popular and scholarly imagination almost a century later.

NOTES

Epigraph: Brainy Quote, http://www.brainyquote.com/.
1 The Canadian monographs are Eileen Pettigrew, *The Silent Enemy: Canada and the Deadly Flu of 1918* (Saskatoon: Western Producer Prairie Books, 1983); and Esyllt W. Jones, *Influenza 1918: Disease, Death, and Struggle in Winnipeg* (Toronto: University of Toronto Press, 2007). International works include Richard Collier, *The Plague of the Spanish Lady: The Influenza Pandemic of 1918-1919* (New York: Atheneum, 1974); Alfred W. Crosby, *America's Forgotten Pandemic: The Influenza of 1918* (Cambridge: Cambridge University Press, 1989); Dorothy A. Pettit and Janice Bailie, *A Cruel Wind: Pandemic Flu in America* (Murfreesboro,

TN: Timberlane Books, 2008); Geoffrey W. Rice, *Black November: The 1918 Influenza Pandemic in New Zealand,* 2nd ed. (Christchurch, NZ: Canterbury University Press, 2005); and Carol R. Byerly, *Fever of War: The Influenza Epidemic in the U.S. Army during World War I* (New York: New York University Press, 2005). The two collections are Howard Phillips and David Killingray, eds., *The Spanish Influenza Pandemic of 1918-19: New Perspectives* (London: Routledge, 2003); and Fred R. Van Hartesveldt, ed., *The 1918-1919 Pandemic of Influenza: The Urban Impact in the Western World* (Lewiston, NY: Edwin Mellen Press, 1992).

2 Guy Beiner, "Out in the Cold and Back: New-Found Interest in the Great Flu," *Cultural and Social History* 3,4 (October 2006): 498.

3 Phillips and Killingray, *The Spanish Influenza Pandemic;* and Van Hartesveldt, *The 1918-1919 Pandemic.*

4 Charles Rosenberg, "What Is an Epidemic? AIDS in Historical Perspective," in *Explaining Epidemics and Other Studies in the History of Medicine,* ed. Charles Rosenberg (Cambridge: Cambridge University Press, 1992), 278-92; Phillips and Killingray, *The Spanish Influenza Pandemic;* Svenn-Erik Mamelund, "A Socially Neutral Disease? Individual Social Class, Household Wealth and Mortality from Spanish Influenza in Two Socially Contrasting Parishes in Kristiania 1918-19," *Social Science and Medicine* 62 (2006): 923-40; and Beiner, "Out in the Cold and Back."

5 Mamelund, "A Socially Neutral Disease?" 938.

6 Rosenberg, "What Is an Epidemic?" 279.

7 On the modernity of the Great War, see Modris Eksteins, *Rites of Spring: The Great War and the Birth of the Modern Age* (Boston: Houghton Mifflin, 1989); and Jay Winter, *Sites of Memory, Sites of Mourning: The Great War in European Cultural History* (Cambridge: Cambridge University Press, 1995).

8 Howard Phillips and David Killingray, "Introduction," in Phillips and Killingray, *The Spanish Influenza Pandemic,* 5. A recent work that argues the virus originated in China is Pettit and Bailie, *A Cruel Wind.*

9 Byerly, *Fever of War;* Mark Osborne Humphries, "The Horror at Home: The Canadian Military and the 'Great' Influenza Pandemic of 1918," *Journal of the Canadian Historical Association,* n.s., 16,1 (2005): 235-60.

10 Maureen Lux, "'The Bitter Flats': The 1918 Influenza Epidemic in Saskatchewan," *Saskatchewan History* 49,1 (1997): 3-13; Mary-Ellen Kelm, "British Columbia First Nations and the Influenza Pandemic of 1918-1919," *BC Studies* 122 (Summer 1999): 23-45; and D. Ann Herring, "'There Were Young People and Old People and Babies Dying Every Week': The 1918-1919 Influenza Pandemic at Norway House," *Ethnohistory* 41,1 (1994): 73-105.

11 This is the conclusion drawn by Mark Humphries in his recent "The Impact of Non-Pharmaceutical Interventions during a Pandemic Crisis: The Canadian Experience, 1918-1919" (paper presented at the 33rd Annual Conference of the Social Science History Association, Miami, 23-26 October 2008).

12 Matthew Heaton and Toyin Falola, "Global Explanations versus Local Interpretations: The Historiography of the Influenza Pandemic of 1918-19 in Africa," *History in Africa* 33 (2006): 207.

13 Megan J. Davies, "Mapping 'Region' in Canadian Medical History: The Case of British Columbia," *Canadian Bulletin of Medical History* 17 (2000): 73; and Peter Twohig, ed., "Written on the Landscape: Health and Regionalism in Canada," special issue, *Journal of Canadian Studies* 41,3 (Fall 2007).

14 Phillips and Killingray, *The Spanish Influenza Pandemic;* and Niall Johnson, *Britain and the 1918-19 Influenza Pandemic: A Dark Epilogue* (London: Routledge, 2006).

15 Jones, *Influenza 1918;* and Magda Fahrni, "'Elles sont partout': les femmes et la ville en temps d'épidémie, Montréal, 1918-1920," *Revue d'histoire de l'Amérique française* 58,1 (2004): 67-85.

16 Jones, *Influenza 1918.*

17 Beiner, "Out in the Cold and Back."

18 Susan D. Jones, "Body and Place," *Environmental History* 10,1 (January 2005): 47.

19 For one effort to examine influenza in the context of the urban environment, see Magda Fahrni, "Influenza and the Urban Environment, 1918-1920," in *Metropolitan Natures: Environmental Histories of Montreal,* ed. Stéphane Castonguay and Michèle Dagenais (Pittsburgh: University of Pittsburgh Press, 2011), 68-81.

PART I

Public Responses to the Influenza Pandemic in Canada

I

The Limits of Necessity: Public Health, Dissent, and the War Effort during the 1918 Influenza Pandemic

MARK OSBORNE HUMPHRIES

Disease and war have always been linked. In the nineteenth century, armies often suffered more casualties from illness than from enemy action.[1] At the outbreak of the Great War, as whole societies mobilized around the globe, doctors worried that the conflict might thrust new diseases on unprepared and malnourished populations. Canadian doctors were no exception. Colonel Guy Carleton Jones, a Nova Scotia physician and veteran of the Boer War, warned his colleagues early in 1914 to heed the lessons of history.[2] "The trail of infected armies leaves a sad tale of sickness amongst the women and children and non-combatants. Laws and regulations may govern the conduct of war, but disease and infections recognise no such laws and refuse to signal [sic] out the combatant only," he wrote. "Thus we see that war forces itself on the civilian, on the innocent child, on the non-combatant who stays at home ... for who can tell, or count up, or even recognise the victims of war when it once places its hand on a country?"[3] Four years after writing these words, Jones was surgeon-general of Canada's military forces. During the summer of 1918, he found himself at the centre of the largest epidemic to hit Canada since the cholera scares of the mid-nineteenth century. He also found himself caught between his obligations to guard the public health and his duty to sustain the war effort.

Historians have been slow to recognize the connection between war and pandemic influenza. Alfred Crosby's *Epidemic and Peace* first linked the transmission of the virus to the movements of soldiers, and in Canada the disease has long been mistakenly associated with Canadians returning from the fighting in Europe at war's end.[4] Yet the physical transmission of viral material is only one facet of the complex relationship between sick armies and the state. Carol Byerly's *Fever of War* argues that in the United States, war and flu were inextricably linked.[5] She acknowledges that the virus spread with the movements of soldiers and suggests that military physicians and government officials were caught between their obligation to protect the public health and their duty to prosecute the war effort. According to her analysis, health and war became competing interests. This was also true in Canada, where the federal public health infrastructure was less developed and the Canadian people more tired from four long years of fighting.

The military defined Canadian life throughout the pandemic period. By 1918, almost 8 percent of Canadians – 16 percent of the male population – had enlisted or been drafted into the Canadian Expeditionary Force (CEF).[6] When the flu struck, tens of thousands of Canadian parents had already grieved for their dead sons. Over a hundred thousand more Canadians had been wounded. Families scraped together donations for the Canadian Patriotic Fund, and society women organized public rallies for victory bonds. Women nursed the injured and dying, both in uniform and at home. Men and women worked side by side in factories and on farms producing goods "essential to the war effort." The front page of every local paper, big or small, was plastered with news from the front, and lists of casualties, medal winners, and pictures of new recruits covered the inside pages. When influenza struck in the autumn of 1918, the military was Canada's largest employer: it controlled the most manufacturing contracts; it administered the largest network of hospitals. Every sphere of Canadian life – public and private – was tinged with khaki.[7]

In the autumn of 1918, the war effort was reaching its height. There were more soldiers in uniform between July and November 1918 than at any time during the previous four years.[8] In the final three months of the war, the Canadian Expeditionary Force suffered staggering casualties of 11,257 killed and 33,478 wounded, more than at the Second Battle of Ypres, Vimy Ridge, and Passchendaele combined.[9] The demand for replacements to sustain the war effort meant that military necessity and public health became competing interests during the pandemic's autumn wave. The failure to properly attend to the health needs of soldiers in the rush to get men overseas led to the uncontrolled spread of the virus to civilian populations. This conflict between perceived national interest, on the one hand, and public safety, on the other, focused disaffection across traditional boundaries of ethnicity and class. Wartime dissent encompassed a public critique of the state's management of a major health crisis.

CIVIL MILITARY COOPERATION AND THE FLU'S FIRST WAVE

The first wave of influenza broke out in the ranks of the Canadian Expeditionary Force in France and Belgium in May 1918, sickening Canadian soldiers stationed in England a month later.[10] The epidemic was noted in hospital war diaries, but it seemed to have provoked no more initial worry than mumps, measles, or diphtheria, all of which were routine among Canadian units.[11] Convalescent soldiers infected with this first wave of influenza sailed for Canada on 26 June. Fears about German U-boats lurking off the northeastern seaboard and the sinking of hospital ships meant that this ship, the *Araguaya,* was the last Canadian vessel to ferry wounded soldiers back across the Atlantic until the end of September.[12] When it arrived in Halifax harbour on 7 July, both the civilian and military authorities were responsible for ensuring that the flu did not make its way into Canada.

In the summer of 1918, Canada's government in Ottawa had little experience in managing national epidemics of contagious disease. Under the British North America Act, 1867 (BNA Act), the provinces were responsible for "the Establishment, Maintenance, and Management of Hospitals, Asylums, Charities, and Eleemosynary Institutions in and for the Province," whereas Ottawa had been given control over "Quarantine and the Establishment and Maintenance of Marine Hospitals."[13] As the role of government and definitions of public health changed during the next fifty years, jurisdiction over unspecified areas of public health became a matter for debate. Federal politicians believed that the residual powers clause of the BNA Act left public health to Ottawa, but in practice the government had allowed the provinces to assume a larger part of the responsibility. Nevertheless, Ottawa still claimed control over questions of public health that concerned the Dominion as a whole.

In Canada, quarantine was handled by the director general of public health. Appointed in 1899 as a deputy minister and "Sanitary Advisor of the Dominion Government," Dr. Frederick Montizambert reported to the Department of Agriculture for eighteen years before his office was transferred to the Department of Immigration and Colonization in the winter of 1918.[14] A giant, broad-shouldered man with a drooping moustache and wild, bushy eyebrows, Montizambert looked more the part of a general than a health official. A careerist who nevertheless bickered often and loudly with his bosses over his salary, rank, title, and holidays, he began his tenure in the civil service at the Grosse Ile, Quebec, quarantine station in 1867 and was able to speak from personal experience about public health management under every government since Confederation.[15] As director general of public health, Montizambert was charged with "administration in all matters pertaining to Quarantine, that is, the dealing [sic] with any infectious disease, on its presenting itself at any of the ports of the Dominion, maritime or inland."[16] When the *Araguaya* arrived in Halifax, it was up to the aging doctor to work with the Canadian military to contain the disease.

When the ship made port at Halifax harbour, 23 percent of its soldier-passengers were infected with an "epidemic of [a] new variety of influenza"; however, the local civilian quarantine authorities disavowed any responsibility for dealing with them.[17] Major General Carleton Jones, the man who had warned of the link between war and disease, recognized that Ottawa had jurisdiction over any sickness onboard ships and immediately wired Montizambert. "Quarantine authorities Halifax disclaim any responsibility respecting troop ships," read his urgent telegram. "This is not according to my understanding of your regulations [stop] desired to meet you in every way consider that coordinated action should be taken."[18] Montizambert agreed with Jones's assessment and demanded that the uncooperative quarantine officer immediately take charge of the ship. He also wanted to see this new disease for himself and boarded an overnight train.[19]

Soon after he arrived in Halifax, two new problems arose with quarantine on the St. Lawrence. On the thirteenth, two empty troopships, the *Nagoya* and *Somali,* passed inspection at Grosse Ile and were sent up the river to Montreal to pick up soldiers scheduled to sail for Europe. But there, the embarkation medical officers – the military doctors in charge of inspecting departing troops and certifying that crossing the Atlantic was medically safe for them – refused to grant permission for either ship to begin loading passengers. The problem was not with the soldiers waiting on the docks, but with the ships' crews, some of whom were now noticeably sick with the flu. The embarkation medical officers demanded that the vessels be sent back to Grosse Ile for disinfection and quarantine; this would mean that the soldiers' departure would have to be delayed.[20] Working together with the military, Montizambert agreed with the army doctors' assessment of the situation and notified his staff at Grosse Ile that, in future, they were to make every effort to keep the disease out of the country and away from Canadian troops.[21]

On the same day, Montizambert asked the minister of immigration and colonization to confirm his provisional ruling that Spanish influenza should be listed as a "quarantinable disease."[22] On the twenty-second, he received the minister's confirmation, and with the problem seemingly in hand on the east coast, he turned his attention westward. He wired his staff in Victoria with details of the situation in the east, and with the stamina of a much younger man, he hopped a cross-country train to prepare William Head quarantine station in Victoria for the epidemic.[23] While visiting British Columbia, he assured the *Vancouver World* that every precaution was being taken to prevent the flu from spreading to the Dominion.[24]

It would seem that civilian-military cooperation had initially succeeded. An examination of military hospital records from Nova Scotia, Quebec, Ontario, and British Columbia shows that the flu was not widespread among Canadian troops – who were its chief vector – during the summer of 1918.[25] At St. Jean Military Hospital, Montreal (which became a flu hotspot during the more fatal wave in September), authorities admitted only 36 patients with influenza-like symptoms between 5 June and 4 September 1918.[26] In contrast, during the pandemic's more deadly wave, the same institution admitted 245 patients between 5 September and 4 December.[27] At the Toronto Base Hospital – another flu hotspot in the autumn – 185 patients were admitted with influenza-like symptoms between 1 July and 24 September, compared with 1,577 between 25 September and 25 October.[28] Even at Camp Hill Hospital in Halifax, where sick soldiers from overseas inflated the number of flu victims in July, a total of 285 cases resembled influenza between 1 July and 29 September (or 13 percent of all admissions).[29] In contrast, during the first two weeks of October alone, the same hospital admitted 249 cases (or 42 percent of all admissions). Although the summer wave was milder and therefore presented a less significant challenge to the military than the more serious second wave, civilian-military quarantine efforts at Canada's ports seemed to work.

In the summer of 1918, there was no conflict between the military's interests and public health, because the army did not perceive attempts to stop the import of the disease into Canada as a threat to the war effort. Injured soldiers returning to Canada were no longer of use to the military, so quarantine was not a hindrance to military effectiveness. In June and

July, the drive to get troops overseas was also not as pressing as it would become only a few weeks later. At the end of June 1918, the German spring offensive – which had nearly won the war for Germany – petered out.[30] The Canadian Corps was never in Germany's line of advance and had avoided the horrendous casualties that decimated many other formations within the British army. The dire predictions of the spring, that the Canadian Corps would be short of replacements by several thousand soldiers, had not come to pass.[31] Thus, when the flu appeared among Canadian soldiers, the military authorities' power to conduct the war effort as they saw fit was not threatened by the efforts of public health officials to prevent its spread.

As the war effort ramped up in late August and Canadian troops went into a long period of sustained combat, the demand for soldiers overseas grew. At that point, accommodating concerns about public health and the health of individual soldiers became increasingly difficult for the military. On 8 August 1918, the Canadian Corps began what we now know was the final campaign of the war. Despite a succession of victories, by mid-September it was far from clear that the war would soon reach an end.[32] Although the German army was falling back, the British Expeditionary Force (of which the Canadians were a part) was running out of fresh recruits.[33] To sustain the momentum of the advance, Canada and the United States had to funnel troops to Europe as quickly as they could get them across the Atlantic, reducing training periods and sending conscripts to the front. To speed up the process, American soldiers from the eastern seaboard travelled to Montreal and Quebec City to fill up space on Canadian ships. Just as the situation was growing more urgent, the second wave of influenza arrived in Canada.

The second and more deadly wave of the flu first appeared among American soldiers at Camp Devens outside of Boston on 8 September 1918.[34] By the month's second week, it had already spread across Massachusetts and into New York State.[35] On 17 September, it broke out among Polish American recruits at a camp outside of Niagara-on-the-Lake.[36] On the other side of Lake Ontario, it spread into Quebec, where, on 20 September 1918, soldiers began reporting sick at St. Jean Military Hospital.[37] The officer in charge of military medicine for the Montreal area, Lieutenant-Colonel F.S. Patch, recorded in his war diary that the "epidemic [was] probably brought to St. Johns [sic] by recruits from the United States, probably Boston, where the epidemic is raging."[38] On 20 September 1918, American recruits also brought the flu to Nova Scotia when an American troop transport in transit between New Jersey and France, the SS *Nestor*, offloaded sick soldiers in Sydney harbour.[39]

Montizambert could not effectively intervene to stop the arrival of the pandemic's second wave.[40] Infected American soldiers crossed into Canada on sealed military trains that were not subject to federal quarantine regulations. Sick soldiers taken off coastwise troopships – vessels destined for a foreign rather than a Canadian port – were not technically subject to quarantine as they fell under provincial jurisdiction.[41] Once the flu entered Canada, Montizambert could do little more than watch. The ball was now clearly in the army's court. But the military's objective was to keep the Canadian Corps fighting in France, which meant keeping it supplied with reinforcements. In this analysis, concerns about individual and collective health became secondary to the war effort.

On 26 September, as the flu spread like wildfire through the military depots and barracks of Quebec, 1,057 soldiers boarded HMT *City of Cairo*, destined for Liverpool, England. At the docks, military medical inspectors examined the ship's sanitary state and hospital facilities, just as they had done with the *Nagoya* and *Somali* in July. Although they noted that several of the units waiting to board the *City of Cairo* came from camps infected with influenza, and that the soldiers had been forced to march to the ship through the cold autumn rain, this time the embarkation medical officer allowed the transport to proceed from port. When it left the pier at Montreal, its hospital had space for only twenty-one patients. While it was still in the St. Lawrence, the hospital began to overflow with the ill. The crew emptied a coal bunker beneath the decks, making room for a further fifty-eight patients, but on 3 October a strong North Atlantic gale began to blow, which continued to rage for five long days. As the ship lurched through tall seas, all the portholes were closed up tight and the hatches sealed. Inside the hull of the heaving ship, 75 percent of the passengers fell sick, vomiting and coughing together below decks with little or no ventilation. There were thirty-two deaths at sea.[42]

Although the Canadian army could not have anticipated the extent of the pandemic's impact, reports from Great Britain and the United States indicated the potential for a significant loss of life. Warning signs went unheeded. HMT *Huntsend* also departed Montreal on 26 September with 649 soldiers from across Canada. Even before it left port, there were fifteen cases of influenza and pneumonia in its hospital. The *Huntsend*'s doctor was concerned about the health of his passengers and asked the Quebec embarkation medical officer to re-evaluate the situation. The officer replied that he was "very busy [and] could not go aboard [as he] thought the cases were only very mild ones," but he could remove three of the more serious cases to hospital in Quebec. Despite the fact that some of the passengers were sick, the ship was allowed to sail. By the second morning at sea, the doctor's concerns proved well founded when 150 men reported ill. Although the ship's smoking rooms, library, reading room, officers' cabins, and any other available space were commandeered, there was only enough bed space for seventy patients. The rest had to make do as best they could. Five percent of the entire complement of 649 Canadians aboard the ship died at sea before it made landfall on 11 October.[43]

Similar events transpired on a third transport vessel, the *Victoria,* which sailed from Quebec on 6 October 1918 with 1,076 Canadian soldiers on-board.[44] While the *Victoria* was still moored at Quebec City, thirty cases of influenza were admitted to its hospital. The ship's doctor later claimed that he, too, had asked the Quebec medical officer in charge of the docks to remove sick soldiers from the vessel before it sailed. This officer, Lieutenant Colonel Kerr, was reported to have said "no" and flippantly remarked "your ship [will] become a hospital ship anyway." The *Victoria* was ordered to cast off.[45]

The *Victoria* left port with a full-fledged epidemic already raging on-board. Again, hospital accommodation was minimal, and medical supplies ran out only a few days into the crossing. When the vessel arrived in England, the Canadian authorities in London sent an angry wire to Ottawa: "Transport Victoria arrived here 18th Oct. 28 deaths confirmed on route from influenza and broncho-pneumonia ... Reported that Victoria left with 30 cases in ship's hospital which ADMS [assistant director of medical services] Québec would not permit to be removed before leaving. Full report will be forwarded to you."[46] Military practice might have dictated that the need for troops overseas outweighed concerns about the health of individual soldiers, but official military policy had to be followed.

With deaths aboard the *Victoria* and a complaint by the ship's doctor, a court of inquiry was called to investigate the incident. The court listened to a month of testimony from seventy-five witnesses before finding three officers partially "culpable" in the tragic series of events. Although officials privately admitted that certain "inefficiencies" had occurred, they were reluctant to blame anyone for doing his duty.[47] The court concluded, "The evidence shows that while it was realised that the boat was not adapted for Trans-Atlantic Troop Transport Service it had been made as [accom-modating], clean and comfortable as possible and it was a question of

Military exigency as to whether it was not in order to use it to transport troops across the Atlantic [or] as to whether steps should have been taken to reduce the number of men placed on board such a ship when an epidemic was known to be prevalent."[48]

The *Victoria* may not have been in ideal condition, but military "exigency" was the decisive factor. Cramped quarters, reduced air space, and shared accommodations all helped the virus spread. "The paramount necessity [was] getting troops to the other side," Lieutenant Colonel Kerr testified at the inquiry. "As a result of the sinking of the better ships it was found necessary by the Admiralty to use almost anything that floats."[49] In mid-October, as the epidemic reached its peak in Quebec, the best that Kerr could do to safeguard the health of departing troops was to ask Ottawa to limit their numbers onboard each vessel and have any sick soldiers deposited on Grosse Ile as the ships travelled down the St. Lawrence.[50] On 15 October, Ottawa agreed to allow sick soldiers to be transferred to the quarantine station, but there is no evidence to suggest that the director general of medical services agreed to limit the number of soldiers actually placed on troop transports.[51]

Doctors knew what would happen when sick men were sealed into crowded, poorly ventilated makeshift transports, but in their estimate, the military situation made it a necessary risk. In his testimony before the court, Kerr explained, "It has been in my mind since that any boats transporting troops during this epidemic would find its hospital beds inadequate and would have patients scattered throughout the ship, much in the way that a hospital ship would be ... We had anticipated the situation and had increased the drug supply and anticipated to the extent that afterwards resulted."[52] His phrase "extent that afterwards resulted" was a euphemism for the numerous deaths at sea. Doctors may have known the consequences of their actions, but they had orders to get as many men across the ocean as quickly as possible.

The fact that the deaths occurred on outgoing troop transports ensured that public outcry was minimal, as no concerned witnesses remained in Canada to rally public indignation. At the same time, it is unlikely that anyone would have seriously ventured to challenge the necessity of shipping soldiers overseas in the autumn of 1918. As casualties mounted in France, new recruits *were* needed. Even those who disagreed with the war on principle had to accept that with an army in the field, dead and injured men required replacements for as long as the war continued. If several dozen soldiers had to die so that the Canadian Corps could receive several thousand replacements, that was the reality of war.[53]

FLU AND CONSCRIPTION IN QUEBEC

When military necessity was not apparent, however, the public was not so willing to make sacrifices. Nowhere were the limits of public support more evident than in the province of Quebec during the months following the passage of the Military Service Act. Conscription was imposed in 1917 to solve the military's problem of dwindling voluntary enlistments and to ensure that a sufficient number of replacements could be found for casualties overseas. Every man between eighteen and sixty was ordered to register for possible military service. Of the 332,000 who had registered by 10 November 1917, 93 percent had asked for exemption from the draft for medical, religious, personal, or economic reasons. Opposition to conscription in Canada ran high, especially in Quebec. Whereas the military believed that the draft was necessary to sustain the war effort, during the 1918 influenza pandemic, many in Quebec came to see it as a threat to public health.[54]

In Quebec, old antagonisms between English and French Canadians ensured that conscription became a source of ethnic conflict. In 1916, there had been "recruiting disturbances" in Montreal, and riots across the province in 1917, but the violence escalated in the spring of 1918.[55] In the early morning hours of April Fool's Day (also Easter Monday), English Canadian troops from Ontario opened fire on a crowd of several hundred civilians protesting conscription in Quebec City. Four civilians were killed and many more injured. Press coverage of the riots was extensive, and Henri Bourassa's *Le Devoir* was accused of inciting the violence.[56] In the aftermath, the government passed Privy Council Order 1241, which tightened its control of the press.[57]

As the second wave of influenza arrived in Canada, the Canadian government was preparing to enforce the Military Service Act with unprecedented vigour.[58] Draftees who had failed to comply with the provisions of the act were granted amnesty until 24 August 1918 when they had to report to a barracks or recruiting centre to be registered or inducted into the service. At the end of August, the government began efforts to apprehend those people who had "defaulted" on their obligation to the state. Although they were pursued across Canada, the military authorities focused on defaulters in Quebec.

Groups of soldiers, varying in size from two dozen to several hundred men and known as special service detachments, were given the task of apprehending the missing conscripts in Quebec.[59] These roving bands were charged with "raiding theatres, pool-rooms and visiting, by night, that part of the [cities] occupied by the labouring class."[60] They rode across the countryside, searching lumber camps and farm fields for draft dodgers.[61] If caught, their quarries could expect harsh treatment: "All deserters and absentees without leave should be punished no matter what their medical category ... Even if they cannot be made use of for strictly military service and even if they ... have never been on duty ... field punishment number two (to twenty eight days when imposed by a Commanding officer, or to three months when imposed by a court martial) will be found a convenient punishment to impose."[62] Field punishment number two involved hard labour while restrained in irons.

When the pandemic hit, the more outspoken elements of the press used it to challenge conscription on the grounds that it presented a danger to public health. *La Patrie* questioned the prudence of sending soldiers door-to-door, street by street, to search for defaulters when an epidemic was in full swing:

> Il semble qu'il n'est guère sage d'arrêter chaque jour sur la rue des centaines de jeunes gens et de les conduire sur la rue Peel ou la rue Guy. Les autorités militaires prétendent que la police ne recherche pas les nouveaux conscrits se contentant de mettre le grappin sur les déserteurs. D'aucuns croiront que dans les circonstances il serait plus sage et plus prudent d'attendre que l'épidémie ait disparu avant de pourchasser les déserteurs. Si l'on veut enrayer les ravages de l'épidémie le plus vite possible il ne faut rien négliger. Les autorités militaires doivent seconder les efforts des autorités municipales et du bureau d'hygiène.[63]

La Patrie accused the military authorities of rounding up young men and sending them to local barracks and police stations despite the fact that the city board of health had banned public gatherings and specifically requested that soldiers remain in barracks.[64] The paper further alleged that these nocturnal raids were needlessly infecting innocent men and their families: "Dans ces arrestations nocturnes d'hommes qui paraissaient être d'âge militaire, certains agents amenaient des conscrits, dont les papiers étaient complètement en règle. On les relâchait vers les 10 heures du soir. Plusieurs passaient la nuit et s'éveillaient le matin complètement 'grippés'; par le contact de leurs compagnons déjà malades."[65]

Bourassa's *Le Devoir* agreed and on 5 November the paper reported, "Plusieurs personnes ... ont protesté contre cette mesure qui exposait les jeunes gens à contracter la grippe aux casernes où la maladie n'est pas encore complètement disparue."[66] With influenza, the papers in Quebec had a new vehicle through which to indirectly resume criticism of conscription. Regardless of the underlying political motivations, these were not baseless accusations. Apprehended men who were sent to barracks often returned home to spread the disease among their families. The military was also refusing to comply with civilian regulations that had banned public gatherings, including all religious services. For the army, the issue was not one of public safety, but of military necessity.

Civilian officials disagreed and argued that regardless of the military situation, public health was of primary importance. On 10 October, a delegation from the Montreal Board of Health met with Major-General G.W. Wilson, the commander of the Montreal military district, to demand that he stop contravening the ban against public gatherings. "Il est tout simplement insensé," the doctors told *Le Devoir*, "pour la police militaire de parquer au poste de police No. 4 dans une salle grande comme la main, une centaine de jeunes gens an moment précis où le bureau d'hygiène défend tout attroupement, il va falloir que cela cesse immédiatement."[67] Provincial politicians weighed into the debate, too. In the third week of October, Arthur Sauvé, leader of the provincial Conservatives, wrote to the military authorities to demand that recruiting under the Military Service Act be suspended for the duration of the influenza pandemic. Sauvé claimed that "the military police continued their work, in the town and throughout the countryside, taking men without mercy to the barracks, where the epidemic was prevalent."[68] Although he did not support conscription, Sauvé was no radical and had earlier in the year publicly opposed the Francœur Motion, a request in the Quebec Parliament to debate the province's place in Confederation.[69] Like *La Patrie* and the Montreal Board of Health, Sauvé believed that conscription in an epidemic context threatened public health, regardless of the military's need for manpower. He was not alone. On 31 October 1918, the Central Board of Health of Quebec passed a resolution that read "Whereas the transport of conscripts is the cause of the dissemination of influenza and is also dangerous to the conscripts themselves as well as to the localities to which they are taken, the Central Board of Health demands that no transport of conscripts shall be made during the prevalent epidemic. This is to include absentees without leave."[70] The board was testing the limits of its power. In theory, the BNA Act gave it authority over matters of health within the province, but the War Measures Act had already endowed Ottawa with extraordinary powers. The general officers commanding the Quebec military districts refused to comply with the provincial government's orders.[71]

The military dealt with public anger by issuing denials and making misleading promises. "Since the epidemic of influenza reached such grave proportions the pursuit of draftees by the military police had been called off," General Wilson assured the *Montreal Gazette* in mid-October. "No more men were being called out by the registrar, nor would be until the epidemic was ended ... The only work being done by the military police since the outbreak of the epidemic had been the securing of deserters and this had been done under great precautions."[72] Despite Wilson's claims, the military never actually ceased its pursuit of absentees, deserters, or defaulters. Although the call for new draftees was temporarily suspended on 4 October, the policy seems to have been inconsistently applied and does not appear to have affected the search for those who had already been called up.[73] For example, on 8 October, the military police turned over seventeen men "of various nationalities" to the Second Quebec Regiment for induction.[74] The next day, the fourth battalion of the Canadian Garrison Regiment sent out a party of more than a hundred men "for the purpose of assisting the Assistant Provost Marshall in enforcing the provisions of the Military Service Act."[75] Despite Wilson's assurances, the hunt for defaulters continued.

Civilian officials and the newspapers also seem to have been correct in their assertions that absentees – not only deserters and defaulters – were being rounded up in the streets of Montreal. An order dated 11 October 1918 from the assistant provost marshal of the Montreal military district shows that routine procedure in the area did not change during the pandemic:

Adverting to our conversation of yesterday regarding men apprehended by Military Police on the streets, and taken to the Depot Battalions, the procedure is as follows: Those whose papers do not satisfy the Officer Commanding of the Detachments operations on the streets are sent to the offices of the Civil Section CMPC No. 4 Detachment, 144 Drummond Street, and I might say in passing that this building has been thoroughly fumigated. There papers are then examined by the Deputy Inspector without delay and those whose papers are satisfactory are released and allowed to go at once. With regard to those whose papers are not satisfactory, or who have not registered at all, our Deputies immediately get in touch with the Registrar's officer ... [and] the Registrar's Dept. then gives a ruling on the case and if the man's registration papers and category are such as to allow his release, he is immediately liberated, otherwise he is sent to the Depot Battalion, as ordered by the Registrar.[76]

The Military Service Act continued to be enforced in a similar way beyond Montreal's city limits in towns such as Ste. Agathe, Valleyfield, and St. Hyacinthe during the month of October.[77] All across Quebec, the search for deserters, absentees, and defaulters persisted throughout the pandemic period. Special Service Detachment Number 1, administered out of Quebec City, was engaged in actively trying to apprehend defaulters throughout October and early November. Between 1 October and 13 November, this small detachment of soldiers dealt with more than three hundred men under the provisions of the Military Service Act. Despite sickness from influenza within the unit itself, groups of soldiers continued to travel across the countryside, searching the woods, lumber camps, and villages of Quebec.[78] These tactics ensured that if the disease did leap from soldiers to civilians, it would disproportionately affect working-class civilians in the villages and towns of the Quebec countryside. On 3 October, soldiers from the detachment stalked the streets of Laterrière and Hébertville; on the eighth, they were in St. Gédéon. On the fifteenth – while influenza was prevalent within the unit itself – two parties went to Lake Edward and St. Fulgence; on the twenty-fifth, they scoured Bagotville. On the twenty-eighth, the detachment returned to Laterrière, where two prisoners were taken. On 1 November, it was in Chicoutimi and on the second, Chambord. On the day the armistice was declared, a party of special service soldiers searched the village of Jonquière and subjected two defaulters to field punishment number two.[79]

The military authorities in Quebec believed that the enforcement of conscription was necessary to sustain the war effort, and it would seem that officials in Ottawa never intended that subordinates should suspend the call for draftees or discontinue operations to apprehend deserters. On 21 October 1918, the adjutant general in Ottawa sent explicit instructions to military district commanders explaining how to administer the Military Service Act during the epidemic: "Registrars not to be requested to discontinue ordering men to report, but you may, at your discretion, after consulting with the Assistant Director of Medical Services, take steps to prevent temporary assembly of men in Barracks."[80] Ottawa's sole concession was to extend the temporary leave that had been granted to enable draftee-farmers to return home to help with the fall harvest, and this seems to have been done to prevent healthy soldiers from becoming infected, not to curtail the spread of the disease among the civilian population. Under Ottawa's instructions, defaulters who were captured or men who reported for duty as required were to be granted temporary leave for the duration of the epidemic but only if "this [could] be done without danger of losing the men."[81] Then, on 25 October, three days before the epidemic peaked in Montreal, the military began to quietly resume calling up draftees for service.[82] In a memorandum titled "Influenza Epidemic," an officer at the headquarters of the Montreal military district asked the military registrar to "please start ordering men to report for duty, at the same rate you were doing immediately before the Epidemic, we can then gradually speed up as you think fit."[83]

Undoubtedly, the administration of the Military Service Act in Quebec during the pandemic period contributed to the spread of influenza. Soldiers from infected barracks harassed individuals on city streets, rounded up absentees, and took them to crowded rooms. The fact that many of these men were released from those same infected barracks to travel back to their families in various parts of the city must have contributed to the dissemination of influenza in Quebec. Public health officials and the newspapers protested even under risk of censorship and fines, but to no avail. Compliance with the act was essential to the war effort, and there were more defaulters in Quebec than in any other province. Across Canada, after all the exemptions had been doled out, 142,680 men were ordered to report (or voluntarily reported) for military duty in 1918. Of that number, 27,631 failed to report as ordered, 18,827 of whom were from the province of Quebec.[84] That province had more than double the number of defaulters in the rest of Canada combined.[85] Regardless of the reason for the high rate of default, the military authorities perceived the prevalence of absenteeism to be a threat to military discipline.

FLU AND THE MOBILIZATION OF THE SIBERIAN EXPEDITIONARY FORCE

While soldiers were being assembled in barracks and piled into overcrowded ships in Quebec, elsewhere in the country efforts were under way to assemble, train, and deploy troops for a different purpose that would again place the interests of the military in conflict with public health. Unlike the mobilization of soldiers for Europe, which moved healthy men from the west to infected camps in the east, this new commitment sent sick soldiers westward. Their ultimate destination was Siberia. The Siberian Expeditionary Force (SEF) was a small multinational body taxed with securing a supply line for tsarist Russian forces in their war against the Bolsheviks. For its part, Canada was asked to furnish an expeditionary force of almost three thousand men to complement contingents from the United States and Great Britain. Soldiers for the SEF began to assemble at camps in New Brunswick, Quebec, and Ontario during the last weeks of August and first weeks of September 1918. The plan was for them to converge in Victoria at the end of September in preparation for transit to Russia.[86]

Just as the military loaded sick soldiers onto crowded ships for the voyage to Europe, trains were packed full of troops in Eastern Canada for their voyage to Asia. On the morning of 27 September 1918, recruits at Sussex Camp, New Brunswick, began their journey westward.[87] On that same day, the camp reported its first cases of flu.[88] Before the train reached Montreal, its passengers began to develop the symptoms of the disease, and some of the worst cases were sent to hospitals in Montreal.[89] As the train left town, forty-two more SEF soldiers who had been drawn from infected barracks in the city (probably the St-Jean barracks) climbed aboard for the journey to the Pacific.[90]

Sick SEF soldiers brought influenza to Western Canada. In Winnipeg, infected troops were transferred from a train to local military hospitals on 28 September 1918.[91] Several days later, the flu began to appear in the city itself.[92] On 29 September, just before midnight, a healthy company of the 260th Battalion boarded that train in Regina.[93] Four hours later, when it reached Calgary, twelve sick soldiers had to be removed and admitted to hospital in the city.[94] The military authorities in Calgary wired ahead to Victoria (headquarters for the BC military district) that the flu was prevalent onboard an incoming troop train.[95] When it pulled into the station in Vancouver, the train brought the first cases of influenza to the west coast.[96] The practice continued well after the epidemic became prevalent, and soldiers from Quebec and Ontario were shipped west from camps infected with influenza throughout the autumn.

The mobilization of the SEF from infected camps did not go unnoticed by the press. As in Quebec, dissent arose from a disagreement between the military and civilians as to what was essential to the war effort and what was reckless. By mid-fall, some of the volunteers who had joined the SEF began to question whether Canada actually had any interests at stake in Russia.[97] Many working-class soldiers had sympathy for the socialist revolutionaries and were reluctant to take up arms against them.[98] The mobilization of the SEF and the arrival of the second wave of flu coincided with a general labour revolt in the autumn of 1918 when workers began to demand a share in wartime profits and job security after the war.[99] In October, when it became clear that the conflict would soon end, the issue came to a head as railway strikes in Western Canada threatened to spread into a larger walkout. General strike votes were taken in Winnipeg and

Calgary.[100] In response, collective action was banned, but few believed that the will of the government could truly be enforced.[101] "The latest federal order, prohibiting strikes for the duration of the war looks like a case in point," noted the *Vancouver Sun*. "It sounds fierce enough, but will anything be done towards enforcing it? Not likely. How could it be enforced, anyway, if a large body of strikers were determined to pay no attention to it?"[102] Working-class soldiers in the SEF, drafted from the factories, felt empowered, and in the aftermath of the epidemic their frustrations erupted in mutiny. Men who had watched their comrades become sick and die from flu on the SEF troop trains rioted in the streets of Victoria in mid-December.[103] As Benjamin Isitt argues, the mutiny "was located at the intersection of class and national cleavages [and] provides a compelling window into persistent tensions in Canadian society, tensions that were amplified in the heat of wartime."[104] Influenza was a crystallizing factor that focused and directed existing dissatisfactions toward the state.

Although class was an important dynamic in the pandemic experience, it must not be overemphasized. Anger at Ottawa's handling of the pandemic and, in particular, the military's role in spreading it was more widespread, blurring across traditional lines of class and ethnicity. In a scathing editorial – even for an anti–Union government paper – Frank Oliver's *Edmonton Bulletin* accused the military of undermining public health and that of individual soldiers without any real military necessity:

> Not only did they do nothing to prevent 'flu entering [the country] but since it has entered the military authorities have shipped hundreds of soldiers for the Siberian Expedition across Canada, starting them from the barracks in the east where 'flu was prevalent and transporting them under the conditions that made the spread of the disease certain and with increased virulence. Within the week two train loads of soldiers for Siberia have passed through Edmonton for Vancouver and Siberia ... A number of 'flu cases were taken off both trains and cared for by the military authorities. But what must have been the condition of the men in both trains on arrival at Vancouver? Every condition for taking the disease had been provided during the long train journey. Either the disease does not need to be taken seriously, – which supposition is directly contrary to the universally accepted facts – or these soldiers of Canada were subjected to disease through the criminal negligence of the military authorities. Every sort of outrage has been justified on the grounds of military urgency. There is no such urgency in the case of the Siberian Expedition now that winter has already set in Siberia. And whatever the urgency, there is nothing gained by shipping men across the continent

under conditions that condemn a large proportion to the hospital and some
to the grave. Men who are layed up [sic] by 'flu or have died because of it
can not fight the Bolsheviki. That is not the way to win the war.[105]

In the fall of 1918, popular and official conceptions of military necessity
were diverging. The intransigence of the military authorities brought latent
feelings of disaffection to the surface. In the estimations of Oliver's newspaper, public health and military necessity were not oppositional interests.
There were limits to public support.

Municipal officials in Eastern Canada expressed similar sentiments.
Toronto's outspoken mayor, Thomas Church, who had a penchant for
melodramatic outbursts, loudly protested the military's handling of influenza and tried to persuade the authorities to change their policy of sealing
soldiers into trains when sickness was already prevalent in their units.
"Certain soldiers," Church spat at the head medical officer of the Toronto
military district, "[have] been murdered by the military authorities and
... as Chief Magistrate [I will] not stand by and see any more of them
murdered."[106] Church alleged that the army's base hospital in Toronto was
overcrowded and unsanitary, and that its facilities were being improperly
used.[107] He was also concerned that the Toronto men at Niagara Camp
– many of whom were destined for the SEF – were being housed in tents
during the wet autumn weather.[108] He sent a number of telegrams to the
Department of Militia and Defence in Ottawa, demanding better care for
Torontonian soldiers. He alleged that they were being poorly looked after
at Camp Niagara and pointed out that most other soldiers had already
moved to winter quarters. He requested that they be housed in warmer,
more hygienic conditions in Toronto itself: "Could you not," he asked in
a telegram, "bring back Siberian draft at Niagara? We have good house
accommodations at Exhibition for them. Two men of this draft died
yesterday from outbreak. Niagara draft really all TO men. Fear further
casualties here owing to heavy outbreak of this epidemic at fort Niagara
and in Polish Camp. See no reason why Siberian Draft should be singled
out and kept there in tents."[109] The military dismissed Church's concerns.
"I notice," wrote an official in the adjutant general's office, "that Mayor
Church takes an intense interest in all troops that are not actually being
fed inside the city limits of Toronto."[110] Instead of addressing his questions,
the army decided to immediately move the draft from Niagara to British
Columbia.[111] The mayor's concerns and public anger were unwelcome
challenges to military authority.

Church, like many others who expressed dissent in this period, was accused of radicalism and anti-war sympathies. The deputy assistant director of medical services in Toronto typed out a report outlining his explanation for Church's conduct:

> What I am really concerned about is that the action of the Mayor is but a continuation of the unjust criticism well-known to have been carried out against the military authorities in [Toronto] since soldiers have been during the War first quartered here ... [This] is in my opinion too important a matter to be lightly passed over. I am of the opinion that it has been the cause of the great unrest among returned men which was recently manifested in a series of riots extending over several days, a few weeks ago. I am also of the opinion that if the character of the criticism carried on by the Mayor is not stopped that the riots we have had in Toronto are but the beginning of what may be expected as the soldiers return in increasing number ... Indeed it seems to me that the propaganda referred to is but a type of Bolshevikism [sic] that should be nipped in the bud if at all possible.[112]

It is unlikely that Church, who served as a Tory MP almost continuously from 1921 to his death in 1950, was a closet communist. Bolshevik or not, the military viewed his attack as dangerous anti-government propaganda. Those who opposed military authority represented a threat to the war effort.

The newspapers tended to take the mayor's side, and the gulf between what the military and the public accepted as genuinely necessary continued to grow, even in loyal Ontario. "The shocking situation, with its tragic toll of soldier lives," read an editorial in the *Toronto Globe,* "brought about by official carelessness, mismanagement, and neglect in connection with the Base Hospital, has thoroughly aroused the indignant and determined Canadianism of the people in all parts of the country ... There is – as there should be – an insistent demand for the dismissal of the [military medical officials], and for the complete renovation and reorganization of that essential branch of the military service which they have shown themselves indisposed or unable properly to administer."[113]

It was not the war effort that the *Globe* opposed, only the way in which the military set its priorities. This opinion was shared by other newspapers. In Montreal, the English-language *Star* printed daily coverage of the inquest into the base hospital, righteously describing its inadequate conditions and the dispute between the military and the mayor; it applauded a coroner's verdict against the military after an inquest into one of the deaths.[114] In Edmonton, a father of two soldiers echoed the *Globe's* protest in a letter to the editor of the *Bulletin:* "We have at least the right to claim something more than sheer neglect of our boys ... We certainly had this promptly and full as to those overseas. This much we should have therefore from medical authorities within this Dominion."[115] Another editorial from the *Toronto Globe* seems to best capture the tone of public indignation. The editor accused the military of being an "arrogant and insolent system which regards the continued interest and concern of civilians in their sons and brothers after they have become part of the military forces as presumptuous and calling for reprimand and punishment. This is the attitude of Prussianism – and there is no home for Potsdam at Ottawa."[116] The rigid, uncaring, ceaseless pursuit of military aims at the expense of civilian health and welfare was the image of Wilhelmine Germany that Canadians had rallied to fight in 1914.[117] By the autumn of 1918, some saw these same characteristics in the actions of the officials representing the Union government.

Conclusion

Army and civilian officials were able to work together when their aims did not conflict, as in the summer of 1918 when they successfully cooperated to bar the first wave of influenza from the country, but military necessity ultimately trumped public and individual health during the pandemic. As the need for replacements grew in the autumn, the military became increasingly focused on getting manpower overseas to Europe. Although it sacrificed the health of individual soldiers by crowding them onto troopships, arguing that reinforcements were not needed at a critical juncture in the war would have been difficult. The public could tolerate some sacrifices, but soon, popular and official definitions of military need began to conflict. As the autumn progressed, military officials came to view civilian public health measures on the home front as a threat to the war effort. Despite high numbers of infections and deaths from influenza, they ignored demands to cease conscription during the pandemic and sent thousands of infected soldiers across the country, spreading the disease. As the war effort widened to include a new commitment to send an expeditionary force to Russia, the military became even less willing to be bound by concerns for the health of individual troops or the general public. As popular and official perceptions of military necessity diverged, opposition to the military's handling of the pandemic increased. Army policy sowed seeds of disaffection across a broad stratum of Canadian society.

Despite censorship regulations, newspapers and politicians confronted the army. "The military authorities seem to take the view that the way to deal with a virulent epidemic is to ignore its existence," wrote one newspaper editor, "and if they can keep the facts from getting into the papers, all is well. The deaths of a few common soldiers – draftees – is neither here nor there."[118] The influenza pandemic brought latent anger to the surface and provided a nucleus around which opposition to the state could coalesce. In 1919, many of the same issues regarding the lack of state commitment to civilian health and welfare would re-emerge in the demobilization riots in England, the controversy over medical care and pensions for veterans, and most prominently in the Winnipeg General Strike.[119] The controversy over the management of the 1918 flu epidemic demonstrated that when military necessity and public interest came into conflict, there were limits to Canadian patriotism.

ACKNOWLEDGMENTS

I wish to acknowledge the support of a Social Sciences and Humanities Research Council Canada Graduate Scholarship, funding from the Department of History at the University of Western Ontario, the financial assistance of the Laurier Centre for Military Strategic and Disarmament Studies, and the Department of Humanities at Mount Royal University. I also thank Jonathan Vance, Tim Cook, Terry Copp, Lianne Leddy, Sarah Cozzi, Karen Scott, and Amy Menary.

NOTES

1 See Richard J. Evans, "Epidemics and Revolutions: Cholera in Nineteenth-Century Europe," *Past and Present* 120,1 (1988): 123-46; and William McNeill, *Plagues and Peoples* (Garden City: Anchor Press, 1976).

2 J. George Adami, *War Story of the Canadian Army Medical Corps* (Ottawa: Canadian War Records Office, 1918).

3 Guy Carleton Jones, "The Importance of the Balkan Wars to the Medical Profession of Canada," *Canadian Medical Association Journal* 4,9 (September 1914): 801-2.

4 On the international impact of Spanish flu and armies, see Richard Collier, *The Plague of the Spanish Lady: The Influenza Pandemic of 1918-1919* (New York: Atheneum, 1974); and Alfred W. Crosby, *Epidemic and Peace, 1918* (Westport, CT: Greenwood Press, 1976). On the Canadian military and influenza, see Janice P. Dickin McGinnis, "The Impact of Epidemic Influenza: Canada, 1918-1919," in *Medicine in Canadian Society: Historical Perspectives,* ed. S.E.D. Shortt (Montreal and Kingston: McGill-Queen's University Press, 1981), 447-78; and Eileen Pettigrew, *The Silent Enemy: Canada and the Deadly Flu of 1918* (Saskatoon: Western Producer Prairie Books, 1983). For a revisionist perspective on the origins of flu

in Canada, see Mark Osborne Humphries, "The Horror at Home: The Canadian Military and the 'Great' Influenza Pandemic of 1918," *Journal of the Canadian Historical Association,* n.s., 16,1 (2005): 235-60.

5 Carol R. Byerly, *Fever of War: The Influenza Epidemic in the U.S. Army during World War I* (New York: New York University Press, 2005). See also John M. Barry, *The Great Influenza: The Epic Story of the Deadliest Pandemic in History* (New York: Viking, 2004).

6 G.W.L. Nicholson, *Canadian Expeditionary Force, 1914-1919* (Ottawa: Queen's Printer, 1964), 519-24.

7 There is an enormous literature on Canada in the Great War. Some of the most important works on the social and political history of the war include Robert Craig Brown and Ramsay Cook, *Canada, 1896-1921: A Nation Transformed* (Toronto: McClelland and Stewart, 1974); Jeff Keshen, *Propaganda and Censorship during Canada's Great War* (Edmonton: University of Alberta Press, 1996); David MacKenzie, ed., *Canada and the First World War: Essays in Honour of Robert Craig Brown* (Toronto: University of Toronto Press, 2005); Desmond Morton, *Fight or Pay: Soldier's Families in the Great War* (Vancouver: UBC Press, 2004); Desmond Morton, *When Your Number's Up: The Canadian Soldier in the First World War* (Toronto: Random House, 1993); Desmond Morton and J.L. Granatstein, *Marching to Armageddon: Canadians and the Great War, 1914-1919* (Toronto: Lester and Orpen Dennys, 1989); Robert Rutherdale, *Hometown Horizons: Local Responses to Canada's Great War* (Vancouver: UBC Press, 2004); and John Herd Thompson, *The Harvests of War: The Prairie West, 1914-1918* (Toronto: McClelland and Stewart, 1978).

8 Nicholson, *Canadian Expeditionary Force,* 521-22.

9 The Second Battle of Ypres in April of 1915 was the site of the first German gas attack of the war. These figures are taken from detailed statistics compiled by Major J.P.S. Cathcart in his investigation of pensions in the 1930s. See Library and Archives Canada (LAC), Record Group (RG) 24, vol. 1844, file GAQ 11-11E, Ottawa.

10 See various war diaries of the assistant directors of medical service for the First, Second, Third, and Fourth Canadian Divisions and the Command Areas in England in LAC, RG 9. These are all found in various volumes in series III d 3.

11 See Andrew MacPhail, *Official History of the Canadian Forces in the Great War, 1914-19: The Medical Services* (Ottawa: Department of National Defence, 1925), 271-74.

12 Adjutant General, Department of the Overseas Military Forces of Canada (OMFC), to Deputy Minister, OMFC, 18 September 1918, LAC, RG 9, series III A 1, vol. 84, file 10-11-1. See also Humphries, "The Horror at Home," 242-44.

13 *British North America Act, 1867* (UK), 30-31 Vict., c. 3, ss. 92(7) and 91(11).

14 Canada, *House of Commons Debates* (28 February 1916), 1233. Geoffrey Bilson, "Dr. Frederick Montizambert (1843-1929): Canada's First Director General of Public Health," *Medical History* 29 (1985): 396.

15 See newspaper clippings and obituaries in LAC, Montizambert Family Fonds, Manuscript Group 29C101, vol. 1.

16 Frederick Montizambert, "Public Health and Quarantine: Practice of the Department of Agriculture, and under What Authority," 12 February 1909, LAC, RG 29, vol. 19, file 10-3-1, vol. 1.

17 Major General Jones to Dr. Montizambert, 8 July 1918, LAC, RG 29, vol. 300, file 416-2-12.

18 Ibid.

19 F. Montizambert to Dr. N.E. MacKay, 8 July 1918, LAC, RG 29, vol. 300, file 416-2-12.

20 W.G. Holloway, Senior Naval Officer, Montreal, to Secretary, Department of Naval Service, 13 July 1918, LAC, RG 29, vol. 300, file 416-2-12.

21 Director General of Public Health (DGPH) to G.J. Desbarats, Deputy Minister, Department of Naval Service, 15 July 1918, LAC, RG 29, vol. 300, file 416-2-12.

22 On the arrival of the other two troopships, see Humphries, "The Horror at Home," 243; DGPH to Acting Minister of Immigration and Colonization, 13 July 1918, LAC, RG 29, vol. 300, file 416-2-12.

23 DGPH to Dr. H. Rundle Nelson, William Head, Victoria, BC, 22 July 1918, LAC, RG 29, vol. 300, file 416-2-12.

24 "Awake to Dangers of Spanish Grippe," *Vancouver World,* 9 August 1918.

25 See Humphries, "The Horror at Home," 245-49.

26 "Influenza-like" is taken to include diagnoses recorded as influenza, grippe, flu, pneumonia, bronchial pneumonia, lobular pneumonia, bronchitis, purulent bronchitis, sore throat, tonsillitis, catarrh, and cold. It does not include diagnoses of tuberculosis. The statistics are compiled from hospital admission and discharge books in "Admission/Discharge Books," 5 June-4 December 1918, LAC, RG 9, books 291-97, series II L 1, vol. 9.

27 Ibid.

28 Ibid., 1 July-25 October 1918, books 61-81B, vol. 3.

29 Ibid., 1 July–29 September 1918, books 394, 398, 399, 404, 406, 407, 408, 411, 412, vols. 11, 12, 13.

30 On the German spring offensives, see, for example, Reichsarchiv, *Der Weltkreig, 1914 bis 1918 Band 13 und Band 14* (Berlin: E.S. Mittler und Sohn, 1942-44). The most recent English-language source is David T. Zabecki, *The German 1918 Offensives: A Case Study in the Operational Level of War* (New York: Routledge, 2006).

31 Nicholson, *Canadian Expeditionary Force,* 323-24.

32 Ibid., 362-429; see also James Edmonds, *Military Operations: France and Belgium, 1918,* vols. 1-3 (London: Macmillan, 1935).

33 On 21 October 1918, Sir Henry Wilson, chief of the imperial general staff, informed Field Marshall Sir Douglas Haig, the commander in chief, that if the war continued into 1919, the strength of the British army would be depleted by 48 percent. See Haig's diary entry for 21 October in Robert Blake, ed., *The Private Papers of Douglas Haig, 1914-1919* (London: Eyre and Spottiswoode, 1952), 331.

34 Byerly, *Fever of War,* 74-75.

35 Barry, *The Great Influenza,* 197-99.

36 Lt. Col. A.T. LePan to the Chief of the General Staff, Department of Militia and Defence, 22 March 1919, LAC, RG 24, vol. 1883A, file "Polish Army Camp."

37 War Diary (WD), Assistant Director of Medical Services (ADMS), Military District (MD) 4 (Montreal), 20 September 1918, LAC, RG 9, vol. 5061, file 976, pt. 1.

38 Ibid., 21 September 1918.

39 Port of East Hoboken, New Jersey, to Chief of E.S., 23 September 1918, entry 2023, National Archives and Records Administration (NARA), RG 92, Washington; Lt. Col. Edward A. Pitzka, Chief Surgeon SS *Nestor,* 22 September and 2 October 1918, entry 2023, NARA, RG 92; WD, ADMS, MD 6 (Halifax), 22 September 1918, LAC, RG 9, vol. 5062, file 978, pt. 3.

40 For all flu-related correspondence of the DGPH, consult LAC, RG 29, vol. 300, file 416-2-12. Although these records contain numerous items from July until the first week of

August, a gap occurs between mid-August and 29 September when correspondence continues.

41 F. Montizambert to A.C. Hawkins, 30 September 1918, LAC, RG 29, vol. 300, file 416-2-12.

42 "Influenza Epidemic: Abstract of Report on Influenza Epidemic on Board HMT 'Huntsend' and 'City of Cairo,'" n.d., LAC, RG 9, series III B 2, vol. 3752, file 3-1-1-5; "Outbreak of Influenza on Troopships," n.d., LAC, RG 24, vol. 1847, file GAQ 11-61.

43 Ibid.

44 "Influenza Epidemic on Troopships," 7 December 1924, LAC, RG 24, vol. 1872, file SF-13-2.

45 Testimony of Lieutenant Colonel Kerr, ADMS Embarkation, 3 December 1918, LAC, RG 24, vol. 2558, file C2529, vol. 2.

46 OMFC to Ottawa, 22 October 1918, quoted in ibid.

47 Assistant Director General Medical Services to General Ashton, 28 January 1919, LAC, RG 24, vol. 2558, file C2529, vol. 2.

48 "Proceedings Court of Inquiry HMT Victoria: Summary of Facts," 21 January 1919, LAC, RG 24, vol. 2558, file C2529, vol. 2.

49 Testimony of Kerr, 3 December 1918, 3.

50 Lt. Col. Kerr to Director-General of Medical Services (DGMS), Ottawa, 11 September 1918, reprinted in ibid., 13.

51 Deputy-Minister of Militia and Defence to DGPH, 15 October 1918, LAC, RG 29, vol. 300, file 416-2-12. The court of inquiry proceedings reprint Kerr's request, not the reply. A search of the relevant DGMS files turned up a response to the request concerning Grosse Ile but nothing in connection with the suggestion that ships carry fewer soldiers.

52 Testimony of Kerr, 3 December 1918, 1.

53 On the meaning of the First World War in Canada, see Jonathan Vance, Death so Noble: Memory, Meaning, and the First World War (Vancouver: UBC Press, 1997).

54 Nicholson, Canadian Expeditionary Force, 321-22.

55 District Intelligence Officer (MD 4) to the Assistant Adjutant General (MD 4), "Anti-Recruiting Disturbances," 24 August 1916, LAC, RG 24, vol. 4479, file 25-1-13; and General Officer Commanding MD 5 (Quebec) to the Secretary of the Militia Council, "Anti Conscription Activities Shawinigan Falls, P.Q.," 12 September 1917, LAC, RG 24, vol. 4517, file C159a 1.

56 Keshen, Propaganda and Censorship, 77.

57 Ibid., 66.

58 Nicholson, Canadian Expeditionary Force, 319-28.

59 See, for example, Brigadier-General J.F. Landry, "Confidential Operations Orders," 13 and 14 September 1918, LAC, RG 24, vol. 4518, file 4170.

60 Canadian Military Police, Civil Section, MD 5, 31 September 1918, LAC, RG 24, vol. 4518, file C170.

61 See various reports in LAC, RG 24, vol. 4518, file C170.

62 Telegram 110 from General Service Officer (unspecified) to Colonel J.A. Beaubien, n.d., LAC, RG 24, vol. 4518, file 4170.

63 "Prudence militaire," La Patrie (Montreal), 10 October 1918, 4.

64 Ibid. For concurrent coverage of civilian public health measures, see "Public Places Closed by City Health Board," Montreal Gazette, 8 October 1918, 1.

65 "Les policiers militaires vont chômer," *La Patrie* (Montreal), 11 October 1918, 3.

66 "Les appels suspendus," *Le Devoir* (Montreal), 5 November 1918, 1.

67 "En guerre ouverte contre l'épidémie," *Le Devoir* (Montreal), 11 October 1918, 2.

68 "Wants Recruiting Stopped Pro Tem," *Montreal Gazette,* 17 October 1918, 3.

69 Richard Ouellet, ed., *Les débats de l'Assemblée législative (reconstitués), 14e législature, 2e session* (Quebec City: Assemblée nationale du Québec, 2002), 154-63, http://www.assnat.qc.ca/.

70 Deputy Minister of Militia and Defence to Deputy Minister of Department of Justice, 31 October 1918, LAC, RG 13, vol. 1939, file 2362-1918.

71 Deputy Minister of Justice to Deputy Minister of Militia and Defence, 5 November 1918, LAC, RG 13, vol. 1939, file 2362-1918.

72 "Wants Recruiting Stopped Pro Tem," 3. See also, for example, "Les appels suspendus," 1.

73 Captain, MSA, DO, MD No. 4, to Registrar D, MSA, Montreal, 4 October 1918, LAC, RG 24, vol. 4498, file MD4-60-1-1.

74 Lieut. Colonel Commanding 2nd Que. Regt. to A.A.G., MD 4, 8 October 1918, LAC, RG 24, vol. 4498, file MD4-60-1-1.

75 WD, 4th Battalion, Canadian Garrison Regiment, 9 October 1918, LAC, RG 9, vol. 5061, file 976, pt. 1.

76 Memorandum by Assistant Provost Marshal, MD 4, 11 October 1918, LAC, RG 24, vol. 4498, file MD4-60-1-1.

77 WD, 4th Battalion, Canadian Garrison Regiment, 20 October 1918.

78 See "Reports on Activities of Troops of Quebec Special Service Detachment Number 1," 15, 17-18, 24, 26 October 1918, LAC, RG 24, vol. 4518, file 4170-2.

79 See various "Reports on Activities of Troops of Quebec Special Service Detachment Number 1," 1 October-13 November 1918, LAC, RG 24, vol. 4518, file 4170-2.

80 "Telegram 15307, Reference Influenza Epidemic from Adjutant General," 21 October 1918, LAC, RG 24, vol. 4498, file MD4-60-1-1.

81 Ibid.

82 S. Boucher, "The Epidemic of Influenza," *Canadian Medical Association Journal* 8, 12 (December 1918): 1087-88.

83 "Influenza Epidemic," Captain, MSA, DO, MD 4 (Headquarters), to Registrar "D," Military Service Act, Montreal, 25 October 1918, LAC, RG 24, vol. 4498, file MD4-60-1-1.

84 J. Castell Hopkins, *The Canadian Annual Review of Public Affairs, 1918* (Toronto: Canadian Annual Review, 1919), 473-75.

85 Ibid. The total for the rest of Canada was 8,804.

86 Nicholson, *Canadian Expeditionary Force,* 490.

87 General Officer Commanding MD 7 (Saint John) to Quartermaster General, Ottawa, 26 September 1918, LAC, RG 24, vol. 4574, file 3-9-47, vol. 2.

88 WD, ADMS, MD 7, 28 September 1918, LAC, RG 9, vol. 4063, file 978, pt. 1.

89 District Records Officer, MD 4, to District Records Officer, MD 7, 7 November 1918, LAC, RG 24, vol. 4574, file 3-9-47, vol. 1; District Records Officer, [MD 7], to ADMS, MD 7, 27 November 1918, LAC, RG 24, vol. 4574, file 3-9-47, vol. 1.

90 WD, ADMS, MD 4, 29 September 1918, LAC, RG 9, vol. 5061, file 976, pt. 1.

91 Acting Provost Marshall, MD 10 (Winnipeg), to the District Casualty Officer, MD 10, n.d., LAC, RG 24, vol. 4607, file MD10-20-102, vol. 1.

92 Esyllt Wynne Jones, "Searching for the Springs of Health: Women and Working Families in Winnipeg's 1918-1919 Influenza Epidemic" (PhD diss., Department of History, University of Manitoba, 2003), 47.

93 WD, Assistant Adjutant General and Quartermaster General, MD 12 (Regina), 29 September 1918, LAC, RG 9, vol. 5065, file 992; and WD, 1st Depot Battalion Saskatchewan Regiment, 29 September 1918, LAC, RG 9, vol. 5065, file 992.

94 ADMS, MD 12 (Calgary), to DGMS, Ottawa, 2 October 1918, LAC, RG 24, vol. 1992, file HW 762-11-15.

95 WD, Assistant Adjutant General in charge of administration, MD 11 (Victoria), 1 October 1918, LAC, RG 9, vol. 5065, file 990, pt. 1.

96 WD, ADMS, MD 11, 3 October 1918, LAC, RG 9, vol. 5065, file 990, pt. 1.

97 See Benjamin Isitt, "Mutiny from Victoria to Vladivostok, December 1918," *Canadian Historical Review* 87,2 (2006): 223-64.

98 Ibid.

99 See Craig Heron, ed., *The Workers' Revolt in Canada, 1917-25* (Toronto: University of Toronto Press, 1998). See also Thompson, *The Harvests of War*.

100 See, for example, "Vote Strongly for a General Strike," *Manitoba Free Press* (Winnipeg), 24 October 1918, 5; "Railroad Strike throughout West Gains Strength," *Edmonton Journal*, 10 October 1918, 21; and "Calgary Outside Employees Are on Sympathy Strike," *Edmonton Journal*, 12 October 1918, 1, 3.

101 See, for example, "Provision for Settlement of Labour Disputes Makes Strikes Illegal Hereafter," *Edmonton Journal*, 12 October 1918, 2; "Full Explanation of New Order Prohibiting Strikes and Lockouts," *Winnipeg Tribune*, 22 October 1918, 1; and "All Strikes and Lockouts Banned by Government," *Vancouver Sun*, 12 October 1918, 1.

102 "Making Another Mistake," *Vancouver Sun*, 14 October 1918, 6.

103 Isitt, "Mutiny from Victoria to Vladivostok," 223-64.

104 Ibid., 227.

105 "Union Government and the Flu," *Edmonton Bulletin*, 25 October 1918, 7.

106 Report from Deputy ADMS Sanitation to ADMS, MD 2, 9 October 1918, LAC, RG 24, vol. 4386, file 34-7-136, vol. 5.

107 Colonel, CAMC for ADMS, MD 2, to DGMS, Ottawa, 14 October 1918, LAC, RG 24, vol. 4386, file 34-7-136, vol. 5; see also T.L. Church to Captain Seymour, RAF, 15 October 1918, LAC, RG 24, vol. 4386, file 34-7-136, vol. 5.

108 T.L. Church to Major-General Logie, Military Headquarters, Toronto, 16 October 1918, LAC, RG 24, vol. 4386, file 34-7-136, vol. 5.

109 T.L. Church to Minister of Militia, 8 October 1918, LAC, RG 24, vol. 1992, file HQ 762-11-15.

110 Brigadier General Gwynne for Adjutant General to Private Secretary of the Minister of Militia and Defence, 10 October 1918, LAC, RG 24, vol. 1992, file HQ 762-11-15.

111 Major General, Canadian General Staff, to Adjutant General, Ottawa, 9 October 1918, LAC, RG 24, vol. 1992, file HQ 762-11-15.

112 Report from Deputy ADMS Sanitation to ADMS, MD 2, 9 October 1918, LAC, RG 24, vol. 4386, file 34-7-136, vol. 5.

113 "Hospitals for Our Soldiers," *Toronto Globe*, 1 November 1918, 6.

114 See various articles on the Ontario page of the *Montreal Star* in late October and early November 1918. See especially 6, 7, and 8 November 1918, 2.

115 Anonymous letter to the editor, *Edmonton Bulletin*, 2 November 1918, 7.

116 "Ottawa – and the Base Hospital," *Toronto Globe,* 30 October 1918, 6.
117 Vance, *Death so Noble,* 12-34.
118 "Fighting Flu with the Censorship," *Edmonton Bulletin,* 31 October 1918, 7.
119 On flu, labour, and the Winnipeg General Strike, see Esyllt W. Jones, *Influenza 1918: Disease, Death, and Struggle in Winnipeg* (Toronto: University of Toronto Press, 2007).

2

"Rendering Valuable Service": The Politics of Nursing during the 1918-19 Influenza Crisis

LINDA QUINEY

A t 9:00 a.m. on 2 October 1918, Gertrude Murphy boarded the train at Calgary station, bound for the small Alberta town of Drumheller. The conductor warned her that the town was under quarantine, with the "worst type of Flu in Alberta." Although no one was to board or disembark there, an exception was made for Murphy because of her Voluntary Aid Detachment (VAD) nurse's badge. As Murphy recalled years later, for the duration of the journey she became an object of curiosity but also fear, as passengers cautiously kept their distance and even avoided passing her to get to the washroom.[1] Gertrude Murphy's experience as a nursing volunteer during the height of the fall 1918 wave of the influenza pandemic highlights two critical aspects of the crisis: first, the pervasive fear of infection, as palpable as any "plague" experience, ancient or contemporary; and second, the assumption that women, in the role of nurses, should be the front-line workers in this early-twentieth-century health crisis.[2] Society expected women's service and sacrifice, whether as volunteers or qualified professionals. Male public figures, such as the mayor of Ottawa, reminded local women that they had a "duty" to volunteer to nurse influenza victims. Conforming to an ideology that accorded women the role of natural caregivers, the mayor declared that they must abandon their patriotic knitting of socks for soldiers and "get into the trenches themselves."[3]

Nursing, in its construction as a natural function of women, quickly became a polemical hotspot on the influenza battlefield. Physicians and health officials were attacking an invisible and unpredictable enemy. A primary mechanism for containment was the constant vigilance of nursing care, which also provided the only effective treatment: bed rest, hydration, and the control of fever.[4] The emergency momentarily blurred professional distinctions in nursing ranks and inadvertently exposed some of the political dimensions of nursing's position in the public health hierarchy of the era. Flu victims could only be grateful for the caring ministrations of the "nurse," but emerging perceptions of female professionalism, with the attendant assumptions of gender and class, surfaced during this unique transitory period of the integration of civilian, military, and voluntary nursing. Thus, the epidemic can be seen as integral to a political and ideological drama that pitted the new professional identity of qualified nurses against that of female volunteers who were socialized by contemporary definitions of gender and class to accept the caregiver role. This healing work, both professional and volunteer, acted as a touchstone for conflicting views of nursing as either a *professionalizing* or a *natural* role for women in the early twentieth century.

WARTIME NURSING

Under normal circumstances, nursing influenza patients at home or in the hospital was a routine task, but the conditions of 1918 were far from normal. As recent scholarship has emphasized, the flu pandemic was intimately interwoven with the prosecution of the war effort. Like other epidemic diseases, it had the propensity to "hitch a ride" on major transportation routes, particularly those used in the mobilization of troops.[5] Mark Humphries demonstrates that the second and deadliest wave of influenza, which crossed Canada during the late summer and fall of 1918, was facilitated in its spread by a broadened war effort and by the movement of fresh troops westward toward the Siberian front in September 1918. This military activity hampered the effectiveness of any public health dictums against rail travel; in Humphries's estimation, military policy was at least partially responsible for spreading the infection from east to west at the height of the pandemic.[6]

The First World War and the influenza epidemic intersected with a critical period in the development of Canadian professional nursing. The war had greatly affected the complement of medical and nursing personnel in hospitals throughout the country. Historian Kathryn McPherson observes that by 1916, some 20 percent of the Winnipeg General Hospital's nursing graduates were engaged in some aspect of military or Red Cross nursing, and shortages of qualified graduates had already existed prior to the war.[7] McPherson argues that the war contributed to a further drain on nursing resources by attracting both graduates and prospective students into more lucrative war work, a situation that was compounded by an ongoing reduction of the number of available nurses due to marriage, possibly encouraged by men going off to war.[8] With just over three thousand nurses recruited for the Canadian Army Medical Corps (CAMC), the nursing reserves were strained, though not entirely depleted. McPherson estimates that some fifty-six hundred nurses or students were listed in the 1911 census, increasing to more than twenty-one thousand by the 1921 census, although not all were active nurses.[9]

The war had provided an unprecedented opportunity for Canadian nurses to demonstrate their skills and training in the visible context of their role as military nurses with the CAMC. Their status as commissioned officers – they were ranked as lieutenants – set them apart from all Allied military nurses.[10] The leaders of the Canadian National Association of Trained Nurses (CNATN) were optimistic about the potential boost to the status and professional aspirations of Canadian nurses.[11] Even the unwelcome advent of "enthusiastic amateurs," like Gertrude Murphy, who trained as VADs with the St. John Ambulance Association (SJAA), seemed unlikely to dim the reputation of the CAMC Nursing Service.[12]

Prior to the First World War, Canadian nursing leaders had begun to organize for provincial registration legislation as a first critical step in regularizing the standards of qualified nursing practice across Canada. The differences between trained graduate nurses and untrained practitioners were still poorly defined by 1914, and prior to the epidemic, only four provinces had enacted registration legislation.[13] Regardless, in the early years of the war, the VADs, who had been created as a "home guard" of auxiliary volunteers, seemed unlikely to constitute a serious threat to the role or reputation of CAMC or civilian nurses. Overseas, the CAMC refused to permit female volunteers to undermine the efficiency and status of the qualified military nurses in its hospitals. Canadian VADs were welcome only in British military hospitals abroad, working in conjunction with their counterparts in the British Red Cross Society (BRCS) VAD nursing organization.[14] As the war ground on, VADs gradually made inroads as auxiliary personnel in the expanding network of military convalescent hospitals at home, until the onslaught of the epidemic, when their help suddenly became essential to both civilian and military nursing needs.

Nursing, as women's work, became contested territory during the war, in part because the distinction between the qualified military nurse and the officially sanctioned VAD auxiliary was largely imperceptible to the public eye. In Canada, both the CAMC and St. John Ambulance unwittingly reinforced the confusion through the similarity in the style of their nursing uniforms, which stressed the military associations of the work while striving to emphasize a respectable image of femininity.[15] The media, captivated by the unprecedented image of women in military dress, further blurred the distinctions by homogenizing the differences. The favoured representation of both Canada's military nursing sisters and VAD nurses was borrowed from the model of the British Red Cross VAD uniform, displaying a prominent red cross emblem on the apron bib.[16] Thus, the generic, idealized, "Red Cross nurse" became symbolic of the "war nurse" for the Allied cause, further confusing popular recognition of the considerable differences in training and experience that distinguished VADs from military nurses. Even the Canadian government propagandized the Red Cross nurse to help with the war effort in a poster commissioned to promote the sale of victory bonds. The poster, whose subject is the June 1918 torpedoing of the hospital ship *Llandovery Castle,* features an enraged Canadian serviceman clutching the lifeless body of one of the fourteen Canadian military nurses who drowned at sea. A prominent red cross is displayed on her apron bib.[17]

As a wartime domestic resource, VAD training was based primarily on the expectation of service in the field, where volunteers would assist only in makeshift emergency hospitals. The VADs were not intended to function as trained nursing graduates. The evolution of domestic military convalescent hospitals was an unanticipated development in a war that was supposed to be over by Christmas, but once the hospitals were established, VAD service was gradually accepted.[18] The differences between nurse and VAD were most evident in their training. The CAMC nurses had earned their qualifications through three years of rigorous hospital training in accredited schools, successfully completing written and practical examinations.[19] The CNATN had also tried to ensure, although not entirely successfully, that only the most qualified and experienced graduates earned the honour of wearing a lieutenant's insignia.[20] As volunteers, the VAD recruits were required to complete two St. John Ambulance courses, in first aid and home nursing, over a six-week period. Each course consisted of approximately twelve hours of lecture and demonstration. Retired nurses and willing physicians were enlisted to give instruction and to administer the final exams, which were primarily verbal and practical. Few VADs obtained any hospital experience during their training, since civilian hospitals wanted no part of "amateurs," and military convalescent hospitals did not begin to develop across Canada until mid-1915.[21] As unpaid nursing aides, VADs gradually became a more cost-effective asset than the military medical orderlies, who were needed for active service. Thus, by 1918, a significant number of VADs had achieved the benefit of some active hospital nursing experience.

Although their education and experience varied considerably, Canada's VAD and trained nursing ranks were very similar in class and cultural origins. Canadian VADs were predominantly young, single, middle class, and of Anglo-Protestant heritage. British scholarship ties VADs to the upper middle and elite classes of wartime society.[22] As a derivative phenomenon, Canadian VADs have long been thought to occupy the same social strata. However, recent research demonstrates that they were related much more closely to the trained nurses in class, culture, and ethnicity.[23] Lyn MacDonald describes British VADs as "gently nurtured girls," and Anne Summers argues that pre-war VADs were "outside the labour market altogether," but the Canadian evidence does not conform to the idealized "Vera Brittain" model of the British VAD.[24] Although contemporary comment promoted Canadian VADs as products of the "highest and best educated class of society," only a few were daughters of the elite. Many pursued gainful employment in schools, offices, or service sector work but volunteered on evenings and weekends at local convalescent hospitals.[25] Some, like teacher Gertrude Murphy, were available for service only after the epidemic had closed her school. Once dressed in full VAD uniform, however, she and countless others were able to assume the generic identity of "nurse."[26]

By the war's end, the nursing leadership in Canada also acknowledged that the young women who had volunteered as VADs might serve equally well as qualified nurses, but only if properly trained. In the fall of 1918, St. John Ambulance was reorganizing the VAD program to provide the military convalescent hospitals with volunteers trained for rehabilitation work. At that time, concerned regarding a projected postwar shortage of nurses to care for invalid veterans, the CNATN was also becoming increasingly uneasy that a pool of some two thousand rudimentarily trained VADs might threaten the status and future job security of qualified nurses. To counter this threat, CNATN president Jean Gunn proposed enrolling VADs as postwar nursing students to help alleviate any potential shortages in the military convalescent hospitals and to simultaneously help counter any future civilian nursing shortages.[27] Her proposal was rejected by both St. John Ambulance and the director of military medical services, though for different reasons. The gesture, however, revealed the truth of Gunn's contention that the VADs had "earned the approval" of their nursing peers, while firmly establishing that the real difference between nurse and volunteer was the level of qualification.[28]

With the war winding down in the autumn of 1918, the readiness with which VADs rallied to the call for nursing aid during the pandemic raised a further red flag for the nursing establishment. Previously, VAD service had been confined primarily to a military setting, with the exception of the December 1917 Halifax explosion, but the pandemic did not recognize the boundaries between civilian and military jurisdictions.[29] In the aftermath of these two domestic crises, Gunn reflected on the meaning for the future of Canadian nursing and the preservation of the quality of nursing care in Canada. The confusion of nursing authority during these medical crises prompted the nursing leadership to reassess the role and identity of qualified practitioners in the postwar period. In a health care emergency, Gunn argued, the public wanted a "nurse," and the origin of nursing care was of little concern. She proposed "some sort" of national organization to meet future health crises with properly trained and certified nurses to counter the uncertain distinctions between trained and untrained nurses, which negated the hard-fought struggle for recognition of nursing as a skilled, scientific, knowledge-based "professional" occupation for women.[30]

ANSWERING THE CALL

During the fall wave of the influenza pandemic, as Gunn correctly understood, whether nurses had professional training seemed largely moot to the public. By the time Gertrude Murphy reported for VAD duty in Calgary, the pandemic had already developed its own dark mythology, with unceasing reports that millions had succumbed worldwide. Rumour hinted that the particularly virulent strain that struck Drumheller was actually "the Black Death."[31] Drumheller in 1918 was still a small mining town, and ironically for Murphy, the only suitable emergency hospital space was located in the schoolhouse. All the patients were miners, most very young, and only one Welsh boy spoke English; the others were from Eastern or Southern Europe, initially twenty in all. Another twenty-three had died before Murphy's arrival and were still awaiting burial because members of the local population were "too sick ... or too scared" to get the job done.[32] Before her arrival, the mine owner and his assistant were the only hospital volunteers, and once Murphy was installed, they concentrated on transporting convalescents back to town, and the dead to the morgue. A trained nurse and second VAD assistant had been promised, but at first Murphy was left alone with twenty critically ill men. Her protests that she was "only a VAD," and did not know what to do, prompted one of the men to observe that they had coped without *any* training. However inadequate she felt, she set to work making beds, emptying bedpans, bathing hands and faces, and feeding any who could manage the soup provided by a local restaurant.[33]

Many female volunteers expressed a sense of duty, as did Montrealer Dorothy MacPhail, who closely resembled the idealized image of the VAD as a member of the privileged classes. The daughter of a prominent pathologist, McGill academic and medical historian Dr. Andrew MacPhail, she was a product of Montreal's upper middle class. Although she was thought to be of a delicate constitution like her late mother, her letters demonstrate that, at twenty-one, she was keen to exercise both her intellectual and physical capabilities. The pandemic struck Montreal just as she had completed her VAD training, and she was eager to heed the calls for help. Letters to her father, who was serving overseas with the CAMC, map her progress toward a more independent adulthood, in large part enabled by the catalyst of the war and the pandemic.[34] MacPhail's VAD training in early 1918 was followed by regular sessions of rolling bandages at the local Red Cross, and by June 1918, she had registered for national service. This was a new regulation for all men and women aged sixteen and older, but shortly thereafter, she was designated the assistant deputy registrar for the St. Antoine District of Montreal.[35]

By mid-October, her letters to her father record that Montreal was "having a bad time" with the flu, now more "a plague than an epidemic," as gathering places were closed and groups of more than twenty-five were banned. On 13 October, MacPhail noted "one hundred deaths a day on average," including family, friends, and neighbours in the exclusive environs of the Golden Square Mile.[36] In Montreal, 3,028 people died during the month of October 1918, 201 of them on 21 October, the worst day of the pandemic.[37] In the midst of this crisis, MacPhail requested her father's permission to sign on for active VAD service. Now a certified VAD nursing assistant, she argued that the city was "crying out for helpers and being young and strong I feel I ought to" – despite the fact that the flu showed no respect for youth.[38] She stated that she had declined a weekend in the country, feeling she should not be away enjoying herself when "everyone else is working," and added that, moreover, "the trains are none too safe."[39]

If trains were sites of contagion, so, too, were the homes and hospitals where women volunteered to care for influenza victims. Medical personnel of all ranks fell prey to the virus in large numbers.[40] The fortunate ones, such as MacPhail, recovered quickly and went back to work, but the overall strain on health care workers rapidly became acute.[41] The CNATN president at the time, Jean Gunn, was also superintendent of nurses at Toronto General Hospital. She was responsible for the training program in an era when most hospital nursing was performed by probationers and students during a three-year program, with only a few qualified nurses on staff as supervisors and teachers. The nursing ranks at Toronto General Hospital had not increased during the war, but the patient load had grown steadily, compounding the strenuous workload of the pupil-nurses. Any days lost to illness increased the burden on the young students.[42] By 16 October 1918, Gunn cited sixty pupil-nurses who had contracted the flu, several of whom ultimately succumbed to it. She enlisted local community volunteers to give them some respite, calling on citizens to take the exhausted nurses out for fresh air and recreation.[43]

Gunn's concerns about untrained nurses in the hospital setting were reflected in the fact that VADs were never considered as potential substitutes for student nurses, or even as auxiliary helpers in Toronto General Hospital during the epidemic. Nevertheless, the lines separating the qualified from the unqualified were blurring. In 1918, the virulence of the disease quickly overtook the availability of qualified nurses.[44] Given the circumstances, the trained nursing establishment could not afford to reject the assistance of volunteer nurses during the epidemic, especially those legitimated by the St. John Ambulance VAD organization. With qualified nurses already working alongside non-licensed practitioners in the military convalescent hospitals, and a nursing shortage, the apparent acceptance of neophyte VADs such as MacPhail at Montreal's Grenadier Guards Armoury Emergency Hospital is thus more readily understood.[45] Similar demands played out in communities throughout the country. Margaret Andrews observes that by January 1919, Vancouver had only 125 graduate nurses available of the 200 normally on call, with some on war service and many others caring for families at home. As elsewhere, the city turned to women from the community, "sending them into wards to assist with a mask, robe, a clinical thermometer and as little as 30 minutes training." Yet, even this was not enough. Newspaper reports described the example of one emergency hospital with only two nurses and two volunteer helpers to care for 203 patients one night.[46]

As the situation became critical across Canada, there was a continuous cry for nursing aid. In Ontario, the provincial board of health created an Emergency Volunteer Health Auxiliary to train nursing volunteers in an abbreviated VAD program designed specifically to aid flu victims. The volunteers were trained and organized throughout the province and authorized with the badge of the Ontario SOS, or Sisters of Service. Recruitment was directed to "young women of education," the demographic most likely to pursue VAD or nurses' training.[47] The program was offered under the auspices of St. John Ambulance, which had given instruction in home nursing and first aid to an estimated sixty thousand Canadians since the war began.[48] It provided an abbreviated version of the VAD home nursing and first aid classes. The *Toronto Globe* also published the full text of the lectures for those who could not attend, on the premise that some knowledge was better than none at all.[49] Official St. John Ambulance accounts maintain that approximately a thousand Canadian families were assisted by SJAB-trained women during the pandemic, including those in Hamilton, just west of Toronto, where the local VAD Nursing Division provided some 740 hours of service to influenza cases. In Ontario's rural regions, many small emergency hospitals benefited from the aid of VADs who replaced stricken qualified nurses, often taking full charge, as Gertrude Murphy did in Drumheller.[50]

Ottawa also had a sizeable cohort of certified VADs eager to undertake war service, particularly overseas. The federal Civil Service Association (CSA) alleged that many of them were unable to do so because they could not be released from their public service jobs, where they were essential replacements for absent men who could not be exempted from service. Unlike CAMC nurses, VADs were not critical to the military, and though some civil service VADs were given leave to serve overseas with the BRCS once this was formally requested in 1916, the CSA's newsletter, the *Civilian,* was adamant that "two or three times as many of our girls would have been in the hospitals overseas had not the departments placed every obstacle in the way of their joining the military service."[51] More positively, this left an estimated 125 Ottawa VADs available to assist in nursing flu victims, many working double duty in federal offices by day and as VADs overnight. Others assisted in the local civic offices, presumably helping with the administration of the emergency efforts, as substitutes for ailing city staff.[52]

At times, VAD nursing went beyond Canadian borders. A group of Halifax VADs offered their services to a Massachusetts hospital for three weeks, in gratitude for its generosity and aid in the aftermath of the 1917 explosion.[53] Further west, Beth Dearden packed her VAD uniform as a precaution when she left Toronto for North Dakota during the pandemic, to help replace ailing workers at her uncle's grain elevator business. She worked a day shift for her uncle, then wore the uniform while on night duty with a stricken family. The uniform may have helped to validate her VAD skills. All her patients survived.[54]

The response to the call for additional nursing aid was unreserved in the autumn of 1918. Not only VADs, but women from the Salvation Army, the CRCS, and the Victorian Order of Nurses (VON) were out in force.[55] The demand for basic nursing expertise during the epidemic subsequently led to new efforts by the CRCS to initiate its own basic home nursing classes during the postwar period, to prepare women in the home to more effectively care for their families. Believing that the CRCS was encroaching on its jurisdiction, St. John Ambulance reacted angrily, a response that paralleled the CNATN attitude to the proposed postwar expansion of VAD service in military convalescent hospitals.[56]

FULFILLING THEIR "DUTY"

In this era, Nancy Bristow argues, there was a presumption that women, whatever their nursing qualifications, would put themselves in harm's way to fulfill their natural caring role.[57] Certainly, many women came forward to nurse influenza victims, despite the risk to themselves. Calculating the number who died as a result is difficult. There are, however, records of some Canadian VADs having been honoured for their sacrifice. Newfoundland was notably the only North American jurisdiction to establish a permanent monument to the sacrifice of a VAD. After three years of VAD hospital work in England, Ethel Dickenson returned to St. John's in August 1918 and despite poor health, recommenced teaching school, but the Newfoundland schools were soon closed to students, reopening as emergency hospitals in early October. Dickenson resumed her VAD role in a local hospital but soon contracted the virus and died in late October 1918. She was respected for her work as both teacher and VAD, and her sacrifice prompted the community to erect a monument to commemorate her service, and by association the wartime service of all Newfoundland military nurses and VADs. Two years to the day after her death, a twenty-six-foot granite Celtic cross was dedicated in Cavendish Square.[58] The British military also honoured VADs, including Dorothy Twist of Shawnigan Lake, British Columbia, who died on active service after succumbing to "pneumonia influenza" and was buried with full military honours at Aldershot Military Hospital in October 1918. At least four other VADs from Canada and Newfoundland are known to have died of the virus.[59] Additional deaths occurred among non-VAD volunteers in communities across Canada, though none were publicly honoured.

The sacrifice of nurses and VADs in the military convalescent hospitals during the pandemic was less likely to garner public attention than the cruel loss of recently returned young veterans. The military hospitals came under intense scrutiny during the epidemic, and the example of young heroes who survived the war only to die from the flu was at times exploited politically. The late summer of 1918 was a particularly difficult time for the military medical services. An ongoing jurisdictional dispute simmered between the CAMC and the civilian Military Hospitals Commission (MHC), turning on which group could better care for veteran convalescents, particularly those who needed to be rehabilitated back into civilian life.[60] By February 1918, the military and the CAMC had prevailed, separating the medical and vocational aspects of rehabilitation. Most of the MHC wartime convalescent hospitals now came under the control of the military and the CAMC, although jurisdictional skirmishes continued between the civilian and military authorities.[61]

Within a few months, the Allies triumphed in the war, but at the cost of an advance described by Desmond Morton and Glenn Wright as causing the "heaviest Canadian casualty toll" of the conflict.[62] The result put an enormous strain on the military hospitals at home and abroad, with the wounded arriving back in Canada during the late summer, just as the epidemic was entering the deadly fall wave.[63] Morton and Wright argue that from the public's perspective, the loss of more young lives to influenza in the convalescent hospitals was due less to the nature of the virus, or the worldwide effect of this virulent strain, than to "military incompetence and neglect" in hospital care, a recurring theme during the war.[64]

Military medical infighting had been ongoing from the late summer of 1916, when the politically charged Bruce Inquiry into the CAMC organization overseas was initiated. As a barely concealed mechanism for settling old scores between members of the military medical hierarchy, the Bruce report, prepared by respected Toronto surgeon Colonel Herbert Bruce, castigated the organizational and financial framework of the CAMC, particularly as it applied to overseas military hospitals. Bruce was especially critical of the 1915 transfer of Imperial VAD hospitals to the CAMC; in his opinion, the hospitals were "staffed by untrained nurses and civilian practitioners" who were "far from satisfactory" by the standards of modern military medical care.[65] The report caused a schism within the CAMC hierarchy. Following the war, Bruce published his interpretation of the rift and amended some of his criticisms, stating that he was censuring the structure of the hospitals, not the primarily BRCS VADs themselves, and he praised the "self-sacrifice and devotion" of the volunteer nurses. He also claimed that, had he been permitted to continue his work of CAMC reorganization, he would have favoured using Canadian VADs in the CAMC hospitals.[66] At the time, however, the public was largely unaware of the restructuring within the CAMC hospitals, and the military medical service was still seen to have much to answer for in the care of the sick and wounded.

The epidemic exacerbated this anger and misinformation. One Toronto military hospital admitted 2,100 influenza cases, of whom 270 developed pneumonia, and 90 died. As Morton and Wright suggest, these numbers were within reasonable limits in a pre-antibiotic era, but Toronto's mayor used them to inflame public outrage. He brought the matter to court, where a grand jury denounced the military for the inadequate care of veterans and for "bad nursing." The CAMC spokesman at the time observed that the accusation simply served to increase the suffering of the bereaved, who were mistakenly led to believe that their loved ones had succumbed to a "lack of care."[67]

In the case of military convalescent hospitals, "bad nursing" implied VADs, a criticism that the civilian nursing establishment employed in its campaign against the continuing postwar service of VADs in military hospitals.[68] Even before the scope of the influenza outbreak was fully realized, Jean Gunn's annual presidential address to the CNATN convention in the summer of 1918 criticized government proposals to make wider use of VADs in military hospitals at home and overseas, primarily for physiotherapy. This plan was highly cost effective, eliminating the need to hire more nurses or trained physiotherapists. Gunn argued that the potential crisis of a nursing shortage, as thousands of convalescent men returned at war's end, should not be permitted to "furnish a loophole for us to lower our standards," which could impede the growing trend toward standardization and registration of nursing qualifications. She emphasized that "we cannot afford to go backwards; we have to go forward."[69] The subsequent reality of dependence on countless unqualified nursing volunteers during the influenza crisis underscored the irony of these comments.

Despite the accusations of bad nursing, and Gunn's more pragmatic concerns for the future of nursing's professional aspirations, first-hand accounts of the VADs' work, both within and beyond military facilities, confirm their essential service in assisting over-burdened military nursing staff during the influenza crisis. Amelia Earhart, the future American aviation pioneer, trained as a VAD late in the war. After a stint in Toronto as a young student, she admitted that she had been largely unaware of "what World War meant" until confronted by men who, no longer marching to brass bands in new uniforms, were now "without arms and legs ... paralyzed and ... blind." As a St. John Ambulance VAD, Earhart served several months in a Toronto CAMC hospital just preceding the armistice, performing tasks that ranged from "scrubbing floors to playing tennis with the patients." During the epidemic, she was one of the few VADs entrusted with night duty, assisting the nursing sisters on a pneumonia ward, helping to "ladle out medicine from buckets in the over-crowded wards."[70] Earhart's voluntary efforts, like those of women volunteers elsewhere, were welcomed by the beleaguered nursing staff, and she was readily accepted into the hospital milieu.

Neither local public health administrators nor their military equivalents could afford to refuse responsible nursing aid during the crisis, regardless of women's qualifications. Ottawa's mayor urged women to do their duty and help care for the sick in their homes, because people were "dying in our midst" from a lack of "proper care" due to the shortage of nursing aid.[71] At Drumheller, there was no public outcry regarding the lack of nursing care; the request for VAD help came from the town's mine operators, who could not get local women to help on-site. Gertrude Murphy's arrival was a great relief, and her lack of experience dismissed as inconsequential, since she was regarded as having more innate nursing proficiency than any male volunteer. As the number of patients steadily rose to more than a hundred, a qualified nurse finally arrived from Edmonton, but she also considered Murphy's expertise more than sufficient and delegated her to "special" the sixteen most critical patients.[72] In this emergency, the qualified practitioner on the ground appears to have had no objection to sharing her responsibilities with a competent VAD volunteer.

"Unqualified" Women

Eileen Pettigrew's overview of the pandemic offers many examples of the selfless work of volunteer nurses across Canada, but she also presents a darker element, including a group of Calgary women who misrepresented their skills and exploited the suffering by advertising themselves as "professional nurses," charging twenty-five dollars a day for their services. At the time, even qualified private duty nurses charged an average of just two dollars for a regular nineteen-hour day.[73] Such opportunism illustrates the desperate need for nursing aid, qualified or otherwise, and although physicians were also in high demand, medical historians appear to concur that competent, or even available, nursing was more valuable overall. Focusing on the American situation, John Barry observes that "nursing could ease the strains on a patient, keep a patient hydrated, resting, calm, provide the best nutrition ... give a victim ... the best possible chance to survive. Nursing could save lives."[74] He adds that in the United States, "nurses were harder to find than doctors during the epidemic." The American nursing establishment had blocked the training of a substantive number of "nursing aides" or "practical nurses" during the war, who, as Barry argues, could have served as a large reserve force. The American nursing leaders echoed the concerns of their Canadian counterparts. Although the creation of thousands of nursing aides had been originally proposed, the Army School of Nursing was established instead; by the time the epidemic peaked, it had only 221 students and no graduates. Simultaneously, due to intensified fighting in France, a thousand qualified nurses were sent overseas for military service.[75] Barry contends that the drive for American Red Cross Society civilian recruits had "stripped hospitals of the workforce" and cites the comment of a recruiter who – on 5 September 1918, three days before the virus "exploded" at Camp Devens – wrote that soon there would be "no nurses left in civil life."[76]

The reliance on unqualified nursing support within the community during the epidemic evoked criticism from within the nursing establishment itself. An editorial in the December 1918 professional journal *Canadian Nurse* decried the lack of preparation for such a crisis on the part of the Canadian nursing establishment. Following the 1917 Halifax explosion, the British Columbia Graduate Nurses' Association had developed an emergency scheme, which it presented to the CNATN convention in the summer of 1918, but it received only minimal acknowledgment at the time. The *Canadian Nurse* editorial subsequently castigated the CNATN membership for "not having an organization to deal with this epidemic," which might have been mobilized and used to advantage, minimizing the reliance on unqualified workers.[77] The BC scheme had proposed an emergency registry of nurses available for any crisis, local or national, to be established as a National Nursing Service Corps, affiliated with both the CNATN and the CRCS, having a roster of experienced nurses who were graduates of large general hospital training schools. Where the stipulation applied, they were to be "registered" nurses, and all would conform to specific parameters that ruled out VAD or other non-qualified applicants.[78]

In 1918, Alberta, Ontario, Quebec, and Prince Edward Island still lagged behind in registration legislation, and Ontario finally complied in 1922.[79] McPherson argues, however, that this early legislation was of varied quality. Educational standards were neither nationally uniform nor guaranteed, even in regulated provinces. Moreover, though registration did prevent unqualified practitioners from advertising themselves as graduates or registered nurses, it did not necessarily stop them "from plying their trade."[80] Thus, the nursing establishment's desire to ensure that VADs and other auxiliary practitioners did not encroach on the domain of qualified graduates became urgent only when both the epidemic and the war were largely concluded. In the midst of the crisis, the leadership was in no position to object to the assistance of volunteers who had a reasonable level of training, experience, and education. Ontario's SOS program seems to confirm that under the circumstances, any training was better than none. Once the situation abated, nursing leaders recognized that the precedents created by the emergency must not become a regularized accommodation for future shortages of qualified practitioners. Gunn's fear of a "loophole" for lowering standards, with regard to the proposed use of VADs for convalescent rehabilitation and physiotherapy in CAMC hospitals, held more urgency by the close of 1918.[81] By then, however, VADs were rapidly returning to civilian life, minimizing their potential threat to the future of Canadian nursing.[82]

In retrospect, Gunn herself acknowledged the value of VAD and unqualified nursing aid during the epidemic and the war years, and she judiciously used it as a platform for reforms to consolidate the status of qualified nursing graduates in the postwar period. In a 1919 address to the CNATN convention, she noted an "indifference on the part of the public" toward nursing and its evolution as a recognized professional occupation for women; Canadians called on a nurse when they were ill, without concern for her background and training. She maintained, however, that the epidemic had galvanized the nation's attention to both the "value" and the "need" of nursing, as well as the urgency to organize nursing reserves to meet future emergencies.[83] During the war, Gunn had been an advisor to the CRCS on nursing issues, and she continued to take a prominent consultative role in the development of postwar Red Cross outreach nursing, concerned that only qualified nurses should be considered for this role.[84] Instead of proposing that the CNATN develop the BC scheme, she implied that the emergency registry should be part of the new peacetime public health mandate of the Canadian Red Cross Society.

CONCLUSION

The influenza epidemic did not initiate the Canadian nursing community's concerns about VADs and unqualified volunteers during the war. Rather, this emergency, in combination with the proposed expansion of the wartime VAD program to fill potential nursing shortages in military convalescent hospitals, helped to underscore the need to promote the qualifications and status of trained graduates.[85] As an ardent supporter of regularized nursing education and standards, Jean Gunn articulated the fears and frustrations of the nursing establishment in being forced to share their position and status at the bedside during the influenza crisis.

By virtue of gender, class, and their affiliation with the military medical services, VADs in particular acquired a new prominence in the hierarchy of volunteer nurses during the crisis. Clad in their distinctive uniforms, with their apparent authority and expertise, VADs presented a reassuring and much needed supplement to qualified nursing care. As a demonstrably essential support service during the epidemic, VADs were readily accepted by patients in the home, as well as those in emergency and military hospitals across Canada. Qualified nurses "on the front lines" of the crisis, who found themselves in command of overcrowded hospitals with too few of their peers to adequately perform the necessary tasks, were grateful for the efforts of VADs and other volunteers who put their own health at risk to help in any way that was useful: administering medicine, changing bedpans, feeding patients, or bathing fevered brows. At the peak of the epidemic, VADs like Gertrude Murphy frequently found themselves acting as substitutes for the unavailable skills of trained and experienced graduate nurses.

As women, however, neither professional nurses nor volunteers were immune to the politics of health. At times, women were criticized for their apparent failure to respond to their feminine duty to offer care, resulting in too few volunteers to meet the overwhelming demand. On the other hand, the necessary substitution of VADs for qualified nursing in the care of war veterans also met with criticism. Nursing became a political touchstone during the influenza crisis. Arguably, the situation was also used to advantage by the nursing establishment to emphasize the professional authority of nursing. The relentless carnage of the war had intensified the atmosphere of panic and despair that accompanied the flu pandemic. This battle on the home front was as deadly as any of the war, and it ultimately exacted an even greater cost in lives. Overseas, the military nurse was seen as a subsidiary support to the men on the battlefields, but on the domestic front, nursing was almost the only defence against a relentless and invisible enemy. VADs were denied access to CAMC hospitals abroad, but they proved their worth through their dedication and selflessness at the bedside of the suffering at home. A crisis that confounded "normal" divisions of labour in health care, and intensified ongoing debates about women's work, the pandemic generated contradictory and often conflicting notions of women's inherent healing capabilities, role in society, and professional advancement.

By July 1919, with both the war and the epidemic behind it, Ottawa was no longer pressing to train VADs for work in the rapidly declining number of veterans' hospitals, and the 106 VADs still on active service soon retired into obscurity as the hospitals closed.[86] The emergencies had abated, both at home and abroad, and Jean Gunn was promoting different avenues of service for veteran CAMC nurses in the growing field of public health nursing, hoping to demonstrate a new level of professional accomplishment for experienced graduates.[87] In her first postwar address to the CNATN, she praised the many VADs who had "rendered valuable service at home" during the war.[88] She made no mention of the epidemic, but the thousands of women who had served as volunteer and VAD nurses during the crisis could share in this measured praise. Like their civilian and military counterparts, few saw their efforts as heroic; that word was reserved for veterans and the soldiers who did not return. These women did their "duty" as volunteer nurses, as gender and class dictated, oblivious to the political and ideological skirmishes that shadowed their essential role in the influenza war.

NOTES

1 Gertrude Charters, "The Black Death at Drumheller," *Maclean's*, March 1979, 20-21. Murphy became Gertrude Charters at the time of her marriage.
2 Maureen Lux, "'The Bitter Flats': The 1918 Influenza Epidemic in Saskatchewan," *Saskatchewan History* 49,1 (Spring 1997): 5.
3 Quoted in Eileen Pettigrew, *The Silent Enemy: Canada and the Deadly Flu of 1918* (Saskatoon: Western Producer Prairie Books, 1983), 101.
4 Rhonda Keene-Payne, "We Must Have Nurses: Spanish Influenza in America, 1918-1919," *Nursing History Review* 8 (2000): 150; see also Lux, "'The Bitter Flats,'" 5; and Janice P. Dickin McGinnis, "A City Faces an Epidemic," *Alberta History* 24,4 (Autumn 1976): 2.
5 Lux, "'The Bitter Flats,'" 4; Mary-Ellen Kelm, "British Columbia First Nations and the Influenza Pandemic of 1918-1919," *BC Studies* 122 (Summer 1999): 31-32; Esyllt Jones, "Contact across a Diseased Boundary: Urban Space and Social Interaction during Winnipeg's Influenza Epidemic, 1918-1919," *Journal of the Canadian Historical Association,*

n.s., 13 (2002): 122; and Janice P. Dickin McGinnis, "The Impact of Epidemic Influenza: Canada, 1918-19," in *Medicine in Canadian Society: Historical Perspectives,* ed. S.E.D. Shortt (Montreal and Kingston: McGill-Queen's University Press, 1981), 123.

6 Mark Osborne Humphries, "The Horror at Home: The Canadian Military and the 'Great' Influenza Pandemic of 1918," *Journal of the Canadian Historical Association,* n.s., 16,1 (2005): 235-60.

7 Kathryn McPherson, *Bedside Matters: The Transformation of Canadian Nursing, 1900-1990* (Toronto: Oxford University Press, 2003), 55-56.

8 Ibid., and 271n2.

9 Ibid., 271n2.

10 G.W.L. Nicholson, *Canada's Nursing Sisters* (Toronto: Samuel Stevens, Hakkert, 1975), 48-99; and Jean Gunn, "The Services of Canadian Nurses and Voluntary Aids during the War," *Canadian Nurse* 15,9 (September 1919): 1975.

11 Ibid., 1976; Natalie M. Riegler, "The Work and Networks of Jean I. Gunn, Superintendent of Nurses, Toronto General Hospital, 1913-1941: A Presentation of Some Issues in Nursing during Her Lifetime, 1882-1941" (PhD thesis, Department of Education, University of Toronto, 1992), 198.

12 Jean Gunn, "Nursing: Address Given before National Council of Women," *Woman's Century,* August 1918, 11.

13 David Coburn, "The Development of Canadian Nursing: Professionalization and Proletarianization," *International Journal of Health Services* 18,13 (1988): 444. The designation of "Registered Nurse" (RN) confirmed a nurse's qualifications. She had trained in an accredited nursing school and passed standardized provincial examinations. However, the designation of "professional" remains a contested identity in nursing scholarship. See McPherson, *Bedside Matters,* 7.

14 Linda J. Quiney, "'Assistant Angels': Canadian Women as Voluntary Aid Detachment Nurses during and after the Great War, 1914-1930" (PhD thesis, Department of History, University of Ottawa, 2002), 274-87.

15 The CAMC uniform dress was a distinctive blue, initiating the term "Bluebirds" as an affectionate reference to the nurses. The VADs wore a grey dress, to emphasize the SJAA colours of black and white. For working dress, both groups wore the traditional starched white aprons, collars, and cuffs of the Nightingale nurse. Both had a formal public dress uniform, coat, and hat. The triangular linen head veil was the common feminine attribute of the working uniform, a feature favoured by both groups. See Sybil Johnson to Mother, "Christmas Day, 1916, 6:45," Centre for Newfoundland Studies, Collection-201, Sybil Johnson Papers, file 201.013, St. John's; and Maude Wilkinson, "Four Score and Ten," *Canadian Nurse* 73,10 (October 1977): 29.

16 The symbol was adopted by at least one Canadian VAD division. The graduation photograph of the Calgary Central Nursing Division, No. 39, shows twenty-six women in their working uniforms with red crosses appliquéd, somewhat unevenly, on the apron bibs. Each woman also wears the black armband with the SJAA Brigade Overseas badge. Glenbow Archives, NA-2267-4, Calgary.

17 In bold type, a caption at the top of the poster proclaims "Victory Bonds Will Help Stop This." A caption below reads "Kultur vs Humanity." The soldier holds the dead nurse with one arm and shakes his fist at a German captain, who sneers from the bridge of his retreating submarine. Copies of the poster are held at McGill University Libraries, Rare Books and Special Collections, Montreal, and Library and Archives Canada (LAC), C-55111, Ottawa.

18   Desmond Morton and J.L. Granatstein, *Marching to Armageddon: Canadians and the Great War, 1914-1919* (Toronto: Lester and Orpen Dennys, 1989), 7; and Annmarie Adams, "Borrowed Buildings: Canada's Temporary Hospitals during World War I," *Canadian Bulletin of Medical History* 16,1 (1999): 25-48.

19   McPherson, *Bedside Matters*, 29-47.

20   Riegler, "The Work and Networks of Jean I. Gunn," 148.

21   G.W.L. Nicholson, *The White Cross in Canada: A History of St. John Ambulance* (Montreal: Harvest House, 1967), 58-59; Christopher McCreery, *The Maple Leaf and the White Cross: A History of St. John Ambulance and the Most Venerable Order of the Hospital of St. John of Jerusalem in Canada* (Toronto: Dundurn Press, 2008); and Quiney, "'Assistant Angels,'" 166-68.

22   The extensive scholarship on the British VAD includes Stella Bingham, *Ministering Angels* (London: Osprey, 1975); Deborah Gorham, *Vera Brittain: A Feminist Life* (Toronto: University of Toronto Press, 2000); Lyn MacDonald, *The Roses of No Man's Land* (London: Penguin, 1993); Sharon Ouditt, *Fighting Forces, Writing Women: Identity and Ideology in the First World War* (London: Routledge, 1994); Anne Summers, *Angels and Citizens: British Women as Military Nurses, 1854-1914* (London: Threshold Press, 2000); and Janet Sledge Kobrin Watson, "Active Service: Gender, Class and British Representations of the Great War" (PhD diss., Department of History, Stanford University, 1996). Regarding Canadian VAD social status, see Desmond Morton and Glenn Wright, *Winning the Second Battle: Canadian Veterans and the Return to Civilian Life, 1915-1930* (Toronto: University of Toronto Press, 1987), 20.

23   Quiney, "'Assistant Angels,'" 110-23.

24   MacDonald, *The Roses of No Man's Land*, xi; and Summers, *Angels and Citizens,* 232. A survey of active VADs during the war suggests that the assumptions for British VADs may also be faulty. See Gorham, *Vera Brittain,* 101; Imperial War Museum, Women at Work Collection, London; and British Red Cross Society (BRCS), file 10.5/4, London. Brittain's memoir of her VAD service perpetuates the image of the ideal VAD as a young, upper-middle class, well-educated, untried worker. Vera Brittain, *Testament of Youth: An Autobiographical Study of the Years 1900-1925* (1933; repr., London: Fontana, 1979).

25   Maude E. Seymour Abbott, "Lectures on the History of Nursing," *Canadian Nurse* 19,2 (February 1923): 87; Linda J. Quiney, "Borrowed Halos: Canadian Teachers as Voluntary Aid Detachment Nurses during the Great War," *Historical Studies in Education* 15,1 (Spring 2003): 78-99; and Quiney, "'Assistant Angels,'" 123-37.

26   Charters, "The Black Death," 20.

27   Gunn, "Nursing: Address Given before the National Council of Women," 11.

28   Gunn, "The Services of Canadian Nurses and Voluntary Aids," 1977. St. John Ambulance rejected the proposal on the grounds that it denied women the opportunity to volunteer their service, which, more than nursing per se, was the objective of their efforts. See Charles Copp, "St. John's Ambulance Brigade," *Canadian Nurse* 14,7 (July 1918): 1166. The military rejected the proposal because the numerous experienced VADs were expected to continue their unpaid service in convalescent hospitals after the war, providing a much more cost-effective solution to nursing shortages than training and housing VAD pupil-nurses would. See CNATN, "Secretary's Report: Canadian National Association of Trained Nurses' Convention, 1918," *Canadian Nurse* 14,8 (August 1918): 1226.

29   Linda J. Quiney, "'Filling the Gaps': Canadian Voluntary Nurses, the 1917 Halifax Explosion, and the Influenza Epidemic of 1918," *Canadian Bulletin of Medical History* 19,2 (2002):

351-74. The extensive literature on the Halifax explosion includes Alan Ruffman and Colin D. Howell, eds., *Ground Zero: A Reassessment of the 1917 Explosion in Halifax Harbour* (Halifax: Nimbus and Gorsebrook Research Institute, 1994); John Griffith Armstrong, *The Halifax Explosion and the Royal Canadian Navy Inquiry and Intrigue* (Vancouver: UBC Press, 2002); and Laura M. MacDonald, *Curse of the Narrows: The Halifax Explosion, 1917* (Toronto: Harper Collins, 2005).

30 Jean Gunn, "President's Address, Canadian National Association of Trained Nurses' Convention," *Canadian Nurse* 15,8 (August 1919): 1920.

31 Charters, "The Black Death," 20.

32 Ibid., 21.

33 Ibid.

34 LAC, Sir Andrew MacPhail Papers, Dorothy MacPhail file, 1918, Manuscript Group (MG) 30, D150, 1/2/8.

35 Dorothy MacPhail to Andrew MacPhail, 18 January 1918, 24 March 1918, 9 June 1918, 16 June 1918, 22 June 1918, LAC, MacPhail Papers, MG 30, D150, 1/2/8.

36 Dorothy MacPhail to Andrew MacPhail, 13 October 1918, LAC, MacPhail Papers, MG 30, D150, 1/2/8.

37 Max Braithwaite, "The Year of the Killer Flu," *Maclean's,* 1 February 1953, 43.

38 MacPhail to MacPhail, 13 October 1918.

39 Ibid.

40 J.T.H. Connor, *Doing Good: The Life of Toronto's General Hospital* (Toronto: University of Toronto Press, 2000); and Keene-Payne, "We Must Have Nurses," 143.

41 Dorothy MacPhail to Andrew MacPhail, 7 November 1918, LAC, MacPhail Papers, MG 30, D150, 1/2/8; and Keene-Payne, "We Must Have Nurses," 151-52.

42 Connor, *Doing Good,* 202.

43 Natalie Riegler, *Jean I. Gunn: Nursing Leader* (Toronto: A.M.S. and Fitzhenry and Whiteside, 1997), 87; and Connor, *Doing Good,* 203-24.

44 Pettigrew, *Silent Enemy,* 94. Pettigrew's account of only two hundred RNs left on the Vancouver roster does not allow for the fact that British Columbia had enacted registration only in 1918, and qualified nurses were not required to register. However, unqualified women were denied registration. See McPherson, *Bedside Matters,* 67; and Gunn, "The Services of Canadian Nurses and Voluntary Aids," 1975.

45 MacPhail to MacPhail, 7 November 1918.

46 Margaret Andrews, "Epidemic and Public Health: Vancouver 1918-19," *BC Studies* 34 (1977): 28.

47 Advertisement, *Toronto Daily Star,* 15 October 1918, quoted in Pettigrew, *Silent Enemy,* 96.

48 Pettigrew, *Silent Enemy,* 95.

49 Ibid., 97.

50 Nicholson, *The White Cross in Canada,* 71-72; and McCreery, *The Maple Leaf and the White Cross,* 80-81.

51 "One More V.A.D.," *Civilian,* December 1919, 23.

52 "The Epidemic Workers," *Civilian,* December 1918, 39; Nicholson, *The White Cross in Canada,* 72; and "1917-1918 Secretary's Report, Ottawa Local Centre," 4, Archives of Ontario, SJAA Administrative Records, 1909-1977, F823/MU6814, Toronto.

53 "St John Ambulance Brigade Overseas," c. 1918, Nova Scotia Archives and Records Management, Red Cross Collection, MG1 321, Halifax.

54 Pettigrew, *Silent Enemy,* 99-100.

55 Ibid., 101-2.

56 St. John Ambulance Association, "For Humanity," *First Aid Bulletin,* April 1924, 7; and CRCS, *Annual Report* (1923), 24. The CRCS argued that the new classes were to compensate for a lack of SJAA equivalents in rural and remote regions. It also emphasized a less "elite" focus for its courses, making them available to "common folk." CRCS, Minute Book 6, 29 March 1922, 45, and 4 April 1923, 151.

57 Nancy K. Bristow, "'You Can't Do Anything for Influenza': Doctors, Nurses and the Power of Gender during the Influenza Pandemic in the United States," in *The Spanish Influenza Pandemic of 1918-19: New Perspectives,* ed. Howard Phillips and David Killingray (London: Routledge, 2003), 58-69.

58 Cavendish Square is just beyond the forecourt of the Hotel Newfoundland. Centre for Newfoundland Studies, Collection-201, Sybil Johnson Papers; St. John's Local Council of Women, *Remarkable Women of Newfoundland and Labrador* (St. John's: Valhalla Press, 1976), 17; Bert Riggs, "What's All the Fuss about Ethel Dickenson?" *St. John's Gazette,* 6 July 1995, 12; J.R. Smallwood, ed., *Encyclopaedia of Newfoundland and Labrador* (St. John's: Newfoundland Book Publishers, 1981), 1:621-22.

59 Wealtha A. Wilson and Ethel T. Raymond, "Canadian Women in the Great War," in *Canada in the Great World War* (Toronto: United Publishers of Canada, 1921), 6:191. Dorothy Twist was thirty years old. Others known to have died were Bertha Bartlett of St. John's, Nora Young McCord, Grace Bolton of Montreal, and Isabel Henshaw of Winnipeg. See "Roll of Honour: Members VAD Died on Active Service," Imperial War Museum, Women at Work, BRCS 25.5.6.

60 Morton and Wright, *Winning the Second Battle,* Chapter 5.

61 Ibid., 90.

62 Ibid., 91.

63 See Gladys Morton, "The Pandemic Influenza of 1918," *Canadian Nurse* 72,12 (December 1976): 34; Keene-Payne, "We Must Have Nurses," 154; and Alfred W. Crosby, *Epidemic and Peace, 1918* (Westport, CT: Greenwood Press, 1976), 206-7.

64 Morton and Wright, *Winning the Second Battle,* 91.

65 Susan Mann, *Margaret Macdonald: Imperial Daughter* (Montreal and Kingston: McGill-Queen's University Press, 2005), 85; Desmond Morton, *A Peculiar Kind of Politics: Canada's Overseas Ministry in the First World War* (Toronto: University of Toronto Press, 1982), 86-87; and Herbert A. Bruce, "Report on the Canadian Army Medical Service," London, England, 20 September 1916, 26, LAC, William Baptie Papers, MG 30 E3, vol. 1.

66 Herbert A. Bruce, *Politics and the Canadian Army Medical Corps* (Toronto: William Briggs, 1919), 54-55; Mann, *Imperial Daughter,* 231n57; and Herbert A. Bruce, *Varied Operations* (Toronto: Longmans, Green, 1958), 101-2. Bruce also notes that he met his future wife, a BRCS VAD, in late 1918.

67 Morton and Wright, *Winning the Second Battle,* 90-91. The authors cite the CAMC historian Major C.V. Currie. Ibid., 260n48.

68 Gunn, "President's Address," 1920.

69 Jean Gunn, "Canadian National Association of Trained Nurses' Convention, 1918," *Canadian Nurse* 14,8 (August 1918): 1211.

70 Amelia Earhart, *The Fun of It: Random Records of My Own Flying and of Women in Aviation* (New York: Harcourt, Brace, c. 1925), 19-20.

71 Pettigrew, *Silent Enemy,* 100-1.

72 Charters, "The Black Death," 21, 27, 29. "Special" meant she was to concentrate on those sixteen specific patients.

73 Pettigrew, *Silent Enemy*, 93-94.

74 John M. Barry, *The Great Influenza: The Epic Story of the Deadliest Plague in History* (New York: Viking, 2004), 319.

75 Ibid.

76 Ibid., 320.

77 Riegler, "The Work and Networks of Jean I. Gunn," 161-62; and Editorial, *Canadian Nurse* 14,12 (December 1918): 1468-69.

78 "Helen Randal Letter," *Canadian Nurse* 14,8 (August 1918): 1237-39.

79 Coburn, "The Development of Canadian Nursing," 444. Newfoundland, as a British colony, did not pass legislation until 1931.

80 McPherson, *Bedside Matters*, 67-68.

81 Gunn, "Canadian National Association of Trained Nurses Convention, 1918," 1211.

82 Quiney, "'Assistant Angels,'" 365-76.

83 Gunn, "President's Address," 1920.

84 Riegler, *Jean I. Gunn*, 87, 93, 237-38; and Gunn, "President's Address," 1922.

85 Gunn, "Canadian National Association of Trained Nurses' Convention, 1918," 1210-13; and "Report of the Special Committee," *Canadian Nurse* 14,8 (August 1918): 1231-35.

86 Gunn, "The Services of Canadian Nurses and Voluntary Aids," 1977. Gunn notes that 150 nursing sisters remained on duty in the hospitals and that the future of their work was as yet undecided.

87 Meryn Stuart, "War and Peace: Professional Identities and Nurses' Training, 1914-1930," in *Challenging Professions: Historical and Contemporary Perspectives on Women's Professional Work,* ed. Elizabeth Smyth et al. (Toronto: University of Toronto Press, 1999), 171-93.

88 Gunn, "The Services of Canadian Nurses and Voluntary Aids," 1977.

3

"Respectfully Submitted": Citizens and Public Letter Writing during Montreal's Influenza Epidemic, 1918-20

MAGDA FAHRNI

Three weeks after pandemic influenza arrived in Montreal during the autumn of 1918, J.-E. Beaudoin, an accountant, sat down to write the mayor. "Monsieur le Maire," he began. "C'est un proverbe reconnu qu'il faut mieux 'PREVENIR QUE DE GUERIR' et c'est au sujet des règlements d'hygiène que je me permets de faire quelques suggestions." Beaudoin then proceeded to enumerate examples of what he considered "l'état malpropre et dégoutant de nos rues." How, he asked the mayor, could the population be expected to observe public health regulations during an epidemic when Montreal was such an unsanitary city even in ordinary times?[1]

Beaudoin's letter, written at the height of Montreal's influenza epidemic, is of interest here in part for what it tells us about one citizen's sense of his relationship with his local government. Also noteworthy is its overriding concern with prevention. In this latter respect, its message echoed that of members of the medical profession and public health authorities who, in the absence of an effective vaccine or a proven cure for influenza, also placed their faith in prevention. These authorities advocated such common-sense precautions as plenty of rest, sunlight, and fresh air, and advised such tried-and-true practices as avoiding crowds, refraining from spitting in public places, covering one's face when coughing or sneezing, isolating the ill, and disinfecting their homes. Not surprisingly, perhaps, alternative practitioners, quacks, and entrepreneurs of all kinds were quick to step into the breach in the fall of 1918, proposing serums, potions, and supposedly sure-fire solutions to this public health catastrophe.

Less well known is the fact that ordinary citizens like J.-E. Beaudoin also proposed strategies and plans of attack. In Montreal, soldiers, merchants, and municipal taxpayers wrote to city hall and to the daily press, offering their thoughts on the ways in which the epidemic might be contained and managed. On the whole, the solutions proposed by those who wrote as citizens differed little from official precautions, suggesting that the public health campaigns of the late nineteenth and early twentieth centuries had indeed had an impact on the population; by 1918, discourses of contagion, transmission, and prevention informed by the germ theory of disease had clearly taken root in Montreal, although traces of older "miasmatic" explanations of disease transmission are also evident in these letters. Many of the letters written to municipal authorities during the epidemic concerned disease prevention, but they also address other aspects of public health, aspects related to the regulation of urban life during this moment of medical crisis, but also in ordinary times. Public discussion of prevention and contagion in the context of the influenza epidemic appears to have stimulated individual reflection on everyday problems of public health and urban life.

HISTORIOGRAPHY

This essay allows us to approach the history of public health in Quebec and Canada from a novel angle: namely, the responses of citizens to health measures adopted by the state. Much of the extensive historiography of public health in Quebec, in particular, details the adoption of health legislation over the course of the nineteenth and twentieth centuries and the creation of institutions such as local boards of health and the provincial Conseil d'hygiène de la province de Québec (CHPQ).[2] In a very early assessment of public health in Montreal, Terry Copp argues that the distressingly poor health of early-twentieth-century Montrealers was attributable to seriously inadequate health provisions at both the municipal and the provincial levels. Copp claims that though the CHPQ had good intentions, it was not able to force municipalities to do its bidding.[3] More recently, a considerable body of work has emerged that insists on the active and dynamic role played by the CHPQ, which was established in 1886 in the wake of Montreal's smallpox epidemic of 1885.[4] These studies, by scholars such as François Guérard, Othmar Keel, and Peter Keating, suggest that the CHPQ was able to establish a public health infrastructure comparable to those of other North American locales, despite the reluctance and sometimes outright hostility of Quebec's municipalities, particularly in rural areas.[5] Some scholars have also attempted to rehabilitate the reputation of Montreal's board of health, arguing that the negative assessments of Copp and others underestimate the extent to which the board was in fact attempting to address the city's major public health problems.[6]

The Quebec historiography has also examined infrastructural innovations such as sewers, water filtration, and the obligatory pasteurization of milk, endemic public health problems such as tuberculosis and infant mortality, and the roles played by doctors, nurses, and civil servants.[7] Almost all of these studies have dealt to some degree with the changing scientific and intellectual context that shaped the public health movement – most notably, the acceptance of the germ theory of disease from the late nineteenth century onward, a theory that ultimately triumphed over competing explanations such as miasmatic or "contingent-contagionism" theories.[8]

Historians agree that, well into the second half of the nineteenth century, the various branches of the Quebec state concerned themselves with questions of health only during outbreaks of epidemic disease.[9] Yet toward the end of the century, in Quebec as elsewhere, medical professionals attempted to convince civil servants of the importance of establishing permanent measures favouring public health and prevention.[10] Historians of Quebec largely agree that the miasma theory of disease causation, which held sway in the 1860s and 1870s, was instrumental in fuelling initial public health campaigns and attempts to sanitize the environment – what Georges Desrosiers and Benoît Gaumer call "l'hygiène du milieu," or "l'hygiène publique." By the 1880s, in contrast, the emerging medical consensus regarding the germ theory of disease led to campaigns that attempted to educate individuals and specific subgroups of the population about the importance of "hygiène privée," or "hygiène individuelle."[11] Valerie Minnett and Mary-Anne Poutanen's study of the "Swat the Fly" competitions held in Montreal and elsewhere during the early twentieth century – contests that enrolled children in the anti-tuberculosis battle – illustrates one concrete example of this sanitary education movement. "Clean-Up Weeks" and contests that demonized common houseflies as "germs with legs" were ways of educating individual citizens about both the germ theory of disease and their own responsibility for maintaining the public health.[12]

Although historians of Quebec have recognized the key roles of social class and ethnicity in determining who tended to contract communicable diseases and those caused by deprivation, the perspective of ordinary citizens on public health has rarely been probed.[13] As Peter Keating and

Othmar Keel observe, for instance, few historians of Quebec have analyzed popular attitudes toward illness, suffering, and epidemics.[14] There are a few important exceptions: Minnett and Poutanen's study, cited above, Denyse Baillargeon's use of oral history to understand the experiences of mothers who frequented the Gouttes de lait (milk stations), and Robert Gagnon's discussion of petitions from Montreal citizens demanding sewers are all successful efforts to undertake bottom-up public health history.[15]

This essay responds to Keating and Keel's appeal, attempting to gauge ordinary Montrealers' reaction to the influenza epidemic by studying the letters they sent to their local government and the press during this public health catastrophe. It thus joins Esyllt Jones's recent book in examining popular reactions to the early-twentieth-century influenza pandemic.[16] My analysis is inspired by an international historiography addressing citizens' letters and petitions to public officials, one that examines not only the content of the letters, but also the self-presentation of their authors and the ways in which they constructed their relationship with the state. Petitions, for instance, have been much studied, particularly for the pre-industrial period and for people who employed these forms of communication as a way of staking a claim in the political realm even in the absence of democratic rights such as the vote.[17] For more recent periods, scholars have examined citizens' letters to public officials in moments and places as diverse as Depression-era Canada and the USSR.[18] Central to the present discussion is historian Sheila Fitzpatrick's notion of "public letter-writing" – that is, "letters written to public figures and institutions."[19] As Fitzpatrick notes, "the 'publicness' of such letters was only partial": whereas missives published in the local press and studied here presumably reached a wide readership, those sent to civil servants enjoyed a more limited circulation. I also employ, albeit with reservations, Fitzpatrick's definition of "ordinary" citizens, as "the people without official power or position sometimes referred to as subalterns."[20] Few of the letter-writers studied here had "official power or position," but the owners of small and large businesses who took it on themselves to write to the municipal government can only with difficulty be considered subaltern.

SOURCES

The principal sources used in this discussion, then, are letters written by Montrealers during the epidemic to various components of their municipal government: the mayor, the administrative commission, and the board of health. The nature of these epistles varied. Some were effectively multi-authored petitions, requesting special permissions or favours. Others were penned by individuals who shared their thoughts on how the pandemic might be managed or controlled. Two correspondents wrote anonymously.[21] Others took advantage of the crisis in an attempt to settle old scores or resolve long-standing annoyances. Many explicitly referred to themselves as citizens, implicitly justifying their intervention. Several genres of letters identified by Sheila Fitzpatrick for the 1930s USSR can be found here, too: "Complaints, denunciations, petitions, requests for assistance ... letters of opinion, threatening letters."[22] Although one might expect the letters of 1918 to differ from those studied by Fitzpatrick, in that they were written during a moment of acute medical crisis, it is clear that many addressed everyday issues of long-standing concern to their authors, not simply immediate problems and emergency measures.

It is no surprise that the letter-writers targeted the municipal government: it was on the front lines of the battle against influenza, and municipal taxpayers had already constructed a relationship with it.[23] In contrast, I found very few letters written by ordinary citizens to the CHPQ.[24] Although much of the Quebec historiography emphasizes the recalcitrance of many municipalities with regard to implementing public health measures, these residents of Montreal nonetheless chose to address their suggestions to the local board of health. One might ask whether they did so despite its perceived negligence or *because* of it, in an effort to spur it to action. Or perhaps – a third possibility – city residents, unlike later historians, did not perceive the Montreal Board of Health as negligent. The number of letters examined here is relatively small (thirty-four written to municipal authorities), but they have been contextualized by a thorough study of the records of the municipal and provincial governments, and of the Catholic archbishopric of Montreal and of the Grey Nuns, along with the daily French-language and English-language press. In addition, I consider ten letters addressed to the editor of *Le Devoir* during the epidemic; another kind of public letter writing, they address topics similar to those found in the municipal archives. It is impossible to determine the degree to which this small number of letters was representative of public opinion. Rather, I would like to suggest that, whether they were sent directly to municipal officials or to local newspapers in the hope of reaching a wider readership, they reveal the range of concerns voiced by ordinary citizens in a moment of medical crisis.

This chapter, then, examines these proposals by citizens in part to understand public perceptions of the prevention and transmission of communicable disease in early-twentieth-century Montreal. In Quebec, the influenza pandemic arrived at what François Guérard has called a transitional moment between "hygiène du milieu" and "médecine prévent-ive," and we see the co-existence of these two theories and practices in the citizens' letters.[25] This essay also probes the ways in which citizens communicated with their municipal government, studying their self-presentation and the relationships they attempted to establish or maintain with city hall. Finally, it assesses the ways in which citizens reacted to the impact of influenza on daily life in what was then Canada's metropolis.

Official Responses to the Epidemic

Montreal reported its first case of pandemic influenza on 23 September 1918.[26] By the end of January 1919, 19,299 cases had been declared in this city of approximately 640,000 people, and 3,639 Montrealers had died of the disease and of secondary infections, notably pneumonia.[27] As else-where, this strain of influenza targeted young adults in their twenties and thirties: the average age of Montrealers who succumbed to it during the fall of 1918 was 25.07 for women and 25.70 for men. Generally speaking, it felled French Canadians and English Canadians at similar rates: official statistics showed 37.52 deaths per 10,000 French Canadians and 35.53 deaths per 10,000 English Canadians. Proportionally fewer Jewish Montrealers died of the disease (16.45 deaths per 10,000), whereas city residents belong-ing to what were called "Other nationalities" were somewhat more at risk (40.82 deaths per 10,000) than French or English Canadians.[28] Montrealers experienced a second wave of epidemic influenza in the winter of 1920: between January and April of that year, 4,336 contracted it and 431 died. Less dramatic than the autumn 1918 wave, that of 1920 was nonetheless serious. It also appears to have been a more "typical" influenza epidemic, in that it was deadlier for infants and the elderly than for young adults.[29]

In the absence of either an effective vaccine or a cure for the disease, civil and medical officials concentrated their efforts on preventing its widespread transmission among citizens. In Quebec, official prevention measures during the epidemic were decided and administered first and foremost by the Conseil d'hygiène de la province de Québec (CHPQ); operations appear to have been relatively centralized, although local boards of health and individual doctors enjoyed a certain measure of autonomy in decision making.[30] The centralized management of the epidemic was a departure from past practice: the cholera epidemics of the 1830s and the smallpox epidemic of 1885 predated a well-established provincial body to oversee regulations. Indeed, the devastation wrought by smallpox in 1885 was one catalyst for the creation of the CHPQ in 1886.[31] In the case of Montreal, coordination between the provincial and municipal bodies was facilitated by the fact that the CHPQ had its offices in Montreal, on Notre-Dame Street, not far from Montreal's board of health and department of health, both of which were lodged at city hall. Nonetheless, the CHPQ found itself having to remind certain municipalities and local health boards to respect provincial regulations regarding the influenza epidemic.[32]

· The recommendations adopted by the CHPQ at the outset of the pandemic included isolating patients in their homes and disinfecting their lodgings once they recovered. Local health boards and attending physicians were given the right to placard the homes of the ill "when they deem it advisable" but were not required to do so. The CHPQ limited the number of people in attendance at public or private functions, and it closed down places – such as schools, theatres, recreation halls, dance halls, and cinemas – where the public might congregate.[33] Several weeks after the flu arrived in Montreal, the CHPQ made it a reportable illness; ensuring that households and attending physicians adhered to this rule, however, was clearly difficult.[34] Although anti-influenza vaccine trials took place in Quebec during the epidemic, vaccines were not widely used among the general public.[35] Instead, the CHPQ proposed such elementary precautions as disinfecting objects in contact with the ill, proper nose blowing, refraining from spitting, and gargling with table salt and hydrogen peroxide.[36]

This reliance on civic courtesy and the basic rules of hygiene was shared by the municipal department of health, responsible for publicizing, applying, and enforcing provincial regulations.[37] Like the CHPQ, the municipal government also placed its faith in fresh air and sunshine: summarizing the impact of the 1920 influenza epidemic, the City of Montreal's *Bulletin d'hygiène* urged, "Let us then help the sun to freely come in our homes; it is the best preservative against epidemics; let us fight dampness in our dwellings, because it favours the spreading of disease germs."[38] The ubiquity of public health proclamations in the city during the months of the epidemic surely helped to shape – and even fuel – citizen interventions such as the letters written by Montrealers to city hall and the press. But the local government also took concrete action, reserving hospital beds for flu victims and setting up emergency bureaux and hospitals in various public buildings. Physicians, nurses, firefighters, police officers, female volunteers, and members of male and especially female religious communities staffed these emergency shelters and hospices; many of them also conducted home visits to the ill and the dying.[39]

Doctors such as Séraphin Boucher and Elzéar Pelletier were very much in the public eye during the epidemic. As Robert Gagnon's work on sewers demonstrates, doctors already played an important role on the municipal stage in the nineteenth century; this role was highly visible during the 1918-20 crisis.[40] The absolute shortage of doctors and nurses, probably especially outside Montreal, was frequently commented on by health authorities.[41] The crisis strained existing resources to their limits; not one of the CHPQ's inspectors, for instance, had time to deal with other public health issues.[42] Yet the shortage of doctors and nurses was also the result of Canada's military needs during the First World War; indeed, the management of the epidemic must be understood in the context of the war. Mark Osborne Humphries has recently highlighted the conflict between health officials attempting to halt the spread of the disease and military officials concerned with sustaining the war effort. This included hunting down defaulters and deserters, enforcing conscription, and holding pro-war rallies – all inimical to public health. Prevention measures adopted by the health authorities were counteracted by the Canadian military's apparent disregard for them.[43] Humphries's argument is confirmed by my research in municipal and provincial records, which demonstrates that in Quebec, the military did in fact ignore the directives of health officials and continued the mobilization of conscripts and defaulters.[44]

Discourses of prevention were clearly well entrenched among both civil and religious authorities; the latter generally agreed to cooperate with the requests of the former to limit religious gatherings or cancel them altogether for the duration of the epidemic.[45] There were exceptions: the CHPQ occasionally received complaints about parish priests neglecting (or refusing) to close their churches.[46] Anglican bishop John Farthing complained to the CHPQ that certain Catholic priests had failed to close their churches; the CHPQ noted in its minutes that Catholic priests were not the only ones at fault in this regard.[47] On the whole, religious communities were primarily concerned with the care of those already taken ill rather than with implementing measures of prevention. Indeed, the health authorities were dependent on the goodwill of Catholic bishops, and particularly Montreal's archbishop, Paul Bruchési, in putting nuns and religious brothers at the service of the influenza cause. Religious communities, both male and, especially, female, constituted a good part of Montreal's influenza labour force, caring for the sick in their homes and in emergency hospitals.[48]

Citizens and Public Letter Writing

In Montreal's municipal archives, I found thirty-four letters from citizens concerned about the influenza epidemic.[49] Some proposed general measures of public health and prevention. Others offered products (serums, disinfectants) that they claimed would be of use, and one or two congratulated municipal officials on their handling of the emergency. Some were written near the end of the outbreak, asking when normal activities might resume. And fourteen, which came from members of the city's business community, focused on the opening hours of shops and workplaces.

Although all the letters made reference to the immediate context of the epidemic, some also targeted sources of dirt and disease, and proposed concrete measures of hygiene that were not specific to the crisis occasioned by influenza. J.-E. Beaudoin, for instance, with whom we opened this discussion, argued that the unsanitary conditions of Montreal's streets could be traced to second-hand stores, rag stores (with their "old mattresses full of bed-bugs"), fish shops, and live-poultry shops.[50] What these businesses had in common, Beaudoin claimed, was that most of their owners were Jewish. Such shops were a nuisance to neighbours, brought down property values (and thus threatened municipal coffers), and caused disease. His solution was to move them to a location where they would not disturb neighbours or adversely affect the cleanliness of the city, and where they would be under the constant surveillance of the municipal board of health.[51] Isidore Crépeau, president of La Compagnie Céramo-Vitrail, located on Boulevard Saint-Laurent at Marie-Anne, voiced complaints suspiciously similar to those of Beaudoin, and one cannot help but think that the two citizens had conferred before writing their respective letters. Crépeau, too, targeted second-hand and rag shops with their "old mattresses" at the doors, as well as poultry shops and fish shops. He, too, argued that municipal officials ought to capitalize on the crisis in order to regulate these everyday problems of public health. Like Beaudoin, Crépeau recommended moving these businesses away from Montreal's principal commercial arteries and placing them under the surveillance of the city's board of health. He also called for legislation to prohibit the displaying of produce in front of grocery stores, as it was exposed to dust. Like numerous other citizens who wrote to city hall, Crépeau urged an end to the overcrowding of streetcars. Finally, he recommended washing the streets as often as possible to eliminate dust, which, he suggested, "was always a source of infection."[52] A third citizen wrote anonymously, signing her letter simply "Hygiène

Générale" (general hygiene), in order to criticize Montreal's everyday in-salubrities. Like other letter-writers, this Montrealer explicitly linked the epidemic to normal conditions in the city: it was all the more important that her public health criticisms be taken into account, she argued, given that they were formulated during a period of epidemic. Her four-page, single-spaced handwritten missive was one of only two anonymous letters found in the municipal archives; the author claimed to be a woman, and though we cannot verify this assertion, the letter's seeming familiarity with the workings of butcher shops and grocery stores suggests that it was true. The writer had specific targets: candy vendors who handled candy and money indiscriminately without washing their hands; butchers who let customers handle the meat before (and sometimes, without) buying; grocers who neglected to wash their hands and who exposed their produce to dust; and, yet again, overcrowded streetcars. The solution, she argued, lay in increased regulation by the board of health and in public education, by way of newspapers and courses in social and domestic hygiene taught in schools.[53]

Whereas the suggestions made by Beaudoin, Crépeau, and "Hygiène Générale" linked the epidemic to commonplace unsanitary conditions in Montreal, other citizens had proposals specific to the pandemic. John Findlay, for instance, wrote to the administrative commission early in the epidemic to suggest "as a preventive against the spread of Grippe 1) that the Tramways Company be requested to immediately saturize every Street Car in use with a strong disinfectant and 2) that you seriously consider as to advising the closing of Picture Houses, and Theatres." Clearly motivated by the immediate medical crisis in which Montreal found itself, Findlay nonetheless took it on himself to add, "While writing you, may I also suggest that you take up with Mr. Tremblay the advisability of a By Law making it compulsory on Autoists to sound their Horn when crossing Streets, those going East or West, giving one Blast and those going North or South two blasts. My experience is that very few use their Horns while crossing Streets, and if they did there would be fewer accidents."[54] Other citizens also wrote to advise ventilating streetcars, arguing that the cars were "little better than hot-beds of disease" and citing the large number of "conductors and motormen" sick with influenza as proof.[55] Father Joseph de Bray, of Montreal's St-Joseph parish, wrote to the mayor to complain that "*rien d'énergique* ne se fait pour empêcher l'épidémie de se propager." Priests visiting the poorer streets of his parish, he claimed, found influenza victims in their homes, abandoned and without medical care. Why not convert Montreal's schools into emergency hospitals, he suggested, where doctors and priests could administer to the sick without having to go from house to house?[56]

Some citizens hoped to profit from the crisis. G. Beaulieu of the Chemical Import Company advised the board of health that he could supply the city, promptly and at a reasonable cost, with two germicides, to be used to disinfect sidewalks, houses, schools, and public buildings. Monocrézole and Tricrézole were, he claimed, "les plus puissants germicides connus, ces deux Cresols tuent les microbes, tous les germes et tous les vibrions septiques de l'air."[57] Meanwhile, the owner of Lyons' Limited Cut Rate Drug Store informed the mayor that he could supply disinfectants and medicine to those stricken with influenza at reasonable prices, "and to very poor people free." Alluding to drugstores that had attempted to profit from the epidemic by raising their prices, Lyons stated, "We simply make this offer to show you, that there is scarcely any necessity from poor people dying from want of a little medicine."[58]

The connection between influenza and the mobilization of troops for the Great War was evident to those letter-writers who insisted on the necessity of disinfecting and ventilating military barracks. One epistle, signed "Un conscrit!" (a conscript), the second anonymous letter among our sources, requested that the board of health disinfect and air out military barracks so that conscripts would not contract influenza. The writer added, seemingly as an afterthought, "et n'oubliez pas les tramways qui sont beau-coup la grande cause de cette maladie."[59] Arthur Sauvé, leader of Quebec's Official Opposition, went further and sent a telegram urging authorities to suspend the mobilization of conscripts "pour aider les autorités médicales à contrôler le fléau."[60]

Some letters pressed authorities to close down places of public meeting, such as schools, churches, movie houses, and theatres. By the end of October, some of the business-owners affected by such measures were writing to request that their institutions be allowed to reopen. On 6 November, H. LeRoy Shaw, alderman and manager of the Life and Accident Departments of the Travelers Insurance Company, wrote to Ernest Décary, chairman of the Administrative Commission of the City of Montreal – and of the board of health during the epidemic – suggesting that business colleges be allowed to reopen before the public schools, as the former "cater to the older Students, and who are really working under very sanitary conditions, and should not be classed with the Public Schools, where a very large number of small children get together."[61]

The municipal archives house a few letters from the organizers of special events, who wondered whether their event could be held despite the epidemic. H.S. Adlington, secretary-treasurer of the Canadian Northern Montreal Land Company, wrote to Décary to inform him that trains were about to run through the new tunnel that burrowed under Mount Royal and that a special excursion to Model City, on the other side of the mountain, had been planned for a Sunday afternoon; could this excursion take place despite the restrictions on public gatherings? "I may mention that although it will entail a congregation of people for a few minutes in the train while proceeding to Mount Royal," wrote Adlington, "we consider that the fresh air of Model City would soon dissipate any danger which the short confinement in the train would entail, and in fact this means of giving a good number of citizens a breath of fresh air may not be a bad thing in itself." The large "NO" handwritten in the margin suggests that Décary was not persuaded by this logic.[62]

A large number of letters concern the opening hours of shops and services such as banks; in an attempt to reduce congestion in stores and streetcars, the board of health had decreed that such businesses close their doors at 4:00 p.m.[63] What we find in the archives are letters of polite protest written by the owners of small and large businesses concerned about losing trade during the epidemic. Although clearly self-interested, these letters are framed in the language of public health and citizenship. R.N. Fairweather and twenty-seven other department store owners and merchants told the administrative commission that they were "convinced that you were actuated by the sole motive of preserving the Public Health, chiefly by avoiding the congestion of traffic on the Street Cars between the hours of 5 and 7."[64] Although these business-owners wrote with due deference to the authorities, their message was clear: "We appreciate the opinions of the Medical and Sanitation Authorities who advised the measure taken; and, although we do not wish to be considered as making protests, we desire to be placed on record as believing that our scheme [later opening and closing hours] is the better for all concerned, and with which we would be glad to have you conform."[65] Representatives of some of Montreal's major department stores – Almy's, the John Murphy Company, and Dupuis Frères – began their letter requesting that store hours be extended until 6:30 p.m. by stating that they "recognize the grave responsibilities of the board and we are sincerely anxious to do all that is reasonable and within our power to help the situation."[66] Another group of retail merchants informed Ernest Décary that four o'clock closings would have a disastrous impact on their business; nevertheless, they wrote, "Nous considérons cependant que eu égard à l'épidémie que nous subissons actuellement, il est de notre devoir de bons citoyens de contribuer de tout notre possible à enrayer le mal." They argued that their proposed solution – keeping stores open until seven in the evening – would help to reduce overcrowding in the streetcars, as the public could space out its shopping over a longer period of time, and employees could return home after the evening rush hour: thus, "l'importante question de l'Hygiène actuelle de la Ville recevra une solution satisfaisante."[67] Other letter-writers likewise justified their own requests on the basis of public health; witness, for instance, the letter from the Bank of Montreal head office that attempted to persuade Décary that "if ... we are obliged to close [the Hochelaga branch] at four o'clock the congestion prior to that hour will obviously be great and the danger of infection proportionately increased."[68] Most letter-writers included at least a perfunctory sentence acknowledging the extent of the public health catastrophe before turning to its impact on their own daily affairs: Montreal merchants whose shops bordered the municipality of Outremont, for example, began their letter to Dr. Boucher by thanking him "avec grand coeur de l'attention que vous portez à enrayer le fléau de la grippe espagnole," before reporting that Outremont merchants were taking advantage of Montreal's early closing hours, keeping their own businesses open later than usual to reap the benefits.[69]

Some of these writers implicitly or explicitly compared their situation to that of other Montrealers, in particular, their business competitors. Shopkeepers in the northern part of the city petitioned the Outremont Board of Health to impose the same opening hours as those in Montreal proper, so that they would not lose business to Outremont store-owners.[70] F.A. Clarke, owner of the Wigwam souvenir shop on Peel Street, likewise wrote to the board of health to protest the early closing by-law:

> Seeing that the Board has granted a special permit to Messrs F.E. Phelan, Foster Brown, and Mr. T.J. Chapman, to remain open until 6 p.m. I am really in a worse position than they are. I employ only one clerk with myself and son. We sell similar goods as the firms alluded to above and depend, to a great extent, on people who do their shopping between the hours of 2 and 6 p.m. ... All we ask is a little kind consideration of our case, as we claim we are in the same category as the firms to whom your Board has granted a special permit. Trusting you will grant me the same kind treatment as my case is similar in every sense of the word.[71]

Comparisons with other North American cities are also present in some of these letters. One group of merchants, for instance, suggested "following the example of the New York authorities who after one day's trial of 4 o'clock closing changed the business hours of the Merchants on their recommendation and request to 9.45 opening and 6.15 closing, thus keeping the staffs of the stores until the greater crush of the industrial places had been carried."[72] Representatives of some of Montreal's major department stores likewise invoked the example of New York and of Boston, "a city noted the world over for quickness to protect its citizens, at all times in matters of health."[73]

It is clear that for many of these letter-writing citizens, the influenza epidemic provided an opportunity to raise with their local government issues that had long been a source of irritation. This body of correspondence testifies to the desire of some ordinary citizens to regulate urban life and to eliminate aspects of urban space that offended their senses and sensibilities. Isidore Crépeau wrote of the "odeur nauséabonde" of poultry shops and fish shops.[74] Henry Irwin of Westmount complained about the stench of streetcars, claiming to Décary that "I do not think that I have been twice *inside* one of the Company's cars during the last three years, the smell being too disgusting to me at least."[75] Ethnic scapegoating and anti-Semitism are evident in the J.-E. Beaudoin letter with which we began this essay; it is perhaps surprising that there are not more examples of ethnic animosities in these sources.

Some of the letters examined here were addressed to the mayor, others to the board of health, and still others to the city's administrative commission and its chairman, Ernest Décary. The writers speak as citizens, often explicitly using the language of citizenship. Like the citizen letter-writers in the USSR whom Sheila Fitzpatrick studied, these, too, are urban and male.[76] Only one of the forty-four letters examined for this chapter appears to have come from a woman, and she wrote anonymously, under the *nom de plume* "Hygiène Générale." Many authors wrote as municipal taxpayers. Some wrote as petitioners, although few as supplicants.[77] None appear to have perceived themselves as asking for special favours; rather, they requested treatment equal to that given to other Montrealers. For the most part, the tone of the letters is polite and reasonable. Conscious of the health catastrophe in which Montreal found itself, the writers surely tempered any impulse to excess. In many cases, letters are signed "Votre respectueux," "Respectfully submitted," "respectueusement soumises," "salutations respectueuses," or "Yours respectfully": forms of address that reflected early-twentieth-century protocol and hierarchies, but also, possibly, the authors' awareness that municipal officials were dealing with a most difficult situation. The formal "vous," it goes without saying, was invariably used by those who wrote in French.[78] Yet there is also a sense in which these Montrealers are writing as equals, as citizens and taxpayers entitled to both their opinion and the right to express it to their municipal government. In the context of the epidemic, they were aware that they were expected to follow municipal regulations, and clearly, some felt free to offer their own advice in turn. One might ask whether these Montrealers were responding to official efforts to control the epidemic: perhaps they saw their letters to city hall as the gestures of responsible citizens, writing out of a sense of duty.[79] Or perhaps they felt compelled to write because they could see that municipal authorities were having difficulty managing the epidemic. These letters to state authorities are thus rather different from those that have been most frequently studied in the Canadian context – correspondence seeking material aid (a job, a loan, a small sum of cash, an increase in benefits), written in times of crisis such as the Great Depression of the 1930s, and in which the authors felt obliged to prove their worthiness as recipients of assistance.[80] The class position of many of these letter-writers – petit bourgeois, as far as can be ascertained from their occupations, their addresses, and the content of their correspondence – and the fact that many of them were small-business owners suggests that they shared the world view of the elected officials and civil servants who ran city hall, where the interests of property-owners were well represented, as historian Michèle Dagenais has demonstrated.[81] This helps to explain the amicable, almost collegial, tone that pervades many of the letters studied here.

The letters discussed in this chapter are surely only a small proportion of the correspondence sent during the epidemic. The evidence shows, for instance, that city hall received numerous offers of serums, disinfectants, and similar products – even though we have few examples of them here.[82] We cannot know how representative these particular letters are; nor can we know whether they were preserved deliberately or by happenstance. Likewise, the municipal archives contain copies of the answers sent to a few of the letters (notably, grateful replies to offers of material assistance during the epidemic, in cash or in kind), but there is no way of knowing whether they were alone in receiving a reply.[83] Generally speaking, then, we have mere one-sided glimpses into what Fitzpatrick calls "two-way communication."[84] And yet there are hints that the letters had an impact.

Probably in response to the citizen complaints about dust discussed above, the Montreal Board of Health resolved on 15 October 1918 "Que défense soit faite d'exposer les marchandises et spécialement les articles d'alimentation sur les trottoirs."[85] As Joseph A. Amato has argued, the targeting of dust by public health reformers merged older concerns about filth with newer battles against germs.[86] The melding of these two strains of thought is evident in the letters written to municipal governments during the epidemic, as well as in the responses of the board of health.[87]

Other citizens used other means of communicating with city hall: we know, for example, that Médéric Martin, mayor of Montreal, received complaints and suggestions by telephone. These included criticisms that streetcars were not sufficiently aired out or disinfected; that soldiers, who were supposed to be confined to their barracks during the epidemic, were still boarding streetcars; and that many merchants were not conforming to the opening hours decreed by the board of health.[88] The mayor himself wrote letters of suggestion to the board of health: on 11 October 1918, he requested that public laundries be disinfected daily, and on 31 October, he urged the board to reconsider its decision to shorten store opening hours, as its policy would mean financial hardship for small businesses.[89]

Other citizens chose to air their opinions by writing to the daily newspaper. An examination of *Le Devoir* from 26 September 1918 to 30 April 1919 turned up ten letters to the editor regarding the epidemic. To some extent, they echo the themes found in the municipal archives: notably, reactions to public health measures and suggested influenza remedies. Doctor Joseph Élie Bélanger, from Hull, wrote to the newspaper to inform the public of the existence of a French pharmaceutical product that, he was convinced, could cure pulmonary complications of Spanish influenza and possibly the initial infection as well.[90] A. Le Moyne de Martigny, secretary of the Baby Welfare Committee, wrote to *Le Devoir* to suggest that though citizens ought to respect the board's preventive measures, they ought equally to take steps to reduce Montreal's shockingly high infant mortality rate – an endemic public health problem in the city.[91] Dr. T.A. Brisson wrote to criticize the decision of the wartime Canada Food Board to allow wheat substitutes in bread. Overpriced bread of poor quality could not maintain the health of the population, he argued, particularly in a period of epidemic.[92] James Whitaker noted that "we have taken every effort to safeguard the public by cancelling meetings and entertainments. Yet we leave the most dangerous factor in our midst to go free. I mean our familiar unscrubbed street cars. I make the cogent argument that our street

cars are the most potent carriers of this and other diseases." Montreal's
streetcars ought to be properly washed, disinfected, and ventilated,
Whitaker advised. His recommendations echoed official pronounce-
ments: "Last of all," he wrote, "people should bear in mind that fresh air
is the most deadly enemy the disease has, therefore, let the fresh air be our
watchword – no overcrowding of street cars, the airing of the home and
care to not let one's self get fatigued."[93] Eugène Roy, a civil engineering
student, wrote to *Le Devoir* on 14 November 1918 to protest the city's decision in which cinemas and theatres were to reopen and public meetings
to be held once more, whereas boarding schools and universities would
remain closed an extra week. According to Roy, university classes normally
consisted of small numbers of students, whereas hundreds of people (including university students with newfound leisure time) were flooding the
cinemas and theatres.[94] Several Montrealers wrote to *Le Devoir* to praise
the devotion of various male and female religious communities – the Sœurs
de la Providence, the Frères des écoles chrétiennes, the Sœurs Franciscaines,
and the Missionnaires de l'Immaculée-Conception – as well as that of lay
nurses who, since the epidemic began, could be found at the bedsides of
the poor and the ill.[95] It was no accident that such tributes were submitted
to a daily newspaper, with its extensive readership, rather than to city hall,
a more private forum.

CONCLUSION

Médéric Martin, mayor of Montreal, was severe in his condemnation of
the city's board of health, arguing at the height of the epidemic that "si
l'on n'avait pas tant retardé à prendre des mesures pour empêcher la pro-
pagation de l'épidémie de la grippe, cette épidémie aurait pu être contrôlée
bien plus facilement, mais, à venir jusqu'au moment où la maladie a fait
des progrès terribles, l'on ne s'est pas occupé de mettre le public en garde
en aucune façon." In his opinion, the board had dawdled in instigating
measures to stop the spread of influenza and had not sufficiently warned
the public of its dangers.[96]

Nonetheless, it is clear that within days of the epidemic's outbreak, the
public was acutely aware of its dangers, and as we have seen here, many
Montrealers had ideas about how best to halt its spread or otherwise manage it. This chapter is in some ways a bottom-up analysis of the 1918-20
influenza pandemic. Although we do not hear from actual flu victims here,
we do achieve some sense of the impact of influenza on daily urban life.

Montrealers worried about contracting this often fatal illness, but they were also concerned about everyday problems of dirt, disease, and public health, and they seized on this occasion to transmit their opinions to municipal authorities. In some epistles – short or long, hastily scribbled or carefully worded, handwritten or typed – we can glimpse signs that miasmatic thinking persisted alongside the germ theory of disease, which had made significant incursions by the time of the First World War. Whereas Isidore Crépeau wrote rather vaguely of "la poussière qui est toujours une source d'infection," the woman who signed her letter "Hygiène Générale" explicitly used the language of germs, arguing that meat handled by customers and later bought by others might contain the "germes de certaines maladies."[97] G. Beaulieu, attempting to sell his germicides to the board of health, likewise wrote of "microbes" and "germs."[98] In some letters, we see that some citizens advocated state intervention: "Hygiène Générale," for instance, requested public health legislation of various sorts.

It is evident from these letters that Montrealers also worried about their livelihoods, and if their desire to keep their businesses open during the same hours as their competitors seems petty in the context of this medical catastrophe, it is nonetheless a useful reminder of the ways in which epidemic disease can determine bread-and-butter issues such as work and pay. Written in the context of total war, these letters suggest that this was also a context of total epidemic: the influenza pandemic of 1918-20 provoked citizen reflections and interventions on questions of public health but also on issues of everyday life in the early-twentieth-century city.

ACKNOWLEDGMENTS

I would like to acknowledge the generous financial support of the Fonds québécois de la recherche sur la société et la culture, as well as of the Université du Québec à Montréal's Programme d'aide financière à la recherche et à la création. This funding allowed me to hire a number of very able research assistants, and I thank Amélie Bourbeau, Martin Croteau, and Mourad Djebabla for their careful work. Finally, my thanks go to my colleague Carl Bouchard for introducing me to Sheila Fitzpatrick's work on public letter writing and to Esyllt Jones and the anonymous reviewers of this collection for their close readings of this chapter and their useful suggestions for revision.

NOTES

1 Archives de la Ville de Montréal (AVM), Fonds de la Commission administrative, VM18, 127-02-06-02, document 68a, J.-E. Beaudoin to M. Médéric Martin, Maire, Montreal, 19

October 1918. Beaudoin's occupation and address can be traced in the *Annuaire Lovell de Montréal et de sa banlieue* (Montreal: John Lovell and Son, 1917-18 and 1918-19).

2 Hervé Anctil and Marc-A. Bluteau, *La santé et l'assistance publique au Québec: 1886-1986* (Quebec City: Ministère de la santé et des services sociaux, Direction des communications, 1986); Peter Keating and Othmar Keel, eds., *Santé et société au Québec XIXe-XXe siècle* (Montreal: Boréal, 1995); François Guérard, "L'hygiène publique au Québec de 1887 à 1939: centralisation, normalisation et médicalisation," *Recherches sociographiques* 37,2 (1996): 203-27; Georges Desrosiers et al., "Le renforcement des interventions gouvernementales dans le domaine de la santé entre 1922 et 1936: le Service provincial d'hygiène de la province de Québec," *Canadian Bulletin of Medical History* 18 (2001): 205-40; and Georges Desrosiers and Benoît Gaumer, "Les débuts de l'éducation sanitaire au Québec: 1880-1901," *Canadian Bulletin of Medical History* 23,1 (2006): 183-207. The CHPQ was also known as the Conseil supérieur d'hygiène and, after 1922, as the Service provincial d'hygiène de la province de Québec.

3 Terry Copp, *The Anatomy of Poverty: The Condition of the Working Class in Montreal, 1897-1929* (Toronto: McClelland and Stewart, 1974), 88-105. Copp's arguments have been echoed by other historians, most recently in Valerie Minnett and Mary-Anne Poutanen, "Swatting Flies for Health: Children and Tuberculosis in Early Twentieth-Century Montreal," *Urban History Review* 37,1 (Fall 2007): 32-44.

4 Peter Keating and Othmar Keel, Introduction, in Keating and Keel, *Santé et société,* 19; Guérard, "L'hygiène publique"; Desrosiers and Gaumer, "Les débuts de l'éducation sanitaire"; and Desrosiers et al., "Le renforcement des interventions gouvernementales."

5 On the resistance of municipalities to the CHPQ's public health efforts, and on the CHPQ's consequent mistrust of municipal authorities, see ibid.; and Guérard, "L'hygiène publique."

6 Michael Farley, Othmar Keel, and Camille Limoges, "Les commencements de l'administration montréalaise de la santé publique (1865-1885)," in Keating and Keel, *Santé et société,* 93-100, 113-14.

7 Most recent discussions of infrastructure include Dany Fougères, *L'approvisionnement en eau à Montréal: du privé au public, 1796-1865* (Sillery: Septentrion, 2004); and Robert Gagnon, *Questions d'égouts: santé publique, infrastructures et urbanisation à Montréal au XIXe siècle* (Montreal: Boréal, 2006). For endemic problems, see Copp, *The Anatomy of Poverty;* Louise Côté, *"En garde!" Les représentations de la tuberculose au Québec dans la première moitié du XXe siècle* (Sainte-Foy: Presses de l'Université Laval, 2000); Minnett and Poutanen, "Swatting Flies"; Denyse Baillargeon, *Un Québec en mal d'enfants: la médicalisation de la maternité, 1910-1970* (Montreal: Éditions du remue-ménage, 2004); and Martin Tétreault, "Les maladies de la misère: aspects de la santé publique à Montréal (1880-1914)," *Revue d'histoire de l'Amérique française* 36,4 (1983): 507-26. On doctors, see Claudine Pierre-Deschênes, "Santé publique et organisation de la profession médicale au Québec, 1870-1918," *Revue d'histoire de l'Amérique française* 35,3 (December 1981): 335-75; and Jacques Bernier, *La médecine au Québec: naissance et evolution d'une profession* (Sainte-Foy: Presses de l'Université de Laval, 1989). On nurses, see, for example, Yolande Cohen, *Profession infirmière: une histoire des soins dans les hôpitaux du Québec* (Montreal: Presses de l'Université de Montréal, 2000).

8 On these competing theories, see Heather MacDougall, "Public Health and the 'Sanitary Idea' in Toronto, 1866-1890," in *Essays in the History of Canadian Medicine,* ed. Wendy

Mitchinson and Janice Dickin McGinnis (Toronto: McClelland and Stewart, 1988), 62-64. See also Gagnon, *Questions d'égouts*, 8, 214, on miasmatic theories.

9   Jean-Claude Robert, "The City of Wealth and Death: Urban Mortality in Montreal, 1821-1871," in Mitchinson and Dickin McGinnis, *Essays in the History of Canadian Medicine*, 25, 34, 37.

10 Heather MacDougall, examining Toronto, traces the origins of the "sanitary idea" to the cholera epidemic of 1866 and argues that "widespread, public acceptance" of preventive medical services had taken root "by the end of the 1880s." MacDougall, "Public Health and the 'Sanitary Idea,'" 62. Jean-Claude Robert argues that public health thinking began to be evident in Montreal during the 1860s-70s. Robert, "The City of Wealth and Death," 37.

11 Guérard, "L'hygiène publique"; and Desrosiers and Gaumer, "Les débuts de l'éducation sanitaire."

12 Minnett and Poutanen, "Swatting Flies."

13 Louise Dechêne and Jean-Claude Robert, "Le choléra de 1832 dans le Bas-Canada: mesure des inégalités devant la mort," in *Santé et société au Québec XIXe-XXe siècle*, ed. Peter Keating and Othmar Keel (Montreal: Boréal, 1995), 61-84; Copp, *The Anatomy of Poverty;* and Tétreault, "Les maladies de la misère."

14 Keating and Keel, Introduction, in Keating and Keel, *Santé et société*, 17, 27.

15 Minnett and Poutanen, "Swatting Flies"; Denyse Baillargeon, "Fréquenter les Gouttes de lait: l'expérience des mères montréalaises, 1910-1965," *Revue d'histoire de l'Amérique française* 50,1 (1996): 29-68; and Gagnon, *Questions d'égouts.*

16 Esyllt W. Jones, *Influenza 1918: Disease, Death, and Struggle in Winnipeg* (Toronto: University of Toronto Press, 2007).

17 For example, Gail G. Campbell, "Disfranchised but Not Quiescent: Women Petitioners in New Brunswick in the Mid-Nineteenth Century," in *Rethinking Canada: The Promise of Women's History,* 2nd ed., ed. Veronica Strong-Boag and Anita Clair Fellman (Toronto: Copp Clark Pitman, 1991), 81-96.

18 L.M. Grayson and Michael Bliss, eds., *The Wretched of Canada: Letters to R.B. Bennett, 1930-1935* (Toronto: University of Toronto Press, 1971); Lara Campbell, "'A Barren Cupboard at Home': Ontario Families Confront the Premiers during the Great Depression," in *Ontario since Confederation: A Reader,* ed. Edgar-André Montigny and Lori Chambers (Toronto: University of Toronto Press, 2000), 284-306; Lara Campbell, "'We who have wallowed in the mud of Flanders': First World War Veterans, Unemployment and the Development of Social Welfare in Canada, 1929-1939," *Journal of the Canadian Historical Association,* n.s., 11 (2000): 125-49; and Sheila Fitzpatrick, "Suppliants and Citizens: Public Letter-Writing in Soviet Russia in the 1930s," *Slavic Review* 55,1 (Spring 1996): 78-105.

19 Ibid., 79.

20 Ibid., and 78n3. Fitzpatrick's definition refers to "ordinary Russians" in the 1930s.

21 As Fitzpatrick states for 1930s USSR, "Patriotic citizens wrote letters of advice on public policy and signed their names. Angry citizens sent letters of abuse and invective anonymously." Ibid., 80.

22 Ibid. The one genre identified by Fitzpatrick and not evident in the archives that I have analyzed is the "confessional letter."

23 Heather MacDougall notes that public health reformers targeted municipal authorities in the late nineteenth century. MacDougall, "Public Health and the 'Sanitary Idea,'" 62.

24 The response of CHPQ secretary-director Elzéar Pelletier to a female schoolteacher who had written to advise the CHPQ that the municipality of St-Jude had not closed its schools during the epidemic suggests that the CHPQ received at least some letters from citizens. Archives nationales du Québec à Québec (ANQQ), Fonds du Conseil d'hygiène de la province de Québec (CHPQ), E88, contenant 15, registre 84, Elzéar Pelletier to Melle Hectorine Cardin, Institutrice, St-Jude, 18 October 1918.

25 Guérard, "L'hygiène publique."

26 For an overview of the 1918 influenza epidemic in Canada, see Janice Dickin McGinnis, "The Impact of Epidemic Influenza: Canada, 1918-1919," *Historical Papers* (1977): 120-40.

27 *Rapport du Service de Santé de la Cité de Montréal 1918 par le Docteur Boucher, Directeur* (Montreal: A.P. Pigeon, 1919), 19, 20. The total number of cases in Montreal was subsequently revised downward to 19,287. Ibid., 20. See also "L'épidémie d'influenza," *Bulletin d'hygiène, Cité de Montréal* 5,1-6 (January-June 1919): 1-6.

28 *Rapport du Service de Santé de la Cité de Montréal 1918*, 26; L.-F. Dubé, "La Grippe: quels enseignements peut-on tirer de l'épidémie 1918-1920?" *L'Union médicale du Canada* (Montreal), November 1920, 574.

29 *Rapport du Service de Santé de la Cité de Montréal 1920 par le Docteur S. Boucher, Directeur* (Montreal: A.P. Pigeon, 1921), 23. The statistics given here are for the months of January, February, March, and April 1920; Montrealers were hardest hit during February and March. On the differing mortality patterns of the flu in 1918 and 1920 respectively, see Dubé, "La Grippe," 574. One municipal official noted at the end of November 1918 that there was "une mortalité presque nulle dans les hôpitaux d'enfants (Saint-Arsène et Sainte-Justine)." Eugène Gagnon to Séraphin Boucher, 29 November 1918, AVM, Fonds du Conseil de Ville, VM1, S3, D5241.

30 For instance, we read in the CHPQ minutes for 17 October 1918, "Le conseil ne croit pas qu'il doive fixer le temps qu'un malade de grippe doit rester isolé. Il laisse aux médecins et aux conseils locaux d'hygiène à en décider." ANQQ, Fonds CHPQ, E88, contenant 1, registre 2 August 1904-3 January 1919, vol. II, Assemblée of 17 October 1918. Similar decisions can be found in ANQQ, E88, Fonds du Service provincial d'hygiène, contenant 1, registre 2 August 1904-3 January 1919, vol. II, Assemblée of 30 October 1918; and ANQQ, Fonds CHPQ, E88, contenant 15, registre 83, E. Pelletier, M.D., to Dr. Landry, Mont Joli, 12 October 1918.

31 Guérard, "L'hygiène publique," 208. On the 1885 smallpox epidemic, see Michael Bliss, *Plague: A Story of Smallpox in Montreal* (Toronto: HarperCollins, 1991).

32 See Elzéar Pelletier to la Corporation municipale de St-Jude, 18 October 1918, and Elzéar Pelletier to l'officier exécutif du Conseil local d'hygiène, St-Jean de Matha, 29 October 1918, both in ANQQ, Fonds CHPQ, E88, contenant 15, registre 84.

33 AVM, Fonds du Conseil de Ville, VM1, S3, D5241-01, "By-Laws of the Central Board of Health of the Province of Quebec, Relating to Influenza." On the non-obligatory nature of placarding during the epidemic, see also ANQQ, Fonds CHPQ, E88, contenant 15, registre 83, Elzéar Pelletier, Secrétaire-directeur, to Monsieur Messier, Secrétaire-trésorier municipal, Victoriaville, 25 September 1918.

34 ANQQ, Fonds CHPQ, E88, contenant 1, registre 2 August 1904-3 January 1919, vol. II, Assemblée of 24 October 1918; and ANQQ, Fonds CHPQ, E88, contenant 15, registre 84, Jos A. Beaudry, Inspecteur général, to Monsieur Louis Saindon, Secrétaire-trésorier, Cacouna village, 26 October 1918.

35 ANQQ, Fonds CHPQ, E88, contenant 1, registre 2 August 1904-3 January 1919, vol. II, Assemblée of 30 October 1918.

36 "By-Laws of the Central Board of Health." Elzéar Pelletier, secretary-director of the CHPQ, wrote to Louis Beaulieu, secretary of the local board of health in Val Brillant, "Nos règlements n'exigent pas de désinfectant; faire bouillir le linge, aérer et ensoleiller les maisons est tout ce qu'il suffit pour les purifier après la grippe." ANQQ, Fonds CHPQ, E88, contenant 15, registre 84, Elzéar Pelletier to Monsieur Louis Beaulieu, Secrétaire du bureau local d'hygiène, Val Brillant, 26 October 1918.

37 AVM, Fonds du Conseil de Ville, VM1, S3, D5241-01, "City of Montreal. Department of Health. Beware of Spanish Influenza." See other circulars in this file.

38 "L'influenza en 1920: Historique et conseils," *Bulletin d'hygiène, Cité de Montréal* 7,7-8 (July-August 1920): 4. For its part, the CHPQ stated in its 1918 influenza by-laws that "the sun is a powerful disinfectant." "By-Laws of the Central Board of Health." In its correspondence with municipalities regarding the disinfecting of patients' rooms once they were cured of influenza, the CHPQ reiterated, "et on favorise le plus possible la pénétration des rayons solaires, car le soleil est un des meilleurs désinfectants." Pelletier to Messier, 25 September 1918.

39 "L'épidémie d'influenza," *Bulletin d'hygiène, Cité de Montréal* 5,1-6 (January-June 1919): 3-5.

40 Gagnon, *Questions d'égouts,* especially 151-211.

41 ANQQ, Fonds CHPQ, E88, contenant 15, registre 84, Elzéar Pelletier to Monsieur J.S. Croteau, Conseil local d'hygiène, Lake Weedon, 23 October 1918; ANQQ, Fonds CHPQ, E88, contenant 16, registre 88, Elzéar Pelletier to Monsieur A.G. Godbout, Risborough and Marlow, 29 October 1918; and E.-M. G. Savard, Inspecteur en chef, Circulaire à MM. les Inspecteurs régionaux, 11 February 1920. Esyllt Jones notes the shortage of nurses in Winnipeg during the influenza epidemic. Jones, *Influenza 1918,* 67.

42 ANQQ, Fonds CHPQ, E88, contenant 15, registre 84, Jos A. Beaudry, Inspecteur général, to Monsieur Vital Chicoine, Verchères, 31 October 1918.

43 Mark Osborne Humphries, "The Horror at Home: The Canadian Military and the 'Great' Influenza Pandemic of 1918," *Journal of the Canadian Historical Association,* n.s., 16,1 (2005): 235-60.

44 AVM, Fonds du Bureau de Santé, VM170, 119-06-05-03, Procès-verbal d'une séance du Bureau de Santé tenue le 10 octobre 1918. Eugène Godin, the registrar responsible for carrying out the requirements of the Military Service Act in Montreal, responded to the CHPQ's admonishments by stating that "si le danger [of influenza] n'est pas assez grand pour empêcher le public de circuler à ses affaires il ne doit pas l'être assez pour empêcher la continuation du travail à une affaire que vous conviendrez être très importante: gagner la guerre." AVM, Fonds du Conseil de Ville, VM1, S3, D5241, Eugène Godin, Registraire, to M. le Président et les Membres du Conseil Provincial d'Hygiène, 17 October 1918.

45 AVM, Fonds du Conseil de Ville, VM1, S3, D5241-0, Ernest Décary, Président du Bureau de Santé de la Cité de Montréal, to Sa Grandeur Monseigneur Paul Bruchési, 18 October 1918. The CHPQ noted that it had the right to close churches during the epidemic but that it preferred to secure cooperation from religious authorities rather than impose its will. ANQQ, Fonds CHPQ, E88, contenant 1, registre 2 August 1904-3 January 1919, vol. II, Assemblée of 17 October 1918. In the words of Elzéar Pelletier, "The Board has expressed its opinion that although local Board [sic] of Health can close churches, they should preferably use extreme means of persuasion before using that power." ANQQ, Fonds CHPQ,

E88, contenant 15, registre 84, Elzéar Pelletier to Mr. M.E. Thomas, Secretary-Treasurer, Foster, 17 October 1918.

46 ANQQ, Fonds CHPQ, E88, contenant 1, registre 2 August 1904-3 January 1919, vol. II, Assemblée of 17 October 1918; contenant 15, registre 84, Elzéar Pelletier, Secrétaire-Directeur, to Sa Grandeur Mgr Bruchési, Archevêque de Montréal, 22 October 1918.

47 ANQQ, Fonds CHPQ, E88, contenant 1, registre 2 August 1904-3 January 1919, vol. II, Assemblée of 7 November 1918.

48 ANQQ, Fonds CHPQ, E88, contenant 1, registre 2 August 1904-3 January 1919, vol. II, Assemblée of 17 October 1918; and Assemblée of 5 December 1918. On the role of nuns during Montreal's influenza epidemic, see Magda Fahrni, "'Elles sont partout': les femmes et la ville en temps d'épidémie, Montréal, 1918-1920," *Revue d'histoire de l'Amérique française* 58,1 (2004): 67-85.

49 The fonds examined were the following: Fonds de la Commission administrative, VM18; Fonds du Bureau de Santé, VM170; and Fonds du Conseil de Ville, VM1.

50 The original reads, "avec des vieux matelas plein de punaises."

51 Beaudoin to Martin, 19 October 1918.

52 AVM, Fonds du Conseil de Ville, VM1, S3, D5241-02, Isidore Crépeau to E.R. Décary, Président, La Commission d'Hygiène [sic], 11 October 1918.

53 AVM, Fonds du Conseil de Ville, VM1, S3, D5241-02, "Hygiène Générale" to Messieurs les membres du Bureau d'hygiène, Montreal, 14 October 1918.

54 AVM, Fonds du Conseil de Ville, VM1, S3, D5241-02, John Findlay to E.R. Décary, Esq., President, Civic Commission, City Hall, 7 October 1918.

55 AVM, Fonds du Conseil de Ville, VM1, S3, D5241-02, H. Irwin to E.R. Décary, Esq., Chairman of the Administrative Commission of City of Montreal, 23 October 1918. Irwin also noted, "I am pleased to see that many citizens are now writing to the papers to the same effect."

56 AVM, Fonds du Conseil de Ville, VM1, S3, D5241-02, Rev. Jos. de Bray, Presbytère St-Joseph, to Monsieur le Maire, 17 October 1918 (emphasis in original).

57 AVM, Fonds du Conseil de Ville, VM1, S3, D5241-02, G. Beaulieu to M. le Secrétaire du Bureau de Santé, 15 October 1918.

58 AVM, Fonds du Conseil de Ville, VM1, S3, D5241-02, H. Lyons to His Worship Mayor Martin, 23 October 1918.

59 AVM, Fonds du Conseil de Ville, VM1, S3, D5241-02, "Un conscrit!" to Mr. Président du Bureau de Santé, 12 October 1918.

60 AVM, Fonds du Conseil de Ville, VM1, S3, D5241-02, Arthur Sauvé to Conseil d'Hygiène, Hôtel de Ville, Montreal, 15 October 1918.

61 AVM, Fonds du Conseil de Ville, VM1, S3, D5241-02, H. LeRoy Shaw to E.R. Décary, Esq., 6 November 1918; see likewise the letter from F.C. Webster, pastor of the Seventh Day Adventist Church, to E.R. Décary, 5 November 1918.

62 AVM, Fonds du Conseil de Ville, VM1, S3, D5241-02. H.S. Adlington to E.R. Décary, 23 October 1918; for a similar request, see R.C. Holden, honorary secretary of the Victory Loan 1918 Committee. to E.R. Décary, Esq., 5 November 1918.

63 On store opening hours as an issue for municipal government, see Michael Dawson, "Leisure, Consumption, and the Public Sphere: Postwar Debates over Shopping Regulations in Vancouver and Victoria during the Cold War," in *Creating Postwar Canada: Community, Diversity, and Dissent, 1945-75,* ed. Magda Fahrni and Robert Rutherdale (Vancouver: UBC Press, 2008), 193-216.

64 AVM, Fonds du Conseil de Ville, VM1, S3, D5241-02, R.N. Fairweather et al. to The Board of Commissioners, 9 October 1918.

65 Ibid.

66 AVM, Fonds du Conseil de Ville, VM1, S3, D5241-02, Almy's Ltd., The John Murphy Co. Ltd., and Dupuis Frères Ltée to Board of Health, Montreal, n.d.

67 AVM, Fonds du Conseil de Ville, VM1, S3, D5241-02, petition from The 5th Avenue Men's Clothing Co. et al. to Mr. Décary, 16 October 1918. An almost identical petition can be found in the same file: Maison Gagnon et al. to Mr. Décary, 16 October 1918. The file also contains an English version of this petition: John Davies et al. to Mr. Décary, 17 October 1918. In the English version, the first quotation reproduced above is translated as follows: "However, owing to the epidemic which our city is doing its utmost to stop, we think it our duty as citizens of Montreal, mindful of the welfare of the Community as a whole, to do our share to combat this dreadful disease."

68 AVM, Fonds du Conseil de Ville, VM1, S3, D5241-02, Head Office, Bank of Montreal, Montreal, to Mr. Décary, 12 October 1918.

69 AVM, Fonds du Conseil de Ville, VM1, S3, D5241-02, Les sousignés [sic] à Dr. Boucher, 15 October 1918.

70 AVM, Fonds du Conseil de Ville, VM1, S3, D5241-02, petition, 14 October 1918.

71 AVM, Fonds du Conseil de Ville, VM1, S3, D5241-02, F.A. Clarke to the Chairman and members of the Board of Health, 17 October 1918.

72 Fairweather et al. to The Board of Commissioners, 9 October 1918.

73 Almy's Ltd., The John Murphy Co. Ltd., and Dupuis Frères Ltée to Board of Health, n.d. Of course, medical, municipal, and provincial authorities were also interested in the ways in which other cities were dealing with the epidemic. ANQQ, Fonds CHPQ, E88, contenant 27, registre "Inspections – Rapports – Décisions du Conseil 1918," Arthur Bernier, Bactériologiste, to M. le Dr. A. Simard, Président du Conseil Central d'hygiène de la Province de Québec, 16 October 1918. On "inter-city cooperation in matters of disease control," see John B. Osborne, "Preparing for the Pandemic: City Boards of Health and the Arrival of Cholera in Montreal, New York, and Philadelphia in 1832," *Urban History Review* 36,2 (Spring 2008): 29-42.

74 Crépeau to Décary, 11 October 1918.

75 Irwin to Décary, 23 October 1918 (emphasis in original).

76 Fitzpatrick, "Supplicants and Citizens," 104.

77 Ibid.

78 Fitzpatrick finds that in 1930s USSR, some letters written to political leaders used "the familiar second person singular *(ty)*." Ibid., 90.

79 Fitzpatrick states that Soviet citizens who wrote to public officials to denounce fellow citizens claimed to be motivated by a sense of duty. Ibid., 91-92.

80 I think particularly of Lara Campbell's work: see "'We who have wallowed'"; and "'A Barren Cupboard at Home.'" See also Grayson and Bliss, *The Wretched of Canada;* and Magda Fahrni, *Household Politics: Montreal Families and Postwar Reconstruction* (Toronto: University of Toronto Press, 2005), especially Chapter 3.

81 Michèle Dagenais, *Des pouvoirs et des hommes: l'Administration municipale de Montréal, 1900-1950* (Montreal and Kingston: McGill-Queen's University Press and the Institute of Public Administration of Canada, 2000), 14-20.

82 The board of health began a proclamation with the words "Par suite des nombreuses offres de remèdes et de désinfectants faites au Bureau de Santé de Montréal, pour la prévention,

le traitement et la cure de la maladie qui sévit actuellement à l'état épidémique." AVM, Fonds du Conseil de Ville, VM1, S3, D5241-02, Proclamation de E.R. Décary, Dr. H. Oertel, Dr. A. Bernier, Montreal, 24 October 1918.

83 For instance, AVM, Fonds du Conseil de Ville, VM1, S3, D5241, E.R. Décary to H.F. McLean, Esq., 24 October 1918; and AVM, Fonds du Conseil de Ville, VM1, S3, D5241-02, E.R. Décary to J.A. McBride, Esq., 24 October 1918.

84 Fitzpatrick, "Supplicants and Citizens," 101-2.

85 AVM, Fonds du Bureau de Santé, VM170, 119-06-05-03, Procès-Verbaux – Bureau de santé, Procès-verbal, Bureau de Santé (Conseil local d'hygiène de la Cité de Montréal), 15 October 1918.

86 Joseph A. Amato, *Dust: A History of the Small and the Invisible* (Berkeley: University of California Press, 2000), especially 102-7, 112-17.

87 The merging of these two interpretive strands is also captured in a *Montreal Daily Star* article that reported on the health board's decision that same day: the *Star* reporter drew a direct link between foodstuffs exposed to dust and the influenza epidemic. "Food Must Not Be Exposed to Dust and Germs," *Montreal Daily Star,* 15 October 1918, 3.

88 AVM, Fonds du Conseil de Ville, VM1, S3, D5241-01, Médéric Martin, Maire de Montréal, to Ernest R. Décary, Président du Bureau de Santé, 11 October 1918.

89 Ibid.; AVM, Fonds du Conseil de Ville, VM1, S3, D5241-01, Médéric Martin, Maire de Montréal, to M. le Président et à MM. les Membres du Bureau de Santé, 31 October 1918.

90 Joseph Élie Bélanger, "La 'grippe espagnole,'" letter to the editor, *Le Devoir* (Montreal), 5 October 1918, 2.

91 A. Le Moyne de Martigny, "La mortalité infantile," letter to the editor, *Le Devoir* (Montreal), 10 October 1918, 2.

92 T-A Brisson, "Le pain de guerre et la santé publique," letter to the editor, *Le Devoir* (Montreal), 11 October 1918, 2.

93 James Whitaker, "Le tramway," letter to the editor, *Le Devoir* (Montreal), 11 October 1918, 2.

94 Eugène Roy, "Universités et théâtres," letter to the editor, *Le Devoir* (Montreal), 14 November 1918, 2.

95 "Les Sœurs de la Providence," *Le Devoir* (Montreal), 18 October 1918, 2; "Hommage au dévouement," *Le Devoir* (Montreal), 30 October 1918, 2; "Hommage," *Le Devoir* (Montreal), 4 November 1918, 2; and "Une page sur l'épidémie," *Le Devoir* (Montreal), 12 November 1918, 2.

96 Martin to M. le Président, 31 October 1918.

97 Crépeau to Décary, 11 October 1918; and "Hygiène Générale" to Messieurs les membres du Bureau d'hygiène, 14 October 1918.

98 Beaulieu to M. le Secrétaire, 15 October 1918. Esyllt Jones notes the co-existence of germ theory with "older miasmatic theories of disease causation" in Winnipeg's ethnic press during the influenza epidemic. Jones, *Influenza 1918,* 136-38.

PART 2

Who Contracted Influenza and Why?

4

The North-South Divide: Social Inequality and Mortality from the 1918 Influenza Pandemic in Hamilton, Ontario

D. ANN HERRING AND ELLEN KOROL

The 1918 influenza pandemic has become the touchstone event for thinking about disease outbreaks in the twenty-first century and for forecasting their potentially damaging effects.[1] It is often assumed that the pandemic was socially neutral and that virtually everyone was susceptible to the new virus that began circulating in 1918, even though mortality rates varied extensively worldwide, and young adults suffered higher mortality than other age groups.[2] The purpose of this essay is to add to the growing literature that suggests that the 1918 influenza outbreak was anything but democratic and that, like other epidemics, it was felt more keenly among less affluent members of society. Drawing on the mortality experience of Hamilton, Ontario, during the flu's autumn wave, we show that residents of the city's more prosperous southern wards had lower influenza mortality rates than those of the less affluent northern wards, laying bare the social and economic fault lines that divided, and continue to divide, the city today.[3]

INEQUALITIES AND INFECTIONS

Emerging diseases, such as influenza in 1918, are usually understood to be "democratic" in the sense that everyone is theoretically vulnerable because no one has antigens that confer resistance to the new pathogen. Infectious diseases, however, are historically anything but evenly distributed within

and between societies, or across the global landscape.[4] The 1918 influenza
pandemic was no different, but the social conditions that framed local
experiences of it are often forgotten because of overwhelming scientific
interest in the genetic structure of the H1N1 virus associated with it.[5] It is
important to remember that some communities completely escaped the
infection, whereas others in the same region were severely stricken.[6]
Recalculations of influenza mortality at national and continental scales
underscore how variable the impact of the 1918 outbreak actually was.
African nations, for example, show mortality estimates that range from
10.7 per 1,000 in Egypt to 445.0 per 1,000 in Cameroon. Estimates for
the Americas are much lower but also show substantial diversity, ranging
from 1.2 per 1,000 in Argentina to 39.2 per 1,000 in Guatemala. The estimated rates for Canada and the USA are about 6.0 per 1,000.[7] The biosocial
underpinnings of this substantial global diversity have barely been explored,
but at the very least, the evidence from mortality rates challenges the notion that the effect of the 1918 pandemic was indiscriminate.

The variability in impact is not limited to mortality rates. The epidemic
also took a disproportionate toll among young adults, males, pregnant
women, tubercular individuals, immigrant and economically disadvan-
taged neighbourhoods, and marginalized communities that lacked access
to health care.[8] Svenn-Erik Mamelund's rigorous analysis of influenza
mortality in the parishes of Kristiania, Norway (now Oslo), provides solid
evidence that death rates from the disease were worse in parishes characterized by low socioeconomic status.[9] Mamelund's findings prompted the
question that forms the basis for this chapter: Was the 1918 influenza
pandemic in Hamilton, Ontario, socially neutral?

HAMILTON

Before we turn to the features of the epidemic, a brief introduction to the
city of Hamilton is in order. It was founded in 1813 and named after a local
entrepreneur, George Hamilton.[10] Bordered on the north by Lake Ontario
and to the south by the Niagara Escarpment, Hamilton's strategic position
at the head of the lake, excellent port, and proximity to the railway and
US markets made it an ideal location for heavy industry. From 1900 to
1911, industrial employment grew by 100 percent, surpassing even the
growth of Toronto at the time.[11] During the two decades between 1901
and 1921, housing stock nearly tripled.[12] In the wake of industrial expansion

and a real estate boom, Hamilton had earned its reputation as "Steel City" by 1918, boasting, among other heavy industries, the headquarters of the Steel Company of Canada. It was an attractive destination for British and European immigrants seeking work.[13]

In the years between 1911 and 1913 alone, some fifteen thousand immigrants entered the city. Hamilton had been expanding its municipal boundaries to cope with the pressures of population growth and by 1910 was divided into eight wards.[14] The new immigrants settled in the mostly industrial working-class areas of Wards 5, 6, 7, and 8 in the low-lying northern part of the city, adjacent to the lake (see Figure 4.1). Close to the busy transportation corridor and Hamilton's factory heartland, and near the sewage outlet to Burlington Bay, these wards were densely populated. Wards 6 and 7, in fact, exceeded Boston's density ratio in 1900.[15] More prosperous members of Hamilton society lived in Wards 1 and 2 in the southern portion of the city, areas of low population density and higher property values. Their backdrop was the picturesque Niagara Escarpment, located at a distance from the mills, factories, transportation corridor, crowded living conditions, and sewage outlet to the north.[16] Hamilton's residential areas were segregated along social, economic, and ethnic lines, a municipal feature that persists today.[17] In view of the disparities in living conditions in the northern and southern portions of the city, should the 1918 influenza pandemic be expected to take an equal toll among its residents? Before turning to this question, let us first examine the main features of the outbreak in Hamilton.[18]

THE AUTUMN WAVE IN HAMILTON

The so-called 'Spanish influenza,' which had been so prevalent in the United States and Eastern Canada, has struck Hamilton, though in a mild form. Several hundred cases have developed within the past few days, but none of them are serious.

– "Hamilton Went to Bed as Killer Sickness
Swept the Land," *Hamilton Herald*

The arrival of the "Spanish flu" in Hamilton in late September 1918 was heralded by the eruption of a large number of cases at the Royal Air Force camp in Hamilton's west end. It is likely that the virus had spread there from the Niagara region, where it had been brought across the border by American recruits training at the Polish infantry camp at Niagara-on-the-Lake. This was one of the first two Canadian locations infected by influenza.[19] On 22 September, the first flu deaths among soldiers from Niagara were recorded in the registered deaths for Ontario.[20]

The subsequent outbreak at the Royal Air Force camp in Hamilton stretched the capacity of the military hospital and medical personnel to care for the sick soldiers and cadets. A strict quarantine was put into effect at the installation.[21] On 28 September, the *Hamilton Spectator* reported on the epidemic at the military camp, but in a manner similar to the reportage in the *Hamilton Herald,* its severity was downplayed and attributed to a mild weather-related flu.[22] The epidemic had spread nonetheless – and quickly – to the civilian population. Several days later, the first influenza death was registered for a resident of the city. Hatty Wirchowsky, a young married housewife of twenty-five years of age, who lived on King Street West, succumbed to the disease on 3 October. Two days later, Harry J. White, a twenty-nine-year-old married driver, born in England, passed away at the Military Hospital after suffering for four days with bronchial pneumonia following influenza.[23]

By then, the situation in Hamilton was understood to be serious and not simply a mild epidemic. With four deaths already attributed to the flu, Dr. James Roberts, Hamilton's medical health officer, was calling for complete closure of the city to contain its spread.[24] A special meeting of the board of health was convened to decide on a plan to be implemented in light of "the certainty of a heavy mortality."[25] Health department officials began a public education campaign conducted primarily through the local press.

The infection continued to spread, however, with sixty new cases reported by 9 October. Schools were particularly hard hit, with some 20 percent of the new cases occurring among children.[26] On 11 October, the *Hamilton Herald* reported that city hospitals were overcrowded and doctors too busy to make reports; by the next day, 518 cases had been added to the list of influenza sufferers.[27]

In an effort to contain the epidemic, the Hamilton Board of Health ordered that schools, theatres, and churches be closed from 20 October to 9 November. After an apparent lull in cases and the illusion that the worst was over, the epidemic resurged, prompting a more stringent ban on public gatherings from 29 November to 17 December.[28] Several temporary hospitals were created to assist with the swelling number of influenza sufferers. Two of the temporary hospitals, the Victoria Convalescent Home and the Jockey Club Hotel, treated 374 of the most serious cases.[29] Registered deaths for Hamilton from October through December indicate that 258 people died at permanent and temporary hospitals, indicative of the important role played by these institutions during the epidemic.[30] A local branch of the Ontario Emergency Volunteer Health Auxiliary coordinated some two hundred volunteer nurses, and church auxiliaries and members of the Imperial Order Daughters of the Empire provided home care, cleaning, cooking, and other vital services to the sick.[31] Cases in Hamilton peaked in late October and early November. On 29 November, after eight weeks of the epidemic, the board of health reported that 4,530 cases had been recorded, 359 of which were fatal.[32] The epidemic spluttered to an end in December of 1918. Although new cases were still being reported, and deaths continued to occur among civilians and soldiers until the end of the year, the board of health announced on 30 December that the epidemic was virtually over.[33]

The autumn wave of influenza was credited with infecting more than eight thousand Hamiltonians and killing more than five hundred of them.[34] The death rate, however, appears to have been lower than that for other cities across Canada and the United States, and congratulatory headlines to that effect appeared in the local press.[35] Hamilton's death rate of 11.9 per 1,000 is about half that of Vancouver's 23.3 per 1,000 but still exceeds the estimated national average of 6.0 per 1,000.[36] These disparities serve to further illustrate the importance of local variability in the experience of the 1918 pandemic.

THE VIEW FROM THE DEATH REGISTER

To explore the distribution of influenza deaths in Hamilton during the autumn wave, it was necessary to transcribe all 965 deaths from all causes registered for the city from October to December 1918. The death registers are held in microfilm format at the Archives of Ontario in Toronto and are available to the public.[37] Each registered death record contains the following information, with varying degrees of completeness: surname, given name, sex, date of death, place of birth, place of death, place of burial, occupation, father's name, mother's maiden name, physician who attended the deceased, informant's name, informant's address, date of return, disease causing death and its duration, immediate cause of death and its duration.[38]

It was necessary to develop a working definition of an influenza death so that the records of each individual who died from the disease could be identified. This process is not as straightforward as it might seem, for at the time of the pandemic, it was understood that influenza acted in concert with other infections, such as staphylococcus and streptococcus, and interacted with pre-existing conditions, such as pregnancy.[39] The virus did not act alone and, in fact, has been identified as a *syndemic* in which not only diseases and other conditions interacted and capacitated each other, but the interaction process itself was further exacerbated by underlying deleterious social conditions.[40] Another question that warrants scrutiny is the extent to which the diagnostic styles of particular physicians may have shaped the view of influenza as recorded in death registers.[41] Cause of death ascriptions, moreover, were affected by the fact that vestiges of humoralism are still present in death records for Hamilton during this time, where causes such as "failure of circulation," convulsions, apoplexy, teething, and senile decay can be found. Finally, research on the pandemic in New York City points to the importance of determining how much of its death toll actually constituted *excess* mortality, calling for longer-term studies that place the "Spanish flu" in deeper historical perspective.[42]

For our purposes here, a death was deemed to have been caused by influenza if either the "disease causing death" or the "immediate cause of death" category, both of which are part of the physician's return, mentioned any of the following, alone or in combination with any other cause of death: flu, influenza, la grippe, Spanish influenza, influenza pneumonia, bronchial pneumonia complicating flu, or bronchial pneumonia after flu. This definition yielded 418 cases of influenza deaths from the register. This approach to case definition is conservative, for it excludes individuals whose death records made no mention of influenza but who may actually have died from it, as, for example, in instances where a death was ascribed to pneumonia or other respiratory illness. Although the outcome of our decision may be an underestimate of influenza mortality, this is preferable to inflating the number of cases by including deaths unrelated to the epidemic or by excluding others, particularly tuberculosis, now emerging as having played a significant role during the pandemic.[43]

In this chapter, therefore, we investigate the contribution of deaths ascribed to influenza. Using this tightly circumscribed definition, we identified and extracted 418 flu deaths from the database of registered mortalities. As expected, this number falls short of the 635 Hamiltonians estimated to have died from influenza during the fall outbreak.[44] Of the 418 influenza death records discussed here, however, 370 also listed pneumonia, bronchitis, and several forms of cardiac illness along with the diagnosis of influenza. Future research aims to broaden the definition of an "influenza death" to include all cases of respiratory disease and to place the findings for 1918 within the context of mortality in Hamilton during the preceding five years.

The next step in our analysis involved locating an address for each of the 418 people identified as having died from influenza. This process was hampered by the fact that the death register does not provide the address of the decedent but, rather, the address of the informant. In many cases, however, the informant's address – if he or she were a parent, in the case of a child, or a spouse of the deceased – made it possible to locate a home address for the deceased. In other instances, it was necessary to search other nominative sources and then assign an address based on a successful link. The city of Hamilton directories proved invaluable for this purpose.[45] Addresses were then cross-checked and verified by consulting funeral records, parish burial registers, and the Hamilton Municipal Assessment Rolls for 1919-20. Through this process, we located addresses for 274 of the 418 influenza deaths (66 percent).

Next, the addresses were plotted on a contemporary GIS road map of Hamilton using ArcView 3.2 software.[46] Because ArcView does not provide exact street addresses, home locations were marked to within roughly one block of the true address location. Some streets that existed in 1918 have since disappeared as the city was redeveloped. In such cases, a map for Hamilton in 1913 was consulted.[47] The results are shown in Figure 4.1, in which each dot represents the location of a single influenza death. Interestingly, even though addresses could be located for only 66 percent of the influenza deaths, dots appear in every residential area of Hamilton, showing that deaths occurred throughout the city.[48]

Andrea Chan and Hagen Kluge plotted the spread of the epidemic through Hamilton, using addresses obtained from the registered deaths.[49] During the first two weeks of the outbreak (1 to 14 October), deaths clustered in the west end of the city, where the first cases emerged. From the second half of October through December, influenza deaths appear to have clustered in the east end of town, especially in Ward 8. The east end of Hamilton was colloquially known as the "foreign part of the city." The *Herald* reported on 29 November that nine out of ten cases were occurring

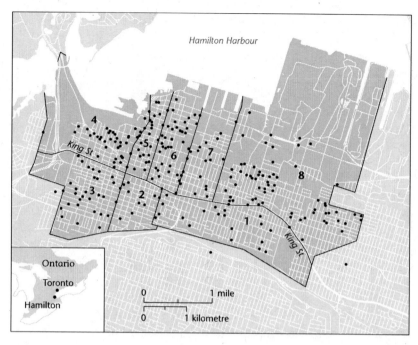

Figure 4.1 Plottable addresses and locations of death in the eight wards of Hamilton, 1 October to 31 December 1918, (n = 274). *Sources:* See footnotes 37, 45, 46, 47, and 52. Adapted by Eric Leinberger

in the east end and that "foreigners" were requesting assistance from the police.[50] Dr. Roberts responded that the disease was spread evenly in the city.[51] Although that may have been true for *cases* of the disease, evidence from the registered deaths suggests that influenza *mortality* was disproportionately focused among people living in the poorer parts of Hamilton.

The North-South Divide

The plotted deaths were used to estimate influenza mortality rates per 1,000 for each of the eight wards in Hamilton (see Figure 4.2).[52] Estimated mortality rates for the three more affluent wards in the south (Wards 1, 2, and 3) ranged from 1.8 to 2.1 per 1,000. The five northern wards (Wards 4, 5, 6, 7, and 8) yielded estimated mortality rates that ranged from 3.3 to 4.0 per 1,000, with the exception of Ward 7, which had the lowest mortality

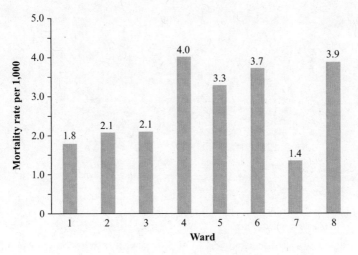

FIGURE 4.2   Estimated influenza mortality rates in Hamilton, by ward, based on plottable addresses(n=274). *Sources:* See footnotes 37, 45, 46, and 47

rate of all (1.4 per 1,000). This is probably an underestimate of Ward 7's true level of influenza mortality because the ward was one of the most impoverished in the city. Close to the port lands and filled with boarding houses, it was often the first place of residence for new immigrants to Hamilton.

When the deaths for the south and north wards are pooled and compared statistically using chi-square (X^2) and odds ratio (OR) analysis, the magnitude of the north-south divide along socioeconomic lines is even more striking (see Figure 4.3). The OR, otherwise known as the "cross-product ratio," is a key parameter in epidemiological analysis.[53] Estimating the OR for the southern and northern wards is not the same as simply comparing their influenza mortality rates; rather, the OR compares the *odds of an outcome occurring* (in this case, dying from influenza) to the odds of an outcome not occurring (not dying from influenza), for individuals exposed to a particular factor (living in the northern wards as opposed to the southern wards).[54]

The OR for influenza mortality for the pooled northern and southern wards is 1.76, with a 95 percent confidence interval (CI) ranging from 1.5 to 2.7.[55] In other words, people living in the northern wards had, on average, one and three-quarter higher odds of dying from influenza than those living in the south. We strongly suspect, however, that influenza mortality

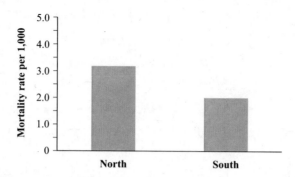

FIGURE 4.3   Estimated influenza mortality rates in Hamilton, south versus north wards (n = 274). *Sources:* See footnotes 37, 45, 46, 47, and 52

was considerably underreported in Ward 7, which would have the effect of *reducing* the magnitude of the gap in mortality between northern and southern wards. For this reason, we removed the Ward 7 data and conducted a second chi-square analysis. As expected, the OR from this analysis was larger at 2.03, with an accompanying 95 percent CI of 1.3 to 2.4.[56] The confidence intervals of both chi-square analyses do not cross 1 (unity) and are therefore statistically significant. Taken together, these analyses suggest that someone living in Hamilton's northern wards had 1.75 to 2.0 times higher odds of dying from influenza than someone living in the more affluent southern wards.

That said, we should recall that it was possible to plot only 66 percent of the flu deaths; consequently, the plottable deaths, those with addresses, underrepresent mortality during the autumn wave. Who, then, is missing? Scrutiny of the registered deaths for Hamilton shows that slightly over one-quarter of those who died during the autumn outbreak did so in hospitals or other institutions. As mentioned above, the Victoria Convalescent Home and the Jockey Club Hotel, for instance, were both temporary hospitals that treated over three hundred of the most serious cases.[57] It was impossible to locate home addresses for many of the people who died in hospital, which precluded assigning their deaths to a specific ward. The ability to find and plot addresses became increasingly difficult as the epidemic progressed from October through December. This reflects, in large measure, the increasing likelihood that sick individuals would die in hospitals during the later weeks of the epidemic when the death toll was higher.[58] Impoverished individuals, or those with a relatively small support group, would also be more likely to have been sent to hospitals for treatment. Typically, middle-class and wealthy people of this era were treated at home, cared for by family physicians, relatives, and servants.[59] More affluent individuals who had the means and necessary connections to be treated at home would also be more likely to have a traceable home address, including a listing in the Hamilton directory. Because of this, the inequality in the odds of dying from influenza, represented by the disparity in mortality between Hamilton's north and south wards, is probably even greater than this study would suggest.

CONCLUSION

This analysis of mappable influenza deaths during the autumn outbreak of the "Spanish flu" in Hamilton indicates that some parts of the city experienced higher mortality rates than others. People living in lower socioeconomic areas, specifically the industrial, working-class, northern wards of Hamilton, were at higher risk of dying from influenza than those who lived in the more affluent southern wards. The findings support Mamelund's argument that mortality from the 1918 pandemic was influenced by social inequality and suggest that the pandemic was not socially neutral in Hamilton; instead, it laid bare the social fault lines that divided the city. In 2004, Howard Phillips observed that insufficient attention has been paid to examining connections between the pandemic and social conditions during the First World War.[60] The story of Hamilton's experience is one small step toward answering Phillips's challenge to develop more social histories and toward addressing Mamelund's important question about the role played by social inequality in the expression of the pandemic.[61]

This is not just a historical problem; it has implications for contemporary public health policy. The 1918 flu is the model against which twenty-first-century pandemics are measured; it is the "mother of all pandemics."[62] Fears about an impending epidemic of H5N1 avian influenza have been anchored to the 1918 outbreak, which has become a key element in popular and scientific narratives about "the next pandemic."[63] In view of recent experience and ongoing concerns about another pandemic of H1N1 (otherwise known as "swine flu"), it is important to explore the complexities of the 1918 experience – a notable contribution of this volume – and to probe the links between clusters of diseases, death, and underlying social inequalities.

ACKNOWLEDGMENTS

We wish to thank the wonderful students in Anthropology 4BB3, Anatomy of a Pandemic, whose research is fundamental to this essay. We are particularly grateful to Andrea Chan and Hagen Kluge for their work on the death registers and initial GIS maps. We also thank Tracy Farmer for her advice and suggestions as this research proceeded. The GIS analysis could not have been completed without the assistance of Cathy Moulder and Lloyd Beck, librarians at the Lloyd Reed Maps Collection, at McMaster's Mills Library. This research was supported by a McMaster University Faculty of Social Sciences Undergraduate Summer Research Award (Korol) and a McMaster University Faculty of Social Sciences Academic Innovation Award (Herring).

NOTES

1   D. Ann Herring, "Viral Panic, Vulnerability and the Next Pandemic," in *Health, Risk and Adversity,* ed. Catherine Panter-Brick and Agustin Fuentes (Oxford: Berghahn Press, 2009), 78-97; Stacy Lockerbie and D. Ann Herring. "Global Panic, Local Repercussions: Economic and Nutritional Effects of Bird Flu in Vietnam," in *Anthropology and Public Health: Bridging Differences in Culture and Society,* 2nd ed., ed. R.A. Hahn and M.C. Inhorn (Oxford: Oxford University Press, 2009), 566-87; and D. Ann Herring and Alan C. Swedlund, eds., *Plagues and Epidemics: Infected Spaces Past and Present* (Oxford: Berg Press, 2010).

2   For the flu and social neutrality, see Svenn-Erik Mamelund, "A Socially Neutral Disease? Individual Social Class, Household Wealth and Mortality from Spanish Influenza in Two Socially Contrasting Parishes in Kristiania 1918-19," *Social Science and Medicine* 62 (2006): 923-40. For mortality rates, see Janice P. Dickin McGinnis, "The Impact of Epidemic Influenza: Canada, 1918-19," in *Medicine in Canadian Society: Historical Perspectives,* ed. E.D. Shortt (Montreal and Kingston: McGill-Queen's University Press, 1981), 447-77; and N.P.A.S. Johnson and J. Mueller, "Updating the Accounts: Global Mortality of the 1918-1920 'Spanish' Influenza Pandemic," *Bulletin of the History of Medicine* 76 (2002): 105-15.

3   See Tracy Farmer, "Putting Health in Its Place: Women's Perceptions and Experiences of Health in Hamilton's North End" (PhD thesis, Department of Anthropology, McMaster University, 2004).

4   Paul Farmer, *Infections and Inequalities: The Modern Plagues,* rev. ed. (Berkeley: University of California Press, 1999).

5   Herring, "Viral Panic, Vulnerability and the Next Pandemic."

6   D. Ann Herring, "'There Were Young People and Old People and Babies Dying Every Week': The 1918-1919 Influenza Pandemic at Norway House," *Ethnohistory* 41,1 (1994): 73-105; D. Ann Herring and L. Sattenspiel, "Death in Winter: Spanish Flu in the Canadian Subarctic," in *The Spanish Influenza Pandemic of 1918-19: New Perspectives,* ed. Howard Phillips and David Killingray (London: Routledge, 2003), 156-72; and D. Ann Herring and L. Sattenspiel, "Social Contexts, Syndemics, and Infectious Disease in Northern Aboriginal Populations," *American Journal of Human Biology* 19,2 (2007): 190-202.

7   Johnson and Mueller, "Updating the Accounts."

8   Johnson and Mueller, "Updating the Accounts"; Esyllt W. Jones, "'Cooperation in all human endeavour': Quarantine and Immigrant Disease Vectors in the 1918-1919 Influenza Pandemic in Winnipeg," *Canadian Bulletin of Medical History* 22,1 (2005): 57-82; and

Maureen Lux, "'The Bitter Flats': The 1918 Influenza Epidemic in Saskatchewan," *Saskatchewan History* 49,1 (Spring 1997): 3-13; Mamelund, "A Socially Neutral Disease?"; and A. Noymer, "Testing the Influenza-Tuberculosis Selective Mortality Hypothesis with Union Army Data," PAA Extended Abstract, 23 September 2995, http://paa2006.princeton.edu/; A. Noymer and M. Garenne, "Long-Term Effects of the 1918 'Spanish' Influenza Epidemic on Sex Differentials of Mortality in the USA," in Phillips and Killingray, *The Spanish Influenza Pandemic,* 202-17; A. Noymer and M. Garenne, "The 1918 Influenza Epidemic's Effects on Sex Differentials in Mortality in the United States," *Population and Development Review* 26,3 (2000): 565-81; and J.K. Taubenberger and D.M. Morens, "1918 Influenza: The Mother of All Pandemics," *Emerging Infectious Diseases* 12,1 (2006): 15-22.

9   Mamelund, "A Socially Neutral Disease?"
10 R. Louis Gentilcore, "The Beginnings: Hamilton in the Nineteenth Century," in *Steel City: Hamilton and Region,* ed. M.J. Dear, J.J. Drake, and L.G. Reeds (Toronto: University of Toronto Press, 1987), 99-118.
11 Farmer, "Putting Health in Its Place," 77.
12 John C. Weaver and National Museum of Man, *Hamilton: An Illustrated History,* History of Canadian Cities (Toronto: J. Lorimer and National Museum of Man, National Museums of Canada, 1982), 99.
13 From 1891 to 1911, Continental Europeans increased from 6 to 15 percent of Hamilton's population. Harold A. Wood, "Emergence of the Modern City: Hamilton 1891-1950," in Dear, Drake, and Reeds, *Steel City,* 119-37.
14 Weaver and National Museum of Man, *Hamilton: An Illustrated History,* 103.
15 Rosemary Gagan, "Disease, Mortality, and Public Health, Hamilton, Ontario, 1900-1914," *Urban History Review* 17,3 (1989): 161-75.
16 Ibid.
17 Michael J. Doucet and John C. Weaver, "Town Fathers and Urban Community: The Roots of Community Power and Physical Form in Hamilton, Upper Canada, in the 1830s," *Urban History Review* 13,2 (1984): 75-90; Wood, "Emergence of the Modern City"; Gentilcore, "The Beginnings: Hamilton in the Nineteenth Century"; and Farmer, "Putting Health in Its Place."
18 For a detailed analysis of many facets of the Hamilton outbreak, see D. Ann Herring, ed., *Anatomy of a Pandemic: The 1918 Influenza in Hamilton* (Hamilton: Allegra Press, 2006), an edited volume of essays written by McMaster University students. Their research forms the foundation for this chapter.
19 Mark Osborne Humphries, "The Horror at Home: The Canadian Military and the 'Great' Influenza Pandemic of 1918," *Journal of the Canadian Historical Association,* n.s., 16,1 (2005): 235-60.
20 Government of Ontario, Lincoln County death registrations, town of Niagara death registrations, 1918-1919, n.pag., Archives of Ontario, M-film MS 935, reel 244, Toronto.
21 Hamilton Board of Health, *Report, 1917-1918,* 4, Special Collections, Hamilton Public Library, Central Library, Ms. 1918, Hamilton.
22 "Influenza Is Reported in West Hamilton," *Hamilton Spectator,* 28 September 1918, 1; and "Spanish 'Flu' Has Made Appearance Here," *Hamilton Herald,* 30 September 1918, 1.
23 Government of Ontario, Wentworth County death registrations, Hamilton death registrations, 1918-1919, n.pag., Archives of Ontario, M-film MS 935, reel 250.
24 "Four Deaths from 'Flu' Reported Here," *Hamilton Herald,* 5 October 1918, 1, 17.

25 Hamilton Board of Health, *Report, 1918-1919,* 4, Special Collections, Hamilton Public Library, Ms. 1918.

26 "'Flu' Epidemic Shows No Sign of Abatement," *Hamilton Herald,* 9 October 1918, 1, 4.

27 "Fifty New Cases," *Hamilton Herald,* 11 October 1918, 1, 4; and "Over 500 Cases of 'Flu,'" *Hamilton Herald,* 12 October 1918, 1.

28 Adam Benn, "Steel City Shutdown: The 1918 Quarantine in Hamilton," in Herring, *Anatomy of a Pandemic,* 120-33.

29 Hamilton Board of Health, *Report, 1918-1919,* 4.

30 Anna Lisowska, "Healing and Treatment: Who Answered the Call of the Sick?" in Herring, *Anatomy of a Pandemic,* 97.

31 Mara Pope, "The Essence of Altruism: The Spirit of Volunteerism in Hamilton during the 1918 Influenza Pandemic," in Herring, *Anatomy of a Pandemic,* 105-19.

32 Brian Henley, "1918 Flu Took More than 500 Lives," [Our Heritage] Scrapbooks, vol. 8, 1996, 77, compiled by Special Collections, Local History and Archives Collection, Hamilton Public Library, Central Library, 917.1351 OUR, Hamilton, Ontario.

33 Government of Ontario, Hamilton death registrations, 1918-1919.

34 Hamilton Board of Health, *Minutes, 1918-1919,* 20, Special Collections, Hamilton Public Library, Central Library, Ms. 1919.

35 Henley, "1918 Flu Took More than 500 Lives," 77; and "Death Rate in Hamilton under Average," *Hamilton Herald,* 20 December 1918, 4.

36 John Rankin, "The Influenza Pandemic of 1918-1921 in Hamilton" (manuscript, n.d.), 32; and Johnson and Mueller, "Updating the Accounts."

37 Government of Ontario, Hamilton death registrations, 1918-1919.

38 During the winter of 2005-06, Andrea Chan and Hagen Kluge transcribed the registered deaths, created the initial Excel database modified for this study, and located many of the addresses for Hamiltonians who died from influenza. Andrea H.W. Chan and Hagen F. Kluge, "The Epidemic Spreads through the City," in Herring, *Anatomy of a Pandemic,* 41-56.

39 "The Need for Conscription of Canadian Doctors," *Canadian Medical Association Journal* 8,10 (October 1918): 933-35; W.H. Frost, "The Epidemiology of Influenza," *Public Health Reports* 34,33 (1919): 1823-35; and R. Pearl, "Influenza Studies. 1. On Certain General Statistical Aspects of the 1918 Epidemic in American Cities," *Public Health Reports* 34,32 (1919): 1743-83.

40 The syndemics approach emphasizes the biosocial nature of health and recognizes that diseases and other health conditions interact synergistically through multiple biological and psychosocial channels and mechanisms. In particular, the syndemics framework calls for investigation of the ways in which deleterious social conditions shape disease processes and channel multiple conditions into particular social groups. The syndemics approach therefore examines both the emergence and nature of disease clusters (multiple diseases and disorders affecting individuals and groups) and disease interactions (the ways in which the presence of one disease or disorder enhances the health consequences of other diseases and disorders). M. Singer and S. Clair, "Syndemics and Public Health: Reconceptualizing Disease in Bio-Social Context," *Medical Anthropology Quarterly* 17,4 (2003): 423-41; and M. Singer, *Introduction to Syndemics: A Systems Approach to Public and Community Health* (San Francisco: Jossey-Bass, 2009).

41 Janjua notes, for instance, that during the Great Depression in Hamilton, some physicians had a disproportionate impact on how causes of deaths were characterized: 13 of the 215

doctors listed in the death register were responsible for registering almost half the death certificates for infants and stillbirths. M.A. Janjua, "Infant Mortality during the Great Depression in Hamilton, Ontario (1925-1935): Trends, Causes and Implications" (Master's thesis, Department of Anthropology, McMaster University, 2009), 37.

42 D.R. Olson et al., "Epidemiological Evidence of an Early Wave of the 1918 Influenza Pandemic in New York City," *Proceedings of the National Academy of Sciences of the United States of America* 102,31 (2005): 11059-63.

43 The extent to which tuberculosis was a significant contributor to influenza mortality during the 1918 pandemic has only recently been revealed. The natural histories of the two diseases were intimately entwined. See Noymer, "Testing the Influenza-Tuberculosis Selective Mortality Hypothesis"; Noymer and Garenne, "Long-Term Effects of the 1918 'Spanish' Influenza"; and Noymer and Garenne, "The 1918 Influenza Epidemic's Effects."

44 Hamilton Board of Health, *Minutes, 1907-1922,* 20, Special Collections, Hamilton Public Library, Central Library, Ms. 1919.

45 *Hamilton City Directory,* 1918, 15, Lloyd Reed Map Collection, Mills Memorial Library, McMaster University, M-Film FC3098.2.V47 (1916-1918), Hamilton, Ontario; *Hamilton City Directory,* 1918, 16, Lloyd Reed Map Collection, Mills Memorial Library, McMaster University, M-Film FC3098.2.V47 (1918-1920), Hamilton, Ontario.

46 Environmental Systems Research Institute, *Getting to Know ArcView GIS: The Geographic Information System (GIS) for Everyone,* 3rd ed. (Redlands, CA: Environmental Systems Research Institute, 1999).

47 J.B. Nicholson, *Map of Greater Hamilton Canada Comprising the Township of Barton – All Present Subdivisions and Proposed Layouts by the City Corporation and Parts of the Townships of Saltfleet – Binbrook – Glanford – Ancaster – West Flamboro – East Flamboro* (Hamilton: Ramsay-Thomas, 1913).

48 The white, apparently empty area in the northwest corner of the map (upper left) is Cootes Paradise, an uncultivated marshland that was uninhabited in 1918. Today, the northeast corner of Hamilton (upper right) is dominated by steel manufacturers and is not a residential zone. Much of the white area, shown empty of dots, is reclaimed land that did not exist in 1918.

49 Chan and Kluge, "The Epidemic Spreads through the City."

50 "Foreigners Ill," *Hamilton Herald,* 29 November 1918, 4.

51 "Fewer Deaths and Fewer Cases of Influenza," *Hamilton Herald,* 5 December 1918, 1.

52 Population sizes for the wards were obtained for 1915 from the Hamilton Population Scrapbook, compiled by Special Collections, Local History and Archives Collection, Hamilton Public Library, Central Library, 304.60971352 HAM, Hamilton, Ontario.

53 H.T. Reynolds, *The Analysis of Cross-Classifications* (London: Collier Macmillan, 1977); and J.J. Schlesselman, *Case-Control Studies* (New York: Oxford University Press, 1982).

54 The interpretation of odds ratio values is relatively straightforward: if the odds are equal in both categories (exposed and unexposed), their ratio will equal 1.0, indicating no relationship. Departures in either direction suggest association; the greater the deviation from 1.0, the stronger the relationship.

55 Uncorrected X^2 = 15.63, p<0.001, df = 2. OR = 1.76, 95 percent CI (1.51<OR<2.73).

56 Uncorrected X^2 = 24.32, p<0.001, dr = 2. OR = 2.03, 95 percent CI (1.31<OR<2.36).

57 Hamilton Board of Health, *Report, 1918-1919,* 4.

58 Chan and Kluge, "The Epidemic Spreads through the City," 46; and Cheryl Venus and Kiran Persaud, "Hamilton's Epidemic Wave," in Herring, *Anatomy of a Pandemic,* 36-37.

59 Edward Arthur Warwick Smith and Ambrose McGhie Medical Museum, *Hamilton's Doctors 1932-1982* (Hamilton: Ambrose McGhie Medical Museum, 2004), 24; and David Paul Gagan and Rosemary R. Gagan, *For Patients of Moderate Means: A Social History of the Voluntary Public General Hospital in Canada, 1890-1950* (Montreal and Kingston: McGill-Queen's University Press, 2002), 13.
60 Howard Phillips, "The Re-Appearing Shadow of 1918: Trends in the Historiography of the 1918-19 Influenza Pandemic," *Canadian Bulletin of Medical History* 21,1 (2004): 130-31.
61 Mamelund, "A Socially Neutral Disease?"
62 Taubenberger and Morens, "1918 Influenza: The Mother of All Pandemics."
63 Herring, "Viral Panic, Vulnerability and the Next Pandemic"; Lockerbie and Herring, "Global Panic, Local Repercussions"; and Herring and Swedlund, *Plagues and Epidemics.*

5

Beyond Biology: Understanding the Social Impact of Infectious Disease in Two Aboriginal Communities

KAREN SLONIM

In 2003, a novel virus named SARS emerged and changed the way people thought about airborne person-to-person transmitted disease. In its wake, it transformed the great influenza pandemic of 1918-20 from "forgotten" to feared, as public and academic interest in the subject was revitalized by a renewed concern with infectious disease and what Nancy Tomes has termed an emergence into an age of viral panic.[1] Alongside an interest in sequencing the virus, another, equally fruitful, endeavour has taken form.[2] This is the task of understanding the political, social, and environmental components that helped to shape the spread and impact of the disease. By combining these elements within the framework of a syndemics approach, this chapter will show that it is sometimes necessary to go beyond the biological components of a devastating epidemic to fully understand its complexities. Using family reconstitution (concatenate information from baptismal, marriage, and burial records to re-create genealogies), this essay will draw out the face of influenza in Norway House and Fisher River, two Aboriginal communities in the Lake Winnipeg region of Manitoba. Exploring the experiences of their inhabitants affords us a unique opportunity to view how a structurally similar virus interacted with two essentially homogeneous populations to produce two rather different outcomes. A syndemics approach emphasizes that diseases co-exist in a host and are integrated into a given social, political, and geographic environment. An examination of these two communities demonstrates how timing, social organization, environmental degradation, and access to informal networks of care can shape the course of an epidemic. Further-more, this chapter will demonstrate that the morbidity and mortality patterns witnessed during the flu pandemic were not simply a byproduct of pathogen virulence but rather were equally shaped by the social environ-ment within which virus and host interacted.[3]

HISTORICAL OVERVIEW OF THE WESTERN WOODS CREE

The communities explored in this study belong primarily to the Swampy Cree, also referred to as Western Woods Cree or Muskegon.[4] Historically, the Cree inhabited the entirety of the boreal forests west of Hudson and James Bays, including portions of Ontario, Manitoba, Saskatchewan, and Alberta. Their subarctic environment is difficult to farm, making hunting and gathering the most reliable mode of attaining sustenance.

The Hudson's Bay Company (HBC), founded in 1670, played a major role in restructuring the social organization and subsistence strategies of the Cree.[5] The year 1682 marked the foundation of York Factory, and the history of Manitoba as an HBC territory was set in motion. According to Arthur Ray (1978), after an initial period of adjustment, the Native people were said to have willingly taken on the specialized roles of provisioners, traders, and trappers.[6] Their position was further enhanced when the French began to expand their St. Lawrence–based fur-trading operation in the 1680s.

In 1713, the Treaty of Utrecht ended the rivalry between the French and the English over control of Hudson Bay, leaving the region, then called Rupert's Land, under the authority of the HBC. This, however, did not end fur trade competition; rather, it provoked the French to more vigor-ously pursue the creation of inland posts in the hope of cutting off the HBC from its hinterland.[7] Although this strategy proved economically successful for the French, the aggressive competition had a devastating ecological impact. Between 1793 and 1830, big game steadily declined, forcing many Cree to become fishermen and small-game hunters.[8]

As the ecological effects began to depress indigenous populations, pol-itical and economic consequences also occurred. The rivalry between the French North West Company and the English HBC, which in many ways had contributed to indigenous autonomy, ceased in 1821 when the two companies amalgamated and a monopoly was created.[9] Competing and unprofitable posts were shut down, causing indigenous groups engaged in the fur trade to become localized and oriented around a specific post.[10]

The HBC also began to marginalize Native trappers "by reducing the buying price of furs and increasing the selling price of trading goods."[11] This strategy succeeded because European trade goods, such as kettles, knives, guns, blankets, and twine, were now necessities, and Aboriginals had become so specialized in trapping and trading that they were obliged to meet their subsistence needs by purchasing supplies from the HBC.[12] The company's implementation of a debt system, in which it issued equipment to trappers during the fall with the expectation that they would repay their debt with furs in the spring, resulted in a state of "company welfarism."[13]

The once autonomous "Indian" was now an unwitting servant of the HBC system. By the 1870s, the Cree way of life was a shadow of what it had once been. Fur yields were no longer abundant after decades of protracted decline, causing Natives to return to the post during winter to beg for provisions, further entrenching them in a cycle of debt with the HBC.[14] Also in the mid- to late nineteenth century, missionary activity began in earnest.[15] Because of its prominent position, Norway House became the district headquarters for the British Wesleyan Methodist Missionary Society, whose aim was to Christianize the northwest Aboriginals.[16] These efforts were so intensified that, nominally at least, the once diverse Cree population was largely Christian by the twentieth century.[17]

The Hudson's Bay Company had served as both the de facto government of Rupert's Land and its chief commercial enterprise until it ceded control over the area to Canada in 1870.[18] This period was marked by the establishment of a number of treaties, with Treaty 5 being of particular importance as it stipulated the creation of Fisher River and introduced treaty annuity payments. A treaty annuity payment of five dollars was given to each registered Indian annually, and in conjunction with this practice, treaty annuity pay lists were compiled by Government of Canada treaty party officials who visited each reserve during the summer.[19] These disbursements further altered indigenous subsistence. They also provided a means by which the government could track populations.

NORWAY HOUSE AND FISHER RIVER PRIOR TO THE INFLUENZA EPIDEMIC

The HBC post at Norway House was established in 1801.[20] Its strategic position at the northern end of Lake Winnipeg and the southern end of the Nelson River trade axis linking the west, northwest, northeast, and south would make it an important district headquarters in subsequent decades, second only to York Factory.[21] Goods that had been shipped from England to York Factory the previous summer were repackaged in the winter and sent to Norway House, where they were stored over the winter, ensuring the availability of supplies during the difficult season; in the spring, they were forwarded to Methye Portage for further distribution.[22] The Norway House post rose to prominence during the nineteenth century, so that by 1820 it had "become the nexus of HBC provisioning activities in the region."[23] However, it was not immune to social upheaval or environmental depletion, and by 1918, as was the case for surrounding communities, its halcyon days were long past.

The annual cycle at Norway House remained similar to post-contact patterns elsewhere in the subarctic, with summer concentration and winter dispersal into traplines in the form of small hunting groups or local bands serving as the primary social unit.[24] However, as James Waldram, Ann Herring, and T. Kue Young note, Norway House was basically trapped out by the mid-nineteenth century, causing some trappers to journey as far as three hundred miles in their hunt for fur-bearing animals.[25]

Fisher River was founded in 1876 when ninety Swampy Cree families moved south from Norway House to escape the hardships that were plaguing them. By 1893, the Hudson's Bay Company had closed its post at Fisher River, and these former traders and trappers shifted to wage labour, working at lumber camps, fisheries, sawmills, and on steamboats.[26] Reports to the Department of Indian Affairs claim that the community was faring well as an agricultural centre. A report for the year ended 30 June 1906 reads, "At Fisher River, the most desirable reserve in the agency, about 300 head of cattle are kept, as well as a number of horses."[27] This contrasts with the few cattle housed on most other reserves. In 1913, the local Indian agent stated, "Many of the homes in the Peguis and Fisher River reserves are a credit to the occupants."[28] Tina Moffat and Ann Herring indicate, however, that although agriculture was practised to some extent, lumberyard work was far more lucrative.[29]

The annual cycle at Fisher River differed from that of communities engaged in the fur trade. As opposed to heavy dependence on trapping and trade networks with the HBC, the Fisher River subsistence strategy relied on a mixed economy with a strong emphasis on wage labour.[30] Tina Moffat also stresses the importance of lumbering and fishing to Fisher River.[31] The primary social consequence of these different modes of subsistence is that Norway House was much more mobile, with trappers travelling long distances in search of game. A report from 1910 records "some very fine timber" in the vicinity of Fisher River, and it can therefore be assumed that the community was much more sedentary.[32]

MANITOBA ENCOUNTERS THE 1918 FLU

It is believed that influenza entered Manitoba on 30 September 1918 when it arrived in Winnipeg via a troop train. By 3 October, two soldiers had fallen ill from the disease, and the province recorded its first civilian death.[33] The virus travelled from Winnipeg to Berens River at the end of October via the passenger steamship *Wolverine*.[34] Figure 5.1 depicts the first influenza death in several Manitoba communities.[35] The death dates indicate that the virus moved from south to north through the province. Ann Herring suggests that it was spread throughout Manitoba along train lines, roads, and water routes.[36]

The first mention of influenza in the Norway House region comes from the Norway House post journal, which was kept by HBC factor William Campbell: its 3 December 1918 entry reads, "'Spanish Flu' was also reported at an Indian camp at Clearwater Lake, some two or three days north of Cross Lake."[37] The next entry confirms the outbreak at Clearwater Lake and mentions seventeen deaths. Between 9 and 15 December, the illness is recorded as spreading through Norway House. The first reported case is the chore boy, Alex Roberts (on the ninth), followed by Mrs. Kirkness (on the thirteenth) and Mary Roberts (on the fifteenth). Neither the post journal nor the Anglican mission parish records indicate that these individuals succumbed to the virus. On 18 December, the HBC post journal reads "Roderick Roberts's wife died today, this being the first death from the 'Flu' here."[38]

The wealth of information for Norway House is not available for Fisher River. This is in large part due to the fact that its HBC post had closed in 1893; therefore, it had no company factor, who would report daily activities in a post journal. Fisher River was also a relatively new community comprised primarily of agriculturalists and loggers, and has not elicited much attention from researchers of the fur trade period. Much of the information available for the community comes from the Fisher River Oral History Project undertaken in 1991 and the well-maintained records and memoirs of Reverend Frederick G. Stevens and his wife Frances E.E. Stevens.[39]

The first influenza death at Fisher River is recorded in the Methodist Church parish records as having occurred on 30 October 1918, about a

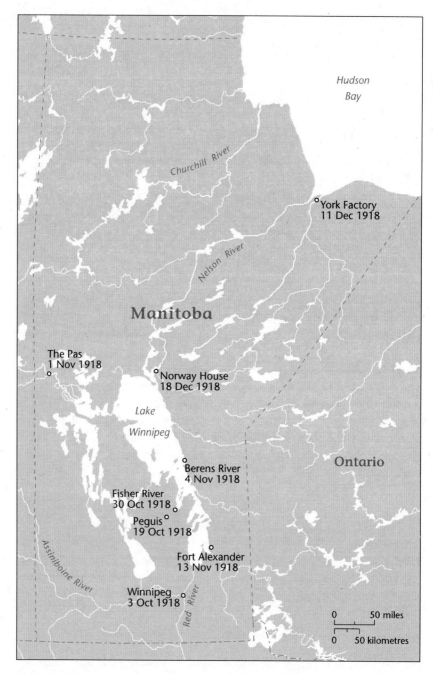

FIGURE 5.1   Date of first flu death in Manitoba communities. Adapted by Eric Leinberger

month before the disease appeared at Norway House or Berens River and Clearwater Lake.[40] It is possible, however, that the flu struck from Berens River, which lay to the north and on the opposite shore of Lake Winnipeg, where it was first reported around the end of October when the *Wolverine* brought more than supplies to the unsuspecting community. There is also a possible connection between the Fisher River outbreak and The Pas, with both locations having experienced their first deaths within a day of one another. We know from the Methodist burial record that the first Fisher River death occurred on 30 October, so the flu must have arrived by 28 October at the latest, taking into account the two-day incubation period.

GAUGING THE IMPACT

There is no statistically significant difference between the overall mortality rates of Anglicans at Norway House (183 deaths per 1,000) and those of Fisher River Methodists (134 deaths per 1,000), both of which numbered 38.[41] However, analysis of historical documents from the region reveals that the pandemic's impact was greater at Norway House than at Fisher River. We can also state with absolute certainty that both communities were disproportionately devastated by the disease: the estimated average for Canadian Aboriginals during the pandemic was 37.7 deaths per 1,000, compared to 6.1 deaths per 1,000 for Canada as a whole.[42]

Newspapers in The Pas gave detailed accounts of the disarray rampant at Cross Lake, Norway House, Pelican Narrows, Beaver Lake, Herb Lake, Lac la Ronge, and Stanley, yet they did not mention the virus plaguing Fisher River. A 7 February 1919 article titled "Heavy Toll of Deaths among Northern Indians" reads,

> Influenza is taking away large numbers of Indians in the outlying tribes. The figures show that there have been 316 carried away in the past month, viz.: Cross Lake 135; Norway House 107; Red Earth 23; Pelican Narrows 30; Cumberland 13; Beaver Lake 8. The disease is raging at Pelican Narrows. In one house there were 20 lying on the floor helplessly sick, with four dead bodies lying in amongst them. The reports coming in say that the conditions at the Narrows are horrible, and every family is down with the flu and helpless. It is thought that, unless relief is given immediately, the entire Indian tribe at Pelican will be wiped out.[43]

With regard to the deaths at Norway House, the paper added that "a letter from Mr. R. Talbot, manager H.B. co. post, Norway House, dated Jan 22nd, states that the Spanish Flu broke out three weeks previously, and at the date of writing there were 107 deaths, representing 12 percent of the population."[44]

The impact of the epidemic, however, is not gauged solely on the basis of newspaper articles; other first-hand accounts and reports made to Indian Affairs have helped establish the difference between Fisher River and Norway House. The Norway House post journal is a daily log of events in the community and therefore contributes valuable insights into its situation. The following excerpts demonstrate the devastating consequences of the outbreak at both the individual and community level:

> Thurs Dec 19 1918
> Adam Dickson, who was to go off with the second mail today, unable to go, having contracted the "Flu" during the night. Tried to get another man in his place, but this was impossible, as every man here that has dogs is unwell.

> Mon Jan 6 1919
> Sent team off again today with wood to Indians on Jack River. Garson around today for first time since taken ill, but not able to do anything. Mrs. Arthurson died during the night. The total deaths at Norway House now amount to 50. Mr. Mercer, who arrived from Cross Lake reports 58 deaths amongst the Indians there.[45]

Because Fisher River was not an HBC post, it had no equivalent daily log. There are, however, two manuscripts from which information can be drawn: written by the Reverend Frederick Stevens and his wife, Frances, they provide a clear indication of how the community was affected by influenza.[46] Stevens spent thirty-three years presiding over the Fisher River Methodist church and demonstrated his dedication through speaking Cree.[47] His devotion was further "corroborated by local Cree resident, Flora Kirkness, who described how Stevens used to make visits around the community, and always visited those who were sick."[48]

His memoir refers to the flu just once: "Soon after our departure from Deer Lake a man was taken sick and could not be cured. All the time some of the older men were just over the border between paganism and Christianity. Other means failing them, they brought out their drums.

The man died. Then they were very much afraid of what they had done. That was the year of the 'flu' and, although they were isolated and none of them took it, they were excited all winter. More or less conjuring went on all the next spring."[49]

Frances Stevens's memoir shows that her husband was at Fisher River at the time of the epidemic, yet he made no mention of its impact there. Her account, which details her everyday life as a minister's wife, demonstrates her interest in documenting and understanding disease patterns. She spoke of her fear that the community might contract diphtheria from her daughter, also named Frances, in 1913. She realized that her daughter had the disease when she noticed that "her throat was covered with a grey film."[50] During the smallpox epidemic of 1915, she comprehensively recorded every aspect of the community's isolation and illness. She wrote, "What was called Smallpox spread like wild fire through out the Reserve and out on the Lake. There were no fatalities nor no marks left and we wondered what it really was. For six weeks, mounties and a couple of visiting doctors and their drivers had to be housed at the Mission. For two weeks the entire family slept in one room in order to accommodate the party. The Indians objected loudly to the Quarantine though they had rationed sufficient food for the duration of the epidemic."[51]

Her accounts of the influenza pandemic, however, seem to lack the vivid detail of the community experience and the conscientious concern displayed during the smallpox outbreak:

The summer had quickly passed and we found ourselves facing the 'Spanish Flu.' As elsewhere, it was a terrible experience. The work in the dispensary never ended while my husband was the first to get it, he kept going. When a doctor arrived in due time, he ordered him to confine his work to dispensary and burying the dead. It was a miracle that he could accomplish that. One day he buried seven, two in one grave. At Berens River thirteen bodies lay in the mission store-house because there was not a sufficient number of men able to dig resting places.[52]

Although this passage does indicate that Fisher River was disrupted by the virus, we can infer from it that the community was nonetheless able to cope. Indeed, rather than focusing on the flu as it affected Fisher River, Frances discussed its deadly results in neighbouring communities, which also suggests that the impact in Fisher River was more moderate than in other communities of the region.

Lastly, the local Indian agent mentioned the epidemic in his 1919 report, which covered both Fisher River and Norway House as the two communities were part of the same district:

> The Indians of Manitoba in common with other sections of the population suffered very severely from the epidemic of influenza, and the mortality among them as a result of this cause was high. The department's medical officers and the agency staff spared no effort in their efficient and energetic efforts to prevent the spread of the disease. Unfortunately it was impossible to secure adequate medical attention for the Indians living in the more outlying parts, a circumstance which is not remarkable in view of the fact that a similar situation existed in the majority of the white communities throughout the Dominion.[53]

The differing experiences of the two communities are best demonstrated in Table 5.1. The expenditures at Norway House speak of a community that is geographically vast and in need of aid. This is represented in both the cost of travel ($656.28) and the high burden of relief supplies ($1,030.33 at Norway House compared to $427.30 at Fisher River). Table 5.1 also indicates differential access or perhaps demand for care. It shows that Norway House relied heavily on the capability of a doctor and his assistants who visited from The Pas. Historical documents show that a temporary hospital had been erected at Norway House in October 1904, after the community suffered a number of epidemics. A Department of Indian Affairs report states that a permanent hospital was to be built there in 1914, where Dr. Norquay, the appointed medical officer, would be provided with a liberal supply of drugs and a trained nurse to care for the "sick and stricken unfortunates."[54] A subsequent report confirmed that the hospital had been constructed, and we can assume that it was fully operational in the years 1918-19. Unfortunately, no records are available as the hospital burned down in 1922 and again in 1952.[55] There are also reports of aid being received by the local resident physician, who became ill for a time during the height of the epidemic. Fisher River's residents seem to have relied on paid medical attendants as well as the local hospital for treatment.

The availability of, or demand for, medical supplies/medicines in the two communities also appears to contrast starkly, as indicated by the disparity in the amount of money allotted to Fisher River ($283.75) and what was afforded to Norway House ($37.15). The dissimilarity in the funds allocated to burials ($93.77 at Norway House and $334.10 at Fisher River) may relate to the timing of the epidemic in each community. The

TABLE 5.1

Expenditures incurred by the Canadian government to manage influenza at Norway House and Fisher River, 1919

Norway House Agency	Cost	Fisher River Agency	Cost
Dr. A. Lorose, services, 60 d. at $15	$900.00	Medical attendance	$132.00
Assistant, 60 d. at $15	$900.00	Medical supplies	$283.75
Assistant, 60 d. at $4	$240.00	Treatment in hospital	$47.25
Travel of Dr. Larose and assistant	$656.28	Relief	$427.30
Sundry services	$95.00	Burials	$334.10
Medicines	$37.15	Freight	$62.80
Rations to men visiting camps	$114.08		
Blankets, 8 pr.	$58.00		
Relief supplies	$1,030.33		
Burials	$93.77		
Total (as recorded in original)	$4,124.61		$1,287.20

SOURCE: General Expenditures "Epidemic of Influenza," in Dominion of Canada, *Annual Report of the Department of Indian Affairs for the Year Ended 31 March 1919* (Ottawa: King's Printer, 1920), I-52

Department of Indian Affairs report consists of information recorded until 31 March 1919; however, it is possible that its listing of burials ended after December 1918. The majority of Fisher River burials had already taken place by this time, whereas the epidemic had not yet truly commenced at Norway House.

Although these informative accounts help to explain how the pandemic was experienced, they throw very little light on the question of why two communities that were merely 715.8 kilometres apart had such diverse encounters with this new strain of influenza. Reviewing the impact of the epidemic within the framework of a syndemics approach aids our understanding of why this disparity existed.

SYNDEMICS

First introduced in 1994 by Merrill Singer, in an anthropology text co-authored with Hans Baer and Ida Susser, syndemics calls for "big picture dialectical thinking in health."[56] The approach encompasses a number of stimulating yet challenging agendas. The first is to view infectious diseases as integrated entities that co-exist in a host and in a given environment. This technique, which has much in common with the ecological idea of synergy, challenges scholars to explore and understand the interactions of disease-causing entities. For example, the biomedical community has clearly demonstrated that HIV-positive individuals who have been exposed to tuberculosis are at an increased risk for developing active and rapidly progressing TB.[57] The syndemics approach also challenges proponents to view these co-infections as a consequence of health-threatening conditions. For example, poverty can result in malnutrition, which has been shown to compromise the immune system.[58] Lastly, syndemics calls for researchers to understand the role of public health systems in delivering and preventing future outbreaks of infectious disease.

Syndemics at the Level of the Microscope

One of the key components in the syndemics framework is the understanding of how different pathogens can influence each other. Ferreting out the elements of an epidemic that are attributable to this complex interaction is a daunting task at best. With this in mind, the following offers a hypothesis to explain the differential age-at-death distribution at Norway

TABLE 5.2

Age-at-death distribution for influenza mortality per 1,000 population at Norway House and Fisher River, 1918-19

Age	N	Norway House % Total mortality	% Overall population at risk (n = 208)	N	Fisher River % Total mortality	% Overall population at risk (n = 284)
0-5	3	7.89%	1.44%	15	39.47%	5.28%
6-15	11	28.95%	5.29%	6	15.79%	2.11%
16 - 20	1	2.63%	0.48%	4	10.53%	1.41%
21 - 65	18	47.37%	8.65%	4	10.53%	1.41%
Over 65	3	7.89%	1.44%	1	2.63%	0.35%
Unknown	2	5.26%	0.96%	8	21.05%	2.82%
Total	38	100.00%	18.26%	38	100.00%	13.38%

Source: Dominion of Canada, *Annual Report of the Department of Indian Affairs for the Year Ended March 31 1917* (Ottawa: King's Printer, 1918)

House and Fisher River, which is plotted in Table 5.2. Influenza deaths at Norway House included very few individuals under the age of six (7.89 percent), whereas the six- to fifteen-year-olds experienced the second-highest death rate, comprising just under 29 percent of the total influenza mortality experienced among Anglicans at Norway House.[59] Of sixteen- to twenty-year-olds, only one person died (2.63 percent). Most deaths occurred among individuals between the ages of twenty-one and sixty-five, comprising just over 47 percent of the total mortality for the Anglican population. The last age category of over sixty-fives also experienced only a few deaths (7.89 percent).

At Fisher River, there appears to be an overrepresentation of deaths among those who were under the age of six (39.47 percent of total mortality). Six- to fifteen-year-olds suffered the second-highest mortality, with six deaths (15.79 percent). Four sixteen- to twenty-year-olds died, leaving only four deaths in the twenty-one to sixty-five age range and one in the over sixty-five category. When these groups are aggregated (so that they are amenable to statistical testing), statistically significant differences are revealed between the distribution of mortality by age and community (see Table 5.3).

Influenza mortality normally takes its highest toll among the very young and the aged. However, a defining characteristic of the 1918-20 pandemic strain was that it caused a peak in mortality among individuals between the ages of twenty and forty.[60] Recent research indicates that this might have been the by-product of a healthy innate immune response that so damaged the lungs as to trigger acute respiratory distress, severe tissue damage, edema and hemorrhaging, and pneumonia in individuals at peak fitness levels.[61]

TABLE 5.3

Chi-square analysis of age at death for Norway House and Fisher River

Location	Age	Observed	Expected	χ^2 value	Adjusted residual
Norway House	0-20	15	22.3	2.4	−1.5
	21-65	25	15.6	3.5	1.9
Fisher River	0-20	25	17.6	3.1	1.8
	21-65	5	12.4	4.4	−2.1

Chi-square value = 13.4
Critical value (0.05, 10) = 3.8

There are several possible explanations for the differential age distributions of flu mortality at Fisher River and Norway House. The dissimilarity may simply be an artifact of the data, although careful scrutiny, utilizing Drake's analysis, of the records and record-keepers suggests that this was not a determining factor.[62]

It is not clear to what extent population size comes into play in this analysis. According to 1917 census data, the Norway House population was 734, of which 208 were Anglicans.[63] Although the entire population at Fisher River was only 493, Methodists accounted for more than half of this number. The age distributions within the two communities are quite similar and would not contribute to the differences expressed in the findings of the analysis.

It is at this point that we may employ a syndemics approach by examining the unique disease profile of the two communities prior to the pandemic in order to fully comprehend how disease interactions play out. For example, according to Moffat, Fisher River typically experienced a high infant mortality rate after the fifth month of age.[64] She adds that approximately 70 percent of all infant deaths at Fisher River between 1910 and 1939 were caused by infectious disease and that almost half of these were caused by acute airborne respiratory infections.[65] These findings help to demonstrate why mortality at Fisher River did not display the common characteristic of the 1918 flu strain – targeting individuals in their prime. Ann Herring and Lisa Sattenspiel also argue that the presence of tuberculosis at Norway House probably "exacerbated the effects of influenza in 1918, contributing to the high proportion of deaths."[66] At a cursory level, there also appears to be a strong association between influenza and tuberculosis mortality at Fisher River, as many families who lost a child to the flu subsequently lost another to tuberculosis.

SYNDEMICS AT THE FAMILY LEVEL: EXAMINING WHO GOT SICK AND ITS IMPACT

Understanding the impact of mortality can be a key determinant in fully comprehending both the long- and short-term effects of an epidemic. With this in mind, the following section will demonstrate the impact of *who* died rather than *how many*.

As a person progresses through the various stages of life, the nature of his or her involvement in the community changes also. An oversimplified way of looking at this is to break the life stages into three general categories: past, present, and future. In this framework, the past consists of a community's elderly members (individuals aged seventy and older). Although they are often involved in its day-to-day functioning, their main contribution occurs at the household level. Elders have also been important keepers of wisdom who provide a wealth of information based on life experience. Joseph Saunderson, a resident of York Factory, stated that elders "stayed home. They often looked after the children while the women were outside working or out hunting."[67] Although they often remained active, their immediate physical impact was usually restricted to the family level.

The future category in this framework encompasses children and preteens; our inquiry includes infants under one year of age and children between two and twelve. The young comprise what a community will be – its future. They do not yet play an autonomous role in its functioning, and like that of the elders, their importance is limited to the family rather than the general populace. In Cree society, puberty often marked the shift from student to hunter, for although a child might make his first kill before reaching puberty, he was usually still in the process of perfecting his skills.[68] Younger children spent their day playing, whereas older children might help with household chores, such as cutting firewood.[69] The death of individuals in these age categories does have an impact on a community, but it lacks the immediacy and severity felt when individuals die in their prime.

Lastly, the third group in this framework consists of those who form the backbone of a community and are responsible for its daily functioning. For our purposes, this group comprises thirteen- to sixty-nine-year-olds. When individuals are removed from this category, the impact is felt immediately, especially in a small community where certain types of expertise are limited to a few people. In normal circumstances, some professions require only a few practitioners, yet their job may be essential for the daily functioning of a community at the time of a disease outbreak. Examples include clergy, doctors, gravediggers, nurses, store clerks, and so on. In addition, individuals in this third group are most likely to have dependants, either children or the elderly, who rely on them as primary caregivers and who become vulnerable to death and starvation when they are removed.

At Fisher River, it was not uncommon for the youngest or close-to-youngest child to perish during the epidemic. Of the nineteen deaths of children under the age of thirteen at Fisher River, twelve were the youngest and four were the second-youngest. In most instances at Norway House, a parent died as a result of the pandemic. Due to the subsistence strategy employed at Norway House, several adults were probably required to support a family, and the loss of a parent would have had detrimental effects on the development and survival of young children. This fact alone could account for the differential impact between these two communities.

Another factor that played a role in determining the impact of the epidemic at Norway House and Fisher River is how the deaths were distributed within and between families. One of the most predominant features of Norway House mortality is that the majority of deaths clustered within particular families. First identified by Herring and Sattenspiel, who examined Treaty Annuity Pay Lists (TAPL), and later supported using family reconstitution, this pattern not only speaks to a community's ability to deal with an epidemic, but is also essential in helping researchers understand the features of mortality in a way that crude death rates cannot.[70] At Norway House, some families remained untouched by the pandemic, whereas others were decimated. The following section explores the effects of this difference.

Figure 5.2 compares the number of deaths in each nuclear family at Norway House and Fisher River. Of the thirty-eight individuals listed in Reverend Stevens's Fisher River burial records, twenty-six (68 percent) can

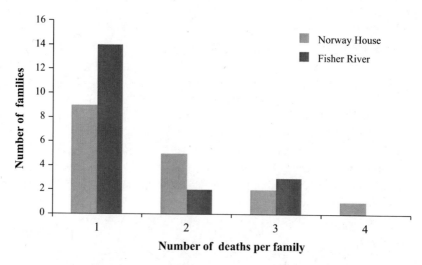

FIGURE 5.2   Distribution of influenza deaths for Norway House and Fisher River per nuclear family, October 1918 to July 1919

be linked to reconstituted families.[71] Of these, the deaths per family break down as follows: one death each in fourteen families, two deaths each in two families, and three deaths each in two families. This equates to 53 percent, 23 percent, and 23 percent of all deaths reported in this community. No families experienced four or more deaths.

Of the thirty-eight individuals included in Reverend Marshall's burial records for Norway House, twenty-nine (76 percent) can be linked to reconstituted families. Of these, the breakdown of deaths per family is as follows: one death each in nine families, two deaths each in five families, three deaths each in two families, and four deaths (or the complete removal) in one family. This equates to 31 percent, 34 percent, 31 percent, and 14 percent of all deaths reported in this community. This figure reveals that Fisher River had the highest proportion of deaths in the one-member-per-family range (53 percent). In contrast, multiple deaths within households appear to be a distinctive feature of Norway House mortality, with just under 50 percent of all deaths taking place within four families.

The Shift from Distress to Disorder

Through further exploration into families that experienced multiple deaths at Norway House and Fisher River, we may begin to ascertain how these collective deaths affected individual families and the communities in which they resided. The goal here is not to report findings of statistical significance; rather, the aim is to put a face on what is sometimes a faceless epidemic. To this end, we examined reconstituted families that lost three or more members to the flu virus.

Figure 5.3 displays the reconstituted data for the Musk family, who lived at Norway House. Prior to the pandemic, it consisted of four members, parents John George and Martha, and their two girls, Madiline and Mary. All died as a result of the epidemic.[72] It is of note that Martha Musk's (Bass) place of birth is listed as God's Lake and that of John George, Oxford House. They were married at Oxford House on 29 August 1898. It is unclear where Madiline and Mary were born, as there are no baptismal records for them at Oxford House, God's Lake, or Norway House. No birth records exist at Norway House, so it is probable that they were born elsewhere. There is no question about the relationships in this family, as they are indicated on the burial record. The children's ages are given as fourteen and eight. The burial record of John George states that he was a trapper, and his marriage record specifies that he was a hunter. It is therefore likely

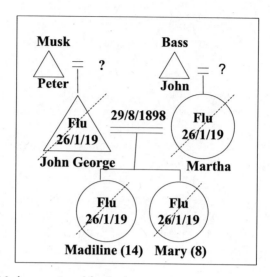

FIGURE 5.3   Musk reconstituted family chart.
Notes: Triangle = male, and a circle = female; equals sign = a marriage; question marks
= missing information or supposition; dashed diagonals = death; dates are burial or
marriage dates

that this family was out on the trapline when they were stricken with
influenza. It is also of note that the Musks collected treaty payments at
Norway House.[73] Their removal from the treaty annuity pay lists in 1919,
coupled with their burial records in the Anglican registry, confirms that
they were struck down during the epidemic.

The second Norway House example is the Robinson family (Figure 5.4),
which consisted of four members, parents William and Flora, and their
two sons, Stanley and Walter James. Stanley and his parents died as a result
of the Spanish flu. There is no marriage record for the parents; nor do birth
records exist for the two boys. Their relationships are established through
notes on the burial documentation as well as their treaty annuity pay list
disbursement for 1918. William was a carpenter for the HBC, which would
have placed him and his family at the post during the pandemic. Stanley
and Flora were among the first to die from the flu, and their burial dates
probably reflect their date of death as both contracted the disease before
Reverend Marshall did.[74] All we know about Walter James is that he was
residing at Norway House at the time of his father's burial.

The Saundersons are the third Norway House family to be explored in
detail (Figure 5.5). On the eve of the pandemic, it consisted of William,

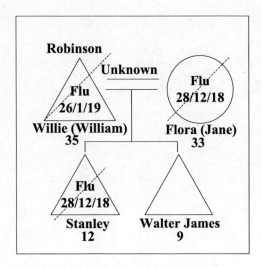

FIGURE 5.4   Robinson reconstituted family chart

his second wife, Edith, and four offspring – a grown married daughter whose name we do not know and three sons, George Albert, Willie, and another boy whose name is not recorded. This boy and Willie, who were aged ten and twelve, perished with their father during the epidemic. William Saunderson married Edith Evanson nearly three years after the death of his wife, Annie. Together, he and Annie had five children, two of whom had married prior to William's remarriage in 1912. There are two possibilities for which family members were cohabiting during the epidemic. First, at the time of William's death, only Willie, George Albert, and the unnamed son were residing with him; second, through the practice of extended kin groupings, he and his mature son were cooperating on the trapline and living together. His first two children are listed as being born at York Factory (1886) and Split Lake (1891), and although none of the remaining offspring have birth records, there is evidence that the family was at Norway House in 1909 (as indicated in Annie Saunderson's burial record) and 1912 (again indicated in the burial record for Jessie Drawrer). The records also indicate that the family remained at Norway House until at least 1929, as suggested by the burial record of George Albert. William's burial record lists him as a trapper, and he may have been out on the trapline with his two youngest sons at the time of their illness and subsequent deaths.

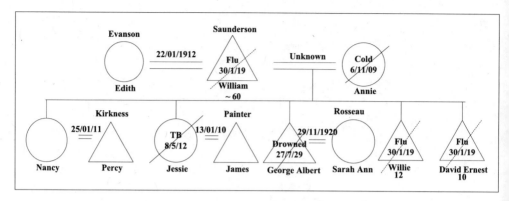

FIGURE 5.5   Saunderson reconstituted family chart

Two other Norway House families experienced more than two deaths: the Gunns and the Basses. Due to a lack of information on the earlier generations, they cannot be definitively linked to a reconstituted family tree and as a result are not included in this discussion.

Only two Fisher River families experienced more than two deaths, and of these, only one – the Boucs – can be reconstituted with confidence (Figure 5.6). It consisted of parents Maurice and Sarah, and their two boys, Alex and Matthew James. Of the four, only Matthew James survived the pandemic. The Boucs were somewhat atypical for Fisher River: most of its families were much larger, and the Boucs represent the only recorded instance in which both parents died of the flu. The virus swept through this family, perhaps after being introduced by Maurice on or around 25 October. Whether Matthew James had grandparents to look after him once his parents died is unknown. He himself died of pneumonia in 1921.

At Norway House, ten spouses were left widowed by the virus, as opposed to three at Fisher River. At both Fisher River and Norway House, one child was orphaned when both parents died. Finally, there was the impact of losing an entire family, which occurred at Norway House but not at Fisher River.

The sheer impact of dealing with numerous families devastated by the pandemic would have greatly influenced the morale at Fisher River and Norway House; as well, multiple deaths within single families speak to a community's ability to deal with an epidemic. The author contends that the differing mortality patterns witnessed at the two communities resulted from a discrepancy in individuals' access to informal networks of care. At Norway House, families were out on their traplines, isolated from each

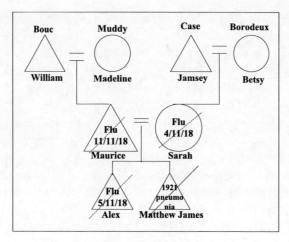

FIGURE 5.6   Bouc reconstituted family chart

other and from extended kin groups, a fact that increased the likelihood of dying of the flu. At Fisher River, families were aggregated within a community structure, which meant that individuals had greater access to internal support systems (especially in the form of extended kin networks). Therefore, although more people may have contracted the flu, these informal networks of care limited subsequent mortality from the disease (or conditions resulting from it, such as the inability to collect firewood or to attain food or water).

SYNDEMICS AT THE ENVIRONMENTAL LEVEL: TRACKING THE TIMING OF THE EPIDEMIC

Parish registry data was utilized to re-create the spread of the epidemic at Fisher River and Norway House. With the omission of six Fisher River and one Norway House deaths, the pandemic seems to have been somewhat more protracted at Fisher River, lasting seven weeks and two days compared to Norway House's five weeks and six days.[75] This appears to support the contention of an epidemic possessing higher morbidity and a lower overall mortality within the stayer (or non-nomadic) communities. Fisher River experienced a fall epidemic that began on 30 October 1918 and tapered off by 19 November, with sporadic deaths after the height of the pandemic. On most days between 4 and 10 November, the community seems to have experienced anywhere from three to five burials daily. The mortality rate peaked on 5 November with five deaths and then again on the ninth with four. It is hard to see the impact of this as anything less than overwhelming. The deaths were distributed throughout many families, suggesting that very few remained untouched by the epidemic. Reverend Stevens's acknowledgment of its disruptive nature and the quick succession of burials is incontrovertible evidence of a society in turmoil.

Norway House's epidemic took hold in the winter, with the first death occurring on 18 December. Two further deaths were recorded on 28 December but no more until 24 January, nearly one month later. During the next seven days, burials peaked, with three on the twenty-fourth, one on the twenty-fifth, eighteen on the twenty-sixth, one on the twenty-ninth, and eleven on the thirtieth.

Herring suggests that burials were suspended between late December and 24 January because the local clergyman, Reverend Marshall, had contracted the flu himself and could not officiate at funerals.[76] This explanation seems very plausible and is supported by a post journal account from 1 January 1919, which reads, "Visited Mr. Marshall, who is down with the 'Flu.'"[77] It can be stated with almost absolute certainty that this entry pertains to Reverend Marshall, as the onset of his illness coincides with the break in burial registration. The date of his recovery, 22 January 1919, is also noted in the post journal, which reads, "Mr. Marshall visited the Fort, this being the first time he has been out since taken down with the 'Flu.'"[78] Two days later, burials resumed at Fisher River.

Scrutiny of Factor William Campbell's post journal reveals further evidence of a delay between death and burial. Of the mortalities mentioned in its pages, three are listed in the Anglican burial register. The first death, that of Effie Roberts, helps to establish the journal's accuracy. According to Campbell, "Roderick Roberts's wife died" on 18 December 1918.[79] Reverend Marshall supports this date by recording that she was buried on 18 December. The second death is that of Jennie Oman Arthurson (Artherson). According to the factor, "Mrs. Arthurson died" on 6 January 1919.[80] Marshall recorded her burial on 25 January, some nineteen days later. Finally, on 15 January, the post journal reads, "John Gunn died," yet the burial record indicates that he was not interred until 24 January.[81]

The impact of mortality at Norway House was staggering. Its immediate effects can be seen in post journal entries and other primary sources. We know from the HBC journal that communication with neighbouring communities had broken down by 19 December as dog teams could no longer be assembled to perform even the most basic services, such as mail delivery. The first mention in the post journal of attempts to get provisions out to Indians on traplines dates from 4 January 1919, when the factor reported sending a "team off to deliver wood."[82] This is seventeen days after the first death at Norway House. Also, the usual Christmas rush did not occur as "most of the people [were] sick" and unable to make the trip to the post.[83] On 29 December, Factor Campbell visited Dr. Norquay (the local physician) and reported that eleven people had died from flu thus far.[84] Three more deaths were reported the next day, and by 6 January, the number had risen to fifty.

Ann Herring's interviews of Norway House residents who experienced the epidemic first-hand reveal the disarray that swept through the community.[85] One of her informants mentioned the "difficulties of burying so many people who died so suddenly, noting that they were brought to a cabin and stacked like wood until it was possible to bury them later."[86] The memoirs of Frances Stevens, "My Experience Living on a Mission," also discuss the problem of finding able-bodied individuals to help prepare and bury the dead. She stated that at "Berens River thirteen bodies lay in the mission storehouse because there was not a sufficient number of men able to dig resting places."[87] Accounts from neighbouring communities describe complete breakdowns in day-to-day functioning as well. At Berens River, Harry Everett recalled that everyone except his father had contracted the flu, and it was all his father could do to ensure that individual residences had adequate food and wood supplies.

First explored in Sattenspiel and Herring, and later expanded in Herring and Sattenspiel, computer modelling based on extensive archival work suggests that the epidemic's seasonal timing not only directly affected the spread of the virus between communities, but also influenced each community's social organization, which structured mortality within families.[88] This leaves us to wonder if mortality and perhaps morbidity at Norway House would have been different had individuals not been participating in a seasonal round and therefore isolated in the countryside without access to informal networks of care.

INCORPORATING POLITICAL, ECONOMIC, AND RELIGIOUS FACTORS INTO THE ANALYSIS

Both Norway House and Fisher River had a hierarchical political and economic structure that fashioned and reshaped the daily lives of residents. It owed a great deal to the early colonial relationships established by Europeans with the indigenous population. The legacy of colonialism can be seen in company welfarism among fur trade families in the central subarctic. Colonial institutions also determined how the influenza virus entered the two communities. At Norway House, its portal of entry appears to have been the Hudson's Bay Company, a contention that is supported by the fact that the first person to show symptoms and the first to die were both HBC employees. At Fisher River, Reverend Stevens seems to have been the first to contract the disease. Therefore, the loci of infection for both communities were institutions that helped to structure social networks and subsistence strategies: the HBC (Norway House) and the church (Fisher River). Furthermore, the conditions created by these colonial institutions may provide clues as to why the impact of the epidemic was more severe at Norway House than at Fisher River, even though the disease was somewhat more protracted at the latter community. We can observe, for example, that the HBC encouraged economic and social competition, whereas the mission fostered a community atmosphere. By examining these institutions as the mainstays of social organization, we can better understand how they moulded community interaction and thus the influenza experience.

At both Norway House and Fisher River, the traditional way of life had been irrefutably altered, and the systems that had once enabled people to deal with hardship or catastrophe had been decimated. Fur trade colonialism had gradually attenuated the intricate social networks that would have created the basis for informal care to cope with the pandemic. At Norway House, the chronic overhunting of fur-bearing animals for the purpose of trade broke down extended-kin-based hunting groups, leaving families alone on their traplines and susceptible to the flu (probably brought back from the trading post). At Fisher River, we see very little evidence of a "traditional" way of life; rather, the community was in the process of redefining itself and its kin networks.

Although they were disproportionately affected by the influenza pandemic relative to non-Aboriginal communities in Canada, Fisher River and Norway House experienced the epidemic quite differently. Their respective populations are too small to provide an accurate idea of age-specific mortality at a precise level, but when very broad categories are developed (zero to twenty, twenty-one to sixty-five and older) a statistically significant difference appears in the age at death of individuals in the two communities.[89] At Norway House, 61 percent of those who died during the epidemic were between the ages of twenty-one and sixty-five or older, whereas mortality at Fisher River disproportionately affected individuals who were twenty and younger (83 percent).[90] The data from Norway House indicate that mortality was clustered in certain families, whereas deaths were distributed throughout families at Fisher River. There is also the strong impression that normal daily functioning ceased at Norway House. Whether this was because a few key individuals became sick (such as Reverend Marshall) or because the entire community was ill at the same time is hard to determine. Also, though a fair amount of disruption occurred at Fisher River, there is very little evidence that its level of turmoil rivalled that of Norway House.

In addressing the question of why influenza affected Norway House and Fisher River differently, this chapter has employed a syndemics approach to explore a number of possible explanations. By looking at the experiences of several families who lost more than one member to the flu, we can trace its impact on family life for those most severely affected by the disease. At Norway House, mortality tended to cluster in specific families, who suffered more than one death; in one case, the disease killed an entire family. This mortality pattern suggests that Norway House trappers and their families lacked access to the care of kin, and it reveals the negative impact of a competitive fur trade colonialism on informal networks of care. Alone on their traplines, with no one to feed them or keep them warm while they suffered from the disease, they perished; without the care of adults, children also died. A different pattern emerges in Fisher River. A more settled community, where many worked in the lumber industry, it seems to have had greater resources to cope with the virus, and as a result, fewer adults died. However, its infants and young children perished at much higher rates than was the norm during the pandemic. The community had a very high rate of infant mortality prior to the appearance of influenza, mostly caused by acute viral respiratory infections, suggesting that certain conditions rendered young children vulnerable to these types of illnesses. Tuberculosis was also a serious health issue among children whose families suffered influenza losses. In general, tuberculosis must be considered as working in tandem with the flu virus.

The influenza pandemic exhibited a diverse set of negative effects in Aboriginal communities, its path shaped in complex ways by local political, social, and economic forces. When we look at Norway House and Fisher River with a historical gaze, it becomes easier to discern why their Cree inhabitants experienced such severe mortality (approximately 18.0 percent and 13.0 percent respectively), in comparison to other North American communities (0.6 percent for all of Canada), during this devastating pandemic.[91]

NOTES

1 Nancy Tomes, *The Gospel of Germs: Men, Women, and the Microbe in American Life* (Cambridge, MA: Harvard University Press, 1998).

2 See, for example, David M. Morens and Anthony S. Fauci, "The 1918 Influenza Pandemic: Insights for the 21st Century," *Journal of Infectious Diseases* 195 (1 April 2007): 1018-28; J.K. Taubenberger et al., "Characterization of the 1918 Influenza Virus Polymerase Genes," *Nature* 437,7060 (6 October 2005): 889-93; and J.K. Taubenberger and D.M. Morens, "1918 Influenza: The Mother of All Pandemics," *Emerging Infectious Disease* 12,1 (2006): 15-22.

3 The present discussion, which is based on family reconstitution, would not have been possible without the scholarship of Ann Herring and her colleagues, who have produced an extensive body of work focusing on this region. See D. Ann Herring, "'There Were Young People and Old People and Babies Dying Every Week': The 1918-1919 Influenza Pandemic at Norway House," *Ethnohistory* 41,1 (1994): 73-105; D. Ann Herring, "The 1918 Influenza Epidemic in the Central Canadian Subarctic," in *Strength in Diversity: A Reader in Physical Anthropology,* ed. D. Ann Herring and Leslie Chan (Toronto: Canadian Scholars Press, 1994), 364-84; D. Ann Herring and L. Sattenspiel, "Death in Winter: Spanish Flu in the Canadian Subarctic," in *The Spanish Influenza Pandemic of 1918-19: New Perspectives,* ed. Howard Phillips and David Killingray (London: Routledge, 2003), 156-172; D. Ann Herring and L. Sattenspiel, "Social Contexts, Syndemics, and Infectious Disease in Northern Aboriginal Populations," *American Journal of Human Biology* 19,2 (2007): 190-202; Tina Moffat, "Infant Mortality in an Aboriginal Community: A Historical and Biocultural Analysis" (Master's thesis, Department of Anthropology, McMaster University, 1992); Tina Moffat and D. Ann Herring, "Historical Roots of High Rates of Infant Death in Aboriginal Communities in Canada in the Early Twentieth Century: The Case of Fisher River, Manitoba," *Social Science and Medicine* 48 (1999): 1821-32; Lisa Sattenspiel and D. Ann Herring, "Structured Epidemic Models and the Spread of Influenza in the Central Canadian Subarctic," *Human Biology* 70,1 (1998): 91-115; Lisa Sattenspiel, Ann Mobarry, and D. Ann Herring, "Modeling the Influence of Settlement Structure on the Spread of Influenza among Communities," *American Journal of Human Biology* 12 (2000): 736-48; and Lisa Sattenspiel and D. Ann Herring, "Simulating the Effect of Quarantine on the Spread of the 1918-19 Flu in Central Canada," *Bulletin of Mathematical Biology* 65,1 (2003): 1-26.

4 Alanson Buck Skinner, "Notes on the Eastern Cree and Northern Saulteaux," in *Anthropological Papers of the American Museum of Natural History,* vol. 9, pt. 1, ed. C. Wissler (New York: American Museum of Natural History, 1912), 9.

5 Conrad E. Heidenreich and Arthur J. Ray, *The Early Fur Trades: A Study in Cultural Interaction* (Toronto: McClelland and Stewart, 1976), 34.

6 Arthur J. Ray, "History and Archaeology of the Northern Fur Trade," *American Antiquity* 43,1 (1978): 26.

7 Ibid., 28.

8 Christopher Hanks, "Swampy Cree and the Hudson's Bay Company at Oxford House," *Ethnohistory* 29,2 (Spring 1982): 109.

9 James G.E. Smith, "Western Woods Cree," in *Handbook of North American Indians,* vol. 6, *Subarctic,* ed. June Helm (Washington, DC: Smithsonian Institution, 1981), 258.

10 Ibid.

11 Frank Tough, "Indian Economic Behaviour, Exchange and Profits in Northern Manitoba during the Decline of Monopoly, 1870-1930," *Journal of Historical Geography* 16,4 (1990): 389.

12 For the nature of trade goods, see Charles A. Bishop, "Demography, Ecology and Trade among the Northern Ojibwa and Swampy Cree," *Western Canadian Journal of Anthropology* 3,1 (1972): 60.

13 For the debt system, see Hanks, "Swampy Cree and the Hudson's Bay Company," 107; for company welfarism, see Tough, "Indian Economic Behaviour," 390.

14 Ibid., 385; and Hanks, "Swampy Cree and the Hudson's Bay Company," 107.

15 Smith, "Western Woods Cree," 259.

16 Herring, "'There Were Young People,'" 75.

17 Smith, "Western Woods Cree," 259.

18 Ibid.

19 Herring and Sattenspiel, "Death in Winter," 168-69.

20 Herring, "'There Were Young People,'" 75.

21 Arthur J. Ray, "Diffusion of Diseases in the Western Interior of Canada, 1830-1850," *Geographical Review* 66,2 (April 1976): 156; and Tough, "Indian Economic Behaviour," 395.

22 Frederick J. Alcock, "Past and Present Trade Routes to the Canadian Northwest," *Geographical Review* 10,2 (August 1920): 71.

23 Herring, "'There Were Young People,'" 75.

24 James G.E. Smith, "Chipewyan, Cree and Inuit Relations West of Hudson Bay, 1714-1955," *Ethnohistory* 28,2 (Spring 1981): 147.

25 James B. Waldram, D. Ann Herring, and T. Kue Young, *Aboriginal Health in Canada: Historical, Cultural, and Epidemiological Perspectives* (Toronto: University of Toronto Press, 2006), 60.

26 Moffat and Herring, "Historical Roots," 1825.

27 Dominion of Canada, *Annual Report of the Department of Indian Affairs for the Year Ended June 30 1906* (Ottawa: King's Printer, 1906), 87, Library and Archives Canada (LAC), http://www.collectionscanada.gc.ca.

28 Dominion of Canada, *Annual Report of the Department of Indian Affairs for the Year Ended March 31 1913* (Ottawa: King's Printer, 1913), 88, LAC, http://www.collectionscanada.gc.ca.

29 Moffat and Herring, "Historical Roots," 1825.

30 Moffat, "Infant Mortality," 10.

31 Ibid.

32 Dominion of Canada, *Annual Report of the Department of Indian Affairs for the Year Ended March 31 1910* (Ottawa: King's Printer, 1910), 97, LAC, http://www.collectionscanada.gc.ca.

33 Eileen Pettigrew, *The Silent Enemy: Canada and the Deadly Flu of 1918* (Saskatoon: Western Producer Prairie Books, 1983), 56-57.

34 Ibid., 79.

35 With the exception of the date for The Pas, which was gleaned from newspaper accounts, these dates were gathered from parish registries.

36 Herring, "'There Were Young People,'" 83.

37 Norway House Post Journal 1918-1939, Archives of Manitoba, Hudson's Bay Company Archives, B. 154/a/87-95, reel no. 1MA46, Winnipeg.

38 Ibid.

39 Frances E.E. Stevens, "My Experience Living on a Mission" (memoirs, photocopy, n.d.), UCA, Frances E.E. Stevens fonds, 80-7, ID 3510.

40 Fisher River burial register, 1918-1951, UCA, 78-27.

41 Mortality rates are calculated from the 1917 census for the Anglican community at Norway House and the Methodist community at Fisher River.

42 Maureen Lux, "Prairie Indians and the 1918 Influenza Epidemic," *Native Studies Review* 8,1 (1992): 25; and N.P.A.S. Johnson and J. Mueller, "Updating the Accounts: Global Mortality of the 1918-1920 'Spanish' Influenza Pandemic," *Bulletin of the History of Medicine* 76,1 (2002): 111.

43 "Heavy Toll of Deaths among Northern Indians," *The Pas Herald and Mining News,* 7 February 1919, 3.

44 Ibid., 1. The present discussion of Norway House confines its scope to Anglican deaths. *The Pas Herald*'s account refers to the community as an integrated whole.

45 Norway House Post Journal 1918-1939, fos. 11, 13.

46 For a detailed discussion of the quality of these sources, see Karen Slonim, "Differences in the Experience of the 1918-1919 Influenza Pandemic at Norway House and Fisher River, Manitoba" (Master's diss., Department of Anthropology, McMaster University, 2004), 41-56; and Moffat, "Infant Mortality."

47 Ibid., 33.

48 Ibid.

49 Stevens, "My Experience Living on a Mission," 89.

50 Ibid.

51 Ibid., 99.

52 Ibid., 103.

53 Dominion of Canada, *Annual Report of the Department of Indian Affairs for the Year Ended March 31 1919* (Ottawa: King's Printer, 1920), 47-48, LAC, http://www.collectionscanada.gc.ca.

54 Dominion of Canada, *Annual Report of the Department of Indian Affairs for the Year Ended March 31 1915* (Ottawa: King's Printer, 1915), pt. II, 151, LAC, http://www.collectionscanada.gc.ca.

55 Larry Krotz, *Indian Country: Inside Another Canada* (Toronto: McClelland and Stewart, 1990), 31.

56 Hans Baer, Merrill Singer, and Ida Susser, *Medical Anthropology and the World System,* 2nd ed. (Westport, CT: Praeger, 2003), 15.

57 For a full discussion, see Zheng W. Chen, "Immunology of AIDS Virus and Mycobacterial Co-Infection," *Current HIV Research* 2 (2004): 351-55.

58 Baer, Singer, and Susser, *Medical Anthropology,* 17.

59 These percentage figures are calculated in relation to the total number of deaths among Norway House Anglicans (thirty-eight), not of the entire population at Norway House.

60 Alfred W. Crosby, *America's Forgotten Pandemic: The Influenza of 1918* (Cambridge: Cambridge University Press, 1989); and Howard Phillips and David Killingray, *The Spanish Influenza Pandemic of 1918-19: New Perspectives* (London: Routledge, 2003).

61 For more information, see John C. Kash et al., "Genomic Analysis of Increased Host Immune and Cell Death Responses Induced by 1918 Influenza Virus," *Nature* 443,7111 (4 October 2006): 578-81; and Darwyn Kobasa et al., "Aberrant Innate Immune Response in Lethal Infection of Macaques with the 1918 Influenza Virus," *Nature* 445,7125 (18 January 2007): 319-23.

62 See Slonim, "Differences in the Experience," 85-90, for a detailed discussion.

63 Dominion of Canada, *Annual Report of the Department of Indian Affairs for the Year Ended March 31 1917* (Ottawa: King's Printer, 1918).

64 Moffat, "Infant Mortality," 84.

65 Ibid., 86.

66 Herring and Sattenspiel, "Death in Winter," 171.

67 Quoted in Flora Beardy and Robert Coutts, eds., *Voices from Hudson Bay: Cree Stories from York Factory* (Montreal and Kingston: McGill-Queen's University Press, 1997), 90.

68 Edwia G. Higgins, *Whitefish Lake Ojibway Memories* (Cobalt: Highway Book Shop, 1982), 83.

69 Beardy and Coutts, *Voices from Hudson Bay,* 44.

70 Herring and Sattenspiel, "Death in Winter"; and Slonim, "Differences in the Experience."

71 Individuals with possible links were not omitted from the sample; for instance, those who lacked a marriage record were included, which is not the norm for family reconstitution techniques. Individuals were also included if there was a strong possibility of a family connection, as, for example, where a family cluster probably existed even though the parents' ages were unknown. For more information, see ibid.

72 All surnames extracted from the Anglican and Methodist parish records are presented as pseudonyms.

73 See Department of Indian Affairs and Northern Development 1862-1959 Treaty Annuity Pay Lists, Norway House Cree First Nation.

74 He is reported to have contracted the disease on 1 January 1919.

75 The six Fisher River deaths occurred on 2 February, 22 April, 27 May, 8 June, 5 July, and 5 November 1919. The Norway House death took place on 8 April 1919. They were omitted because so much time elapsed between them and the pandemic's start date and subsequent period of heightened mortality. The trajectory for the pandemic is based on the time period between the first and last burial in each community.

76 Herring, "'There Were Young People.'"

77 Norway House Post Journal 1918-1939, fol. 12.

78 Ibid.

79 Ibid., fol. 8.

80 Ibid.

81 Ibid.

82 Ibid.

83 Ibid., fol. 9.

84 Ibid.

85 Herring, "The 1918 Influenza Epidemic."

86 Ibid., 376.

87 Stevens, "My Experience Living on a Mission," 107.

88 See Sattenspiel and Herring, "Structured Epidemic Models"; and Herring and Sattenspiel, "Death in Winter."

89 At the time of the epidemic, 208 Anglicans lived at Norway House, and approximately 250 Methodists lived at Fisher River.

90 Slonim, "Differences in the Experience."

91 Johnson and Mueller, "Updating the Accounts," 111.

6

A Geographical Analysis of the Spread of Spanish Influenza in Quebec, 1918-20

FRANCIS DUBOIS, JEAN-PIERRE THOUEZ, AND DENIS GOULET

Throughout the world, the 1918-20 Spanish influenza pandemic killed great numbers in a very short time.[1] Despite its impact, however, little is known about how the disease spread in Quebec. This chapter attempts to remedy this lack by presenting the geographical patterns of the epidemic in Quebec, especially in Montreal, using data provided by the Superior Board of Health of the Province of Quebec (SBHPQ) in 1918 and 1920, which are sufficiently detailed to allow us to analyze the phenomenon (see Appendices A and B). In the first part of our discussion, we employ two documentary sources – the daily Montreal newspaper *Le Devoir* and the annual reports of the SBHPQ – to describe the spread of the virus across the province. In the second part, we present a statistical and geographical analysis by county of the incidence and mortality of the Spanish influenza of 1918. We conclude by examining the mortality caused by the 1920 wave of influenza.

STATISTICS AND METHODS

The statistics concerning Spanish influenza cases and deaths in Quebec are included in the SBHPQ annual reports for 1918 and 1920, and the context for the pandemic's diffusion is provided by contemporary articles from *Le Devoir*. The SBHPQ statistics for Quebec have never before been analyzed. Like other researchers, we discovered that the data have certain weaknesses. In addition, the province had no standard method of collecting health data before 1918. Nor can we assume that the statistics provide a completely reliable count of influenza cases or deaths. However, such problems with data are common in the history of the pandemic, and though we acknowledge the limits of the data, we argue that they are nonetheless useful as they provide best estimates. As for our choice of newspaper, we selected *Le Devoir* because, according to J.-Y. Gravel, it was independent and non-partisan.[2]

We studied the incidence and mortality of the illness in Quebec's sixty-nine counties as given by the SBHPQ for 1918. We adjusted the SBHPQ data so that new cases and deaths by months were compatible with the total numbers by county. We gathered population statistics from municipal data for 1918 and 1920, and from the Canadian census of 1921. Also, we adjusted the SBHPQ statistics to make them compatible with the geographical limits of the municipalities and counties. These data allowed us to calculate the standardized rates of incidence and mortality at the county level for 1918 and 1920. In addition, we used the 1915-17 SBHPQ reports to better understand the extent of the problem of influenza at the county level in the period leading up to the pandemic. Bilateral tests were conducted to establish the differences in frequency before and during the epidemic. Pearson correlations were chosen to establish the differences between urban and rural milieus.[3]

NATURAL HISTORY OF SPANISH INFLUENZA IN QUEBEC

We do not know exactly where or when the Spanish flu entered Canada.[4] According to health department publications, a first wave of influenza arrived on 15 September 1918.[5] It travelled from east to west via all means of communication. An estimate published in 1919 by the SBHPQ asserts that 530,704 Quebecers contracted the illness during the autumn of 1918 and that 13,880 died.[6] Here, as elsewhere, influenza was particularly prevalent in young adults and caused a high incidence of pneumonia in affected patients. Nevertheless, the underreporting of cases and the inaccurate classification of cause of death suggest that the number of mortalities was higher than reported. Provincial officials observed the following: "We are convinced that the deaths caused by this disastrous illness [Spanish influenza] were considerably higher than that [13,880] because the deaths from pneumonia, bronchial pneumonia, congestion of the lungs, meningitis, convulsions etc. are much more frequent in 1918 than in the preceding years."[7]

Quebec does not appear to have experienced the notable spring 1919 wave that affected other parts of Canada. However, in certain regions of the province, a second wave of the epidemic, much less virulent than the previous one, occurred during the early months of 1920.[8] The SBHPQ annual report for 1920 states, "We have had another epidemic of influenza this year (February, March, April 1920) although it has been less severe than that of 1918." During this wave, 9,346 Quebeckers contracted the disease, and 1,855 died.[9]

THE 1918 WAVE: THE VIRUS ADVANCES

The first manifestation of Spanish influenza in Quebec, in late spring 1918, affected military personnel exclusively.[10] Only on 8 September 1918 was the virus reported in the civil population at the College of Victoriaville, in the county of Arthabaska, where twelve professors and 398 students (of 410) fell ill.[11] Two weeks after the college was quarantined, on 23 September 1918, *Le Devoir* printed its first coverage of the Quebec epidemic, relaying statistics from the Quebec City morgue that nine sailors had died in the port of Quebec, apparently of influenza. The next day, the paper published an article presenting the spread of the epidemic in the province. The disease moved rapidly, and the colleges of Arthabaska, Nicolet, and Trois-Rivières were closed. Quebec City noted its first civilian mortality, which occurred on 25 September 1918: "Spanish influenza which has ravaged the region of Quebec for several days appeared yesterday in the population of our city. The first case reported to the authorities occurred at Hôtel-Dieu, and the victim, a young man, died yesterday evening. It has been reported that the nun who treated him is now ill and in danger. Four other cases have broken out in families of the Belvedere neighbourhood."[12]

On 25 September, military authorities ordered that the soldiers in the St-Jean barracks in St-Jean City be quarantined. *Le Devoir* stated that "Major General Wilson declared yesterday that there were actually 355 patients among the 2,500 soldiers in the base."[13] On 26 September 1918, influenza appeared simultaneously at the Sherbrooke Seminary and the Montreal Seminary. *Le Devoir*'s headline read, "First Cases in Montreal: Spanish Influenza Sends Five Victims to the General Hospital."[14] On 30 September, the flu appeared for the first time in the military barracks of Montreal, and the epidemic intensified at the St-Jean barracks. On 1 October, it reached the county of Frontenac: "We hear from St-Sebastian, in the county of Frontenac, that the terrible illness has just appeared in several families."[15] Then, on 3 October, it spread into the Eastern Townships.[16]

The first weeks of the epidemic reveal a relatively slow but constant development. Cases identified at the beginning of July among military personnel coming from England, as well as the presence of the virus on ships in the port of Quebec, are without doubt the principal vectors that ignited the Quebec pandemic. In addition, because of the sudden appearance of the illness, demobilized soldiers who showed symptoms after returning home were often sent to public hospitals, where they infected the civilian population.[17] Thereafter, the phenomenon was amplified by the closing of the College of Victoriaville and the return of its students to their families at the end of September.[18] This explains the particularly high incidence of influenza cases in Arthabaska County. Thereafter, events accelerated and in less than one week, the largest cities of the province were infected: Montreal, Quebec City, Sherbrooke, and Trois-Rivières. During the following days, nearby cities and villages would in turn be stricken.

On 15 October 1918, *Le Devoir* published a table showing the "march of the illness" since 1 October.[19] Next day, the paper stated that "thirty municipalities have been infected by the epidemic and that deaths have already been recorded for several days."[20] Then, on 17 October, it noted that fifty-five municipalities had reported cases of the illness. This edition of the paper clearly indicated "that there is not a municipality in the province which has not been infected with influenza."[21]

THE 1918 WAVE: THE VIRUS RETREATS

The retreat of the epidemic is more difficult to describe. The statement of Dr. Séraphin Boucher, director of the Montreal Department of Health, reported by *Le Devoir* on 13 November 1918, tells the story: "I have always said ... that the epidemic would not cease abruptly and that there would be variations, certain days, in the number of deaths."[22] When one attempts to analyze the diminishment of the epidemic at the city and municipal level, establishing its precise dates of retreat becomes difficult. However, the SBHPQ affirmed that the flu continued to rage until at least 18 December 1918.

The information taken from *Le Devoir* allows us to identify two indicators of the pandemic's retreat in the various parts of the province: namely, the absence of new flu deaths and the lifting of the emergency measures imposed by the SBHPQ. In fact, the cities and municipalities that were first attacked by the disease were also the first to see it disappear. In the case of Montreal, we know that on 23 November 1918, the city's last emergency hospital, so designated by the SBHPQ, closed its doors. This occurred a few days after the repeal of the restrictions imposed on the city.

THE 1920 WAVE: EMERGENCE AND RETREAT

In Quebec, the flu did not reappear in any significant way until early 1920. The first mention in *Le Devoir* of a new epidemic in the United States (in Chicago and the Great Lakes region) dates from 21 January of that year.[23] A few days later, the paper stated that the virus had arrived in Montreal: "Yesterday doctors reported eight cases of influenza, most with complications of pneumonia and bronchial pneumonia: two persons died of the latter illness yesterday."[24] Nonetheless, it had not yet reached epidemic proportions.[25]

Even so, the direct link between influenza, pneumonia, and bronchial pneumonia confirms the presence of an abnormal situation in the metropolis; *Le Devoir* of 29 January 1920 noted that thirty people had died from pneumonia between 20 and 27 January.[26] Only on 4 February did the provincial health authorities confirm that Montreal was affected by influenza: "The city of Montreal is alone in suffering from a wave of influenza which came to us from the United States."[27] By 11 February, Montreal hospitals were overwhelmed, and twelve municipalities had reported cases of the flu.[28] During the next few days, eight other municipalities followed suit. By 13 February, the situation in Montreal had been declared an epidemic.[29] Despite this fact, the spread of the virus was relatively less severe than in the fall of 1918, and the number of affected municipalities remained low. According to the SBHPQ, some 251 municipalities reported signs of the disease. By the beginning of March, conditions had improved in Quebec City and Montreal, and our sources clearly indicate that the epidemic was progressively reaching an end as of 15 March 1920.

COMPARATIVE ANALYSIS OF INFLUENZA IN 1915 TO 1917 VERSUS 1918 AND 1920

The influenza pandemic attacked the province of Quebec on two occasions. The first serious incursion occurred between September and December

1918 and the second between February and April 1920. We undertook
bilateral tests to establish the differences between influenza deaths before and during the epidemic. The following pairs of variables were
compared:

1 Death caused by influenza (DCI) in 1918 with the average DCI score
  of 1915 to 1917
2 DCI in 1920 with the average DCI score of 1915 to 1917
3 DCI in 1918 with DCI in 1920
4 Death caused by influenza, pneumonia, and bronchial pneumonia
  (DCI, P, and BP) in 1918 with the average DCI, P, and BP score of
  1915 to 1917
5 DCI, P, and BP in 1920 with the average DCI, P, and BP score of 1915
  to 1917
6 DCI, P, and BP in 1918 with the average DCI, P, and BP score of 1920
7 DCI in 1915 with DCI in 1916
8 DCI in 1915 with DCI in 1917.

Table 6.1 presents the results obtained.

As we can see, pairs 1 to 6 lie outside the 95 percent confidence interval,
which confirms that they are distinct from each other for all the periods

TABLE 6.1

Results for the comparison of means

Pairs	Mean	Standard deviations (σ)	Standard error	Lower tail	Upper tail	T	Degrees of freedom	Sig. (bilateral)
1	-187.03	409.52	49.30	-285.41	-88.66	-3.79	68	.000
2	-17.70	45.64	5.49	-28.66	-6.74	-3.22	68	.002
3	169.33	365.53	44.01	81.52	257.14	3.89	68	.000
4	-204.19	506.77	61.01	-325.93	-82.45	-3.35	68	.001
5	-33.74	96.60	11.63	-56.95	-10.54	-2.90	68	.005
6	170.45	412.78	49.69	71.29	269.61	3.43	68	.001
7	-8.04	16.30	1.96	-11.96	-4.13	-4.10	68	.000
8	-1.12	4.96	0.60	-2.31	.08	-1.87	68	.066

(Difference between pairs; 95% confidence interval)

analyzed. In addition, the years 1915, 1916, and 1917 are similar, but they differ from 1918 and 1920. This means that the periods of the epidemic depart significantly from random expectation. We employed the analysis of pairs 7 and 8 to analyze the 1918 and 1920 influenza waves (see Appendices A and B).

SOCIODEMOGRAPHIC ANALYSIS OF THE 1918 WAVE

The autumn 1918 wave of influenza had a devastating impact on Quebec. It struck with phenomenal swiftness, and according to Dr. Boucher was one of the "most serious epidemics ever noted in the history of Montreal."[30]

The international literature clearly reveals the sociodemographic aspects of Spanish influenza: the epidemic was especially associated with young men at their peak (aged twenty to forty), and it concentrated in densely populated areas. It would therefore be interesting to know whether these characteristics occur in the data relating to Quebec. Of the 8,888 Quebec males who died of flu-related disease in 1918, 6,812 (or 76.6 percent) succumbed to flu alone. The figure for females is similar: of the 8,427 who died, 6,638 did so of flu alone (78.7 percent). This pattern repeats itself for deaths caused by pneumonia and bronchial pneumonia: mortality for males totalled 2,076 (23.3 percent) and 1,789 for females (21.2 percent). In addition, deaths for twenty- to thirty-four-year-olds represented 39.72 percent of flu deaths and 14.84 percent of those caused by the related illnesses pneumonia and bronchial pneumonia.

Table 6.2 shows the number of deaths from Spanish influenza, pneumonia, and bronchial pneumonia by age group.[31] These results allow us to say that the analysis of deaths by age group is similar to what we find in the literature. However, the very slight variation in the differing rates of mortality by sex does not permit us to conclude that more males died than females.

Population density and whether one lives in an urban or a rural milieu are indicators of contact between individuals. Close proximity can favour the dissemination of a virus and increase its incidence in urban counties or wherever population density is high. The correlations obtained suggest that population density was a pertinent variable relative to the diffusion of the virus (see Table 6.3).

However, if the data for the city of Montreal are subtracted from the analysis, the association between the variables is considerably reduced. This is difficult to analyze. Ideally, our analysis should have included the

TABLE 6.2

Deaths according to age and cause, Quebec 1918

Age at death	Influenza	Pneumonia	Bronchial pneumonia	Total
0-4	2,672	402	1,510	4,584
5-19	2,387	236	102	2,725
20-34	5,378	476	98	5,952
35-44	1,145	205	33	1,383
45-59	672	224	31	927
60 and older	617	424	92	1,133
Unknown	668	27	8	703
Total	13,539	1,994	1,874	17,407

TABLE 6.3

Pearson's correlations for influenza mortality based on population density and environment, Quebec 1918

		Measured correlation	
		Including Montreal	Excluding Montreal
Population density		0.456[a]	0.281[b]
Environment	Urban	0.479[a]	0.711[a]
	Rural	0.311[b]	0.376[a]

Notes: a   significant at $\alpha = 0.01$
       b   significant at $\alpha = 0.05$

spatial organization related to population density, but we do not have that information. On the other hand, we know that more than a quarter of Quebec's population (26.2 percent) lived in Montreal. Table 6.4 presents the data for Montreal and compares these data with those for the province as a whole. The table reveals that the incidence of recorded influenza cases was low in Montreal but that the city nonetheless experienced a death rate proportional to its population. Four scenarios might help to account for these results. First, Montreal may have had a younger population than the rest of the province, which would explain why its death rate was higher than its number of cases would lead us to expect: the virus most significantly targeted persons between the ages of twenty and thirty-four. Second,

TABLE 6.4

Population and epidemiological data for influenza: Montreal compared
with Quebec, 1918

	Montreal (%)	Quebec (province)
Population	589,186 (26.2)	2,248,684
Population density	8,546.36 inhabitants per km	13.72 inhabitants per km
Morbidity	19,613 (4.84)	404,940
Deaths	3,566 (26.34)	13,539

the data could be biased by an underreporting of influenza cases despite
the obligatory declarations imposed by the SBHPQ. Third, infected individuals from other regions of the province may have come to Montreal,
where they died in hospital, which could create an apparent over-mortality.
Fourth, it is possible that the anti-epidemic measures established by the
SBHPQ were effective and diminished the spread and incidence of the
flu. Finally, the evidence demonstrates that Montreal was an important
port of entry for the disease on the North American continent.

INCIDENCE AND MORTALITY OF INFLUENZA BY COUNTY

According to the SBHPQ data, the 1918 wave of influenza produced
404,940 new cases and killed 13,539 people. The diffusion of cases and
deaths varied little throughout most of the sixty-nine provincial counties.
Indeed, in the majority of counties, total morbidity and mortality were
below the provincial average. This situation suggests that certain places
significantly influenced the portrait of the epidemic in Quebec. As we can
notice, frequency of infection was higher in urban districts than in rural
areas. However, it is true that the counties of Arthabaska and Lac St-Jean
had an elevated incidence of the disease and that the death rate was also
high in Sherbrooke, Hull, and Arthabaska Counties.

Counties with the lowest incidences of flu morbidity and mortality were
situated around the Island of Montreal and along the Canada-US border.
Likewise, Brome, Iberville, and Napierville, located on the South Shore
of the St. Lawrence River near the American border, seem to have largely
escaped the impact of influenza. This suggests that the less urban counties
and the agricultural ones were spared, relatively speaking, from the
epidemic.

It is interesting to add to these statistics the mortality caused by pulmonary complications (pneumonia and bronchial pneumonia): 17,407 deaths, or 3,868 more than from influenza alone. This considerable increase in mortality does not lead to a variation in the influenza diffusion level throughout the province. Counties with the highest death rate were Montreal, Quebec City, Jacques-Cartier, and Hull (Ottawa). This is not surprising, because these counties were the most populated in 1918. On the other hand, morbidity and mortality patterns in Sherbrooke, Nicolet, and Arthabaska Counties were peculiar. These three counties form an aggregate that seemed to favour emergence of the virus and higher-than-average mortality.

The provincial rates of incidence and mortality were respectively 1,800.79 and 60.21 per 10,000 inhabitants. Next highest was Montreal, with an incidence rate of 332.88 per 10,000 and a mortality rate that was comparable to the provincial total. Even some of the densely inhabited counties such as Jacques-Cartier and Quebec City had a lower mortality rate than the province itself (Table 6.5). However, the counties localized at the periphery of Arthabaska show rates of incidence and mortality higher than the provincial average (Table 6.6).

We have standardized the incidence and mortality rates for the 1918 influenza wave and calculated the chi-square at the 95 percent confidence interval associated with the statistical significance of the difference. As shown in Table 6.7, the rates obtained for the incidence, the mortality, and the ensemble of standardized rates are significant.

The results obtained correspond with the raw data for cases and deaths. Only two counties – Montreal and Lotbinière – differ from the others. Montreal experienced 19,613 influenza cases during the 1918 epidemic. The standardization of cases shows that the city should have declared about

TABLE 6.5

Influenza mortality and incidence rates per 10,000 inhabitants in the most populated cities and counties, Quebec 1918

Cities and counties	Mortality rate	Incidence rate
Hull (Ottawa)	72.51	2,086.86
Jacques-Cartier	50.73	1,433.55
Montreal	60.52	332.88
Quebec City	49.97	2,757.65
Province	60.21	1,800.79

TABLE 6.6

Influenza mortality and incidence rates per 10,000 inhabitants on the periphery of Arthabaska County, 1918

Cities and counties	Mortality rate	Incidence rate
Arthabaska	136.49	6,098.29
Bagot	79.18	4,488.82
Drummond	101.46	3,108.87
Nicolet	114.57	3,426.80
Richmond	101.26	3,222.78
Sherbrooke	112.85	3,912.00
Wolfe	102.22	3,443.26
Yamaska	97.12	4,809.84
Province	60.21	1,800.79

TABLE 6.7

Chi-square calculated for influenza, Quebec 1918

SIR standardized incidence rate	189,614.45[a]
SMR standardized mortality rate	1,598.11[a]
SMR global	1,531.96[a]

a Significant at α = 0.01

4.5 times this number, for a total of 88,258. However, this low incidence rate was not accompanied by low mortality. It is therefore possible to say that, compared to the province, Montreal had an underreporting of flu cases or an over-mortality. As discussed earlier, this phenomenon can be explained in several ways: Montreal's death rate may have been inflated by people from other counties, or it may be attributable to the youth of its population. The low morbidity could result from efficient emergency services required by the SBHPQ. Like those for Montreal, the statistics for Lotbinière depart from pattern. This county registered 8,434 cases, more than 2.25 times higher than the expected number. Nevertheless, the excessive incidence is not reflected in the statistics for mortality.

The standardization indicates a low incidence of cases and deaths for counties with larger populations. However, counties situated between Montreal and Quebec City on the South Shore show the most extreme standardized rates in the province (see Table 6.8).

Table 6.8

Counties with high standardized incidence and mortality, South Shore of the St. Lawrence River, Quebec 1918

Counties	Number of cases	SIR	Number of deaths	SMR
Arthabaska	14,431	3.39	346	2.27
Bagot	7,710	2.49	161	1.32
Drummond	5,914	1.73	228	1.69
Nicolet	9,631	1.90	377	1.90
Richmond	7,288	1,79	250	1.68
Sherbrooke	11,682	2.17	394	1.87
Wolfe	5,962	1.91	183	1.70
Yamaska	8,271	2.67	180	1.61

The results obtained by calculating lethality differ from the preceding statistics. The counties on the South Shore of the St. Lawrence have a lethality equal to or lower than that of Quebec as a whole, where the value is 3.34 deaths per 100 people. These counties are not alone in dropping below the Quebec average, for only fourteen counties have a higher lethality rate than the province itself. Montreal, with a lethality rate of 18.18 percent, certainly influences the provincial average for this measurement. Global lethality (influenza, pneumonia, and bronchial pneumonia) does not provide a more precise explanation of the lethality statistics in spite of the fact that it increases to 4.3 percent. Including all the causes of mortality increases lethality in Montreal: to 28.10 percent. This perspective again presents a situation where the data for Montreal and those for the province itself differ markedly from each other.

At 3.3 percent deaths for recorded cases, influenza lethality was well above the 0.1 percent engendered by epidemics today, but this death rate was not high compared to other epidemic diseases of the early twentieth century.[32] If we include deaths caused by pneumonia and bronchial pneumonia, the lethality, province-wide, was 4.3 percent. These rates, although high, do not compare with those for Montreal. Indeed, for every five Montrealers who contracted the flu, about one died; if we include pneumonia and bronchial pneumonia, this figure rises to about one in three. Even taking into account the unexpectedly low number of reported cases for Montreal, the data suggest the city's experience differed from that of most other communities in the province.

SOCIODEMOGRAPHIC ANALYSIS OF THE 1920 WAVE

The second wave of the pandemic appeared in Quebec between February and April 1920. However, its diffusion was limited and its strength was not comparable to that of 1918. Indeed, according to SBHPQ data, this wave resulted in only 9,346 influenza cases and 1,855 deaths – 5,646 deaths if we include those caused by pneumonia and bronchial pneumonia. Interestingly, mortality outnumbered incidence in thirty-one of the sixty-nine provincial counties, ten of which reported no cases at all. In all likelihood, the low incidence figure is caused by underreporting of nonfatal cases. This leads to an epidemiological portrait that is both unrepresentative and difficult to describe.

The international literature suggests that the sociodemographic characteristics of the 1920 influenza wave are similar to those of 1918: most victims were men between the ages of twenty and thirty-five. Only the development of the illness in crowded areas is different. According to the SBHPQ statistics, 48.5 percent of those who died from influenza were male, a figure that rises to 51.5 percent when pneumonia and bronchial pneumonia are taken into account. Thus, Quebec's 1920 death rate for males differs very little from that for females. In addition, 24 percent of Quebeckers who died from influenza were between the ages of twenty and thirty-four. When pneumonia and bronchial pneumonia are included, this figure increases to 34 percent. These results are ambiguous, and we cannot confirm that the 1920 wave follows the morbidity pattern described in the literature. Two elements add difficulty to the interpretation of these data. The first is an elevated mortality rate for bronchial pneumonia among those who were five years old and younger. Indeed, about 29 percent of the total deaths reported in the province fall into this category. The second element concerns the ensemble of deaths caused by pneumonia and bronchial pneumonia. Unlike in 1918, mortalities due to these related diseases far outnumbered those caused by influenza alone and represent 67.14 percent of the deaths in 1920. This proportion differs totally from that of 1918, in which 22.23 percent of deaths were caused by pneumonia and bronchial pneumonia. Because of this, we suggest that the analysis of 1920 flu cases should not include data for deaths from pneumonia and bronchial pneumonia.

As in 1918, population density seems to be a pertinent variable in the diffusion of Spanish influenza. Again, if we remove the statistics for Montreal, we see a diminution of the association between the variables.

These results suggest that the factors mentioned for the 1918 wave had an impact on the emergence of flu cases in Montreal.

MORTALITY ASSOCIATED WITH INFLUENZA IN 1920

The epidemiological portrait of Spanish influenza in 1920 is less complete than that of 1918 because it is impossible to analyze all epidemiological parameters related to the incidence of cases. Thus, we are limited to using mortality to outline the epidemiological portrait for 1920.

As in 1918, the most populated and urbanized counties come to the fore in the analysis of influenza in 1920. However, we notice that counties with the highest or slightly above-average mortality were the least seriously affected by the 1918 pandemic. This phenomenon is more evident when we consider the rate of mortality. It is also interesting that Arthabaska, Nicolet, and Sherbrooke Counties were all spared by the 1920 wave. With reference to the analysis of standardized mortality rates, these add no new elements to the analysis of influenza in 1920, even though they are statistically significant. Nevertheless, they allow us to confirm that counties where the mortality rate was higher than the median were those spared by the 1918 wave.

FLU IN 1918 AND 1920 COMPARED TO ITS INCIDENCE IN 1915-17

A comparative analysis of flu-related deaths from 1915 to 1917 with those from 1918 and 1920 reveals that the latter produced respectively 21.37 and 2.93 times more mortalities than the former. Therefore, taking into consideration the average number of flu deaths for pre-epidemic years, which reported an average of 630 per year, we can see that the high incidence of death in 1918 is for the most part transformed into a moderate or low incidence in 1920. We need to remember that influenza was not a reportable illness before 1918. Thus, the statistics for that period do not provide us with a means of measuring actual flu morbidity. This problem persists in some of the statistics from 1918.

The most surprising point concerns deaths caused by pneumonia and bronchial pneumonia: the mortality rate attributable to these diseases during the epidemic years differs very little from the average for 1915-17. Certainly, we have noted that such cases rose abnormally in 1920, but they do not appear to be related to the epidemic landscape of Spanish influenza in Quebec.

IDIOSYNCRASIES OF THE SBHPQ DATA

As mentioned above, our epidemiological data come from the SBHPQ, an official organization that claimed to have been apprised of 530,704 influenza cases and 13,880 deaths. Nevertheless, our per county tabulation of the incidence and mortality rates given in the same data does not confirm these figures. In fact, we have been unable to retrace the number of cases mentioned by the SBHPQ. Rather, we found that cases totalled 404,940 and that mortality, at 13,539, was slightly lower than the SBHPQ figure. Our chi-square tests confirmed that the difference is not significant for the total number of deaths (8.38) but that it is significant for the number of cases (29.82). The finding of such a large difference is odd and cannot be explained in an epidemiological analysis such as this one. However, we suggest that the number of cases mentioned in the official publications of 1918 and even 1919 was based on a global estimate and approximated the values obtained from preliminary SBHPQ reports. We think that, there-after, these values were preferred to the correct data, which were obtained only after the epidemic had ended, leaving the truth of the epidemiological portrait to be forgotten over time. With regard to the non-significant dif-ference of 341 deaths, we suspect that, during the epidemic, mortality was more accurately recorded than morbidity and thus that the preliminary portrait was truer to reality.

DISCUSSION AND CONCLUSION

Data analysis enables us to affirm that the increase in Spanish influenza deaths was not coincidental and that the pandemic struck with as much severity in Quebec as elsewhere in the world. The exceptional pathogenic power of the 1918 virus was a factor in the diffusion of the illness, which killed large numbers of people. Moving from the eastern part of the province via military installations and transportation routes, it initially attacked military personnel and educational establishments before spread-ing throughout the civilian population. We tend to agree with Mark Humphries, who wrote that "the disease was not deliberately spread by the Canadian military, but the movements of the soldiers were intentional, calculated movements designed to further the war effort."[33]

It is important to remember that the SBHPQ statistics were obtained during a time of crisis. Numerous biases can be found in the health statistics compiled throughout this period. For example, some counties under-reported their flu cases in 1920, with the result that mortality apparently outstripped morbidity (see Appendix B).

The impact of the 1918 wave was considerable: 404,940 cases and 13,539 deaths for an impressive lethality of 3.34 percent and a mortality 21.37 times greater than that of the pre-epidemic period, which reported an average of 630 flu deaths per year. It is important to keep in mind that the epidemiological data published by the SBHPQ during the 1918 epidemic differ from those published post-epidemic. The former claimed 530,704 new cases and 13,880 deaths. Regardless, the 1918 wave was without a doubt more serious than that of 1920. In 1918, almost all the province's 1,158 municipalities reported having contact with the virus, whereas only 251 did so in 1920. The 1920 wave killed 1,855 people and resulted in 9,346 cases of influenza, for a mortality rate 2.93 times greater than the average for flu deaths registered from 1915 to 1917. Less severe than the preceding wave, the 1920 epidemic has also been much less thoroughly documented. Therefore, constructing its geographical and epidemiological portrait is challenging.

This analysis allows us to affirm that the locales hardest hit during 1918 were spared in 1920 and that the pattern of diffusion was about the same for both waves. Mortality was most severe in urban centres, Montreal in particular. Flu mortality in Quebec was unusual in two ways: unlike in the rest of the world, sex was not a pertinent variable, and the low incidence of diseases related to the flu (pneumonia and bronchial pneumonia) does not seem to have modified the epidemiologic profile of the pandemic.[34]

Although the circumstances of the Spanish influenza pandemic differ from those of contemporary viruses such as H1N1, a comparison of the two can be an essential tool for understanding the epidemiology of pandemic influenza. In fact, the historical data can assist us in developing contemporary methodologies and policies for prevention in the field of modern public health.

NOTES

1 Alfred W. Crosby, *America's Forgotten Pandemic: The Influenza of 1918* (Cambridge: Cambridge University Press, 1989); J.K. Taubenberger, A.H. Reid, and T.G. Fanning, "Le virus retrouvé de la grippe espagnole," *Dossier pour la science* 50 (2006): 52-59; and M.T. Osterholm, "Preparing for the Next Pandemic," *Foreign Affairs* 84,4 (2005): 24-37.

2 J.-Y. Gravel, *Le Québec et la guerre, 1867-1960* (Montreal: Éditions du Boréal Express, 1974), 57.

3 We used SPSS (Statistical Package for Social Science) "Crosstabulation" to analyze in a tabular format the relationship between two or more categorical variables. This program can also be used with continuous data, but only if such data are divided into separate categories. The purpose of a chi-square (x^2) test of independence is to determine whether the observed values (O) for cells deviate significantly from the corresponding expected values (E) for those cells. If there is a large discrepancy between the observed and the expected values, the chi-square will be large, suggesting a significant difference between O and E values. The significance (or p value) represents the likelihood that a certain result will occur by chance. A significance of less than .05 (p<.05) means that there is less than a 5 percent probability that this relationship occurred by chance. We used a bilateral test when we had little idea of the direction of the correlation. If, however, we had prior expectations about the direction of correlations (positive or negative), the statistic for one-tailed significance was used. A correlation is frequently called the "Pearson product-moment correlation." With the SPSS "Correlation," Pearson r is selected by default if the data are approximately normally distributed. See G. Darren and P. Mallery, *SPSS for Windows Step by Step*, 8th ed. (Boston: Allyn and Bacon, 2008).

4 Eileen Pettigrew, *The Silent Enemy: Canada and the Deadly Flu of 1918* (Saskatoon: Western Producer Prairie Books, 1983).

5 E. Pelletier, *Vingt-cinquième rapport annuel du Conseil Supérieur d'Hygiène de la province de Québec* (Quebec City: E.E. Cinq-Mars, 1919).

6 Ibid., 32.

7 Ibid., 162.

8 Pettigrew, *Silent Enemy.*

9 E. Pelletier, *Vingt-sixième rapport annuel du Conseil Supérieur d'Hygiène de la province de Québec* (Quebec City: Ls-A. Proulx, 1920), 47.

10 Andrew MacPhail, *Official History of the Canadian Forces in the Great War, 1914-19: The Medical Services* (Ottawa: Department of National Defence, 1925).

11 Pettigrew, *Silent Enemy.*

12 "La grippe espagnole est à Québec," *Le Devoir* (Montreal), 26 September 1918, 3. All quotations from *Le Devoir* have been translated into English by the authors.

13 "Précautions nécessaires," *Le Devoir* (Montreal), 26 September 1918, 4.

14 "Premiers cas à Montréal," *Le Devoir* (Montreal), 27 September 1918, 2.

15 "La situation à Saint-Jean," *Le Devoir* (Montreal), 1 October 1918, 4.

16 "Ravages de l'influenza dans les Cantons de l'Est," *Le Devoir* (Montreal), 3 October 1918, 3.

17 Soldiers were treated in military hospitals if they contracted influenza before they were demobilized. After demobilization, they returned to civilian life and were treated in public hospitals for all health conditions. Pettigrew, *Silent Enemy.*

18 "L'influenza à Victoriaville," *Le Devoir* (Montreal), 23 September 1918, 6.

19 "Le Bilan des Mortalités," *Le Devoir* (Montreal), 15 October 1918, 5.

20 "Nouvelles mesures pour combattre le fléau," *Le Devoir* (Montreal), 16 October 1918, 4.

21 "L'épidémie reste à l'état stationnaire," *Le Devoir* (Montreal), 17 October 1918, 4.

22 Quoted in "Opinion du Dr Boucher," *Le Devoir* (Montreal), 13 November 1918, 6.

23 "Plus de victimes que l'an dernier," *Le Devoir* (Montreal), 21 January 1920, 7.

24 "La grippe s'implante lentement," *Le Devoir* (Montreal), 30 January 1920, 3.

25 "Les victimes de la grippe," *Le Devoir* (Montreal), 29 January 1920, 4.

26 Ibid.

27 "Il n'y a de mal qu'ici," *Le Devoir* (Montreal), 4 February 1920, 8.

28 "Les victimes de la grippe," *Le Devoir* (Montreal), 11 February 1920, 4.

29 "L'épidémie est légère," *Le Devoir* (Montreal), 13 February 1920, 3.

30 *Rapport du Service de Santé de la Cité de Montréal 1918.*

31 Although Table 6.2 shows 17,407 males and females who died of flu, pneumonia, and bronchial pneumonia, we related gender to only 17,315 deaths. Thus, 92 deaths from flu, pneumonia, and bronchial pneumonia were not related to gender.

32 Y.-M. Loo and M. Gale, "Fatal Immunity and the 1918 Virus," *Nature* 445,7125 (18 January 2007): 267-68.

33 Mark Osborne Humphries, "The Horror at Home: The Canadian Military and the 'Great' Influenza Pandemic of 1918," *Journal of the Canadian Historical Association*, n.s., 16,1 (2005): 254.

34 Crosby, *America's Forgotten Pandemic;* and Barry, *The Great Influenza.*

TABLE 6.9: APPENDIX A

Statistics used to analyze influenza, Quebec 1918

Counties	New cases of influenza	Deaths due to influenza	Deaths due to influenza, pneumonia, and bronchial pneumonia	Influenza per 1,000 inhabitants		SMR	SIR
				Mortality rate	Incidence rate		
Argenteuil	1,929	35	49	21.41	1,180.03	0.36	0.66
Arthabaska	14,431	323	346	136.49	6,098.29	2.27	0.39
Bagot	7,710	136	161	79.18	4,488.82	1.32	2.49
Beauce	10,377	129	158	33.61	2,703.26	0.56	1.50
Beauharnois	2,888	112	147	59.13	1,524.82	0.98	0.85
Bellechasse	4,658	138	170	66.43	2,242.23	1.10	1.25
Berthier	3,048	47	76	24.06	1,560.52	0.40	0.87
Bonaventure	2,878	72	86	25.99	1,038.76	0.43	0.58
Brome	1,158	29	40	22.76	908.73	0.38	0.50
Chambly	3,093	89	121	42.63	1,481.39	0.71	0.82
Champlain	10,412	308	366	59.68	2,017.48	0.99	1.12
Charlevoix	7,655	183	198	92.79	3,881.65	1.54	2.16
Châteauguay	1,525	53	75	41.05	1,881.16	0.68	0.66
Chicoutimi	10,559	236	258	65.95	2,950.51	1.10	1.64
Compton	3,812	112	131	51.08	1,738.58	0.85	0.97
Deux-Montagnes	1,930	61	82	44.76	1,416.31	0.74	0.79
Dorchester	6,202	114	134	44.68	2,431.01	0.74	1.35
Drummond	5,914	193	228	101.46	3,108.87	1.69	1.73
Frontenac	8,148	168	186	73.23	3,551.56	1.22	1.97
Gaspé	7,064	266	283	69.18	1,837.14	1.15	1.02
Hull (Ottawa)	10,936	380	456	72.51	2,086.86	1.20	1.16
Huntingdon	1,824	50	58	39.85	1,453.85	0.66	0.81
Iberville	970	23	35	25.97	1,095.30	0.43	0.61
Jacques-Cartier	8,477	300	433	50.73	1,433.55	0.84	0.80
Joliette	2,794	65	113	26.34	1,132.18	0.44	0.63
Kamouraska	3,527	81	125	38.64	1,682.33	0.64	0.93
Labelle	9,356	241	280	54.67	2,122.22	0.91	1.18
Lac St-Jean	14,076	232	244	68.55	4,158.84	1.14	2.31
Laprairie	1,810	91	104	79.16	1,574.46	1.31	0.87
L'Assomption	4,050	61	80	44.70	2,967.47	0.74	1.65
Laval	1,782	60	86	25.48	756.69	0.42	0.42
Lévis	8,918	202	263	63.65	2,810.15	1.06	1.56
L'Islet	3,777	102	132	59.97	2,220.72	1.00	1.23
Lotbinière	8,434	129	140	62.03	4,055.59	1.03	2.25
Maskinongé	2,677	75	108	48.45	1,729.44	0.80	0.96

▶

◀ TABLE 6.9: APPENDIX A

Counties	New cases of influenza	Deaths due to influenza	Deaths due to influenza, pneumonia, and bronchial pneumonia	Influenza per 1,000 inhabitants		SMR	SIR
				Mortality rate	Incidence rate		
Matane	6,305	211	234	61.03	1,823.68	1.01	1.01
Mégantic	8,145	177	215	55.26	2,542.93	0.92	1.41
Missisquoi	3,711	75	93	44.47	2,200.42	0.74	1.22
Montcalm	2,555	118	127	88.58	1,918.02	1.47	1.07
Montmagny	5,295	49	83	23.39	2,527.57	0.39	1.40
Montmorency	5,087	119	125	89.21	3,813.34	1.48	2.12
Montreal (city)	19,613	3,566	5,503	60.52	332.88	1.01	0.18
Napierville	1,080	31	47	40.72	1,418.63	0.68	0.79
Nicolet	9,691	324	377	114.57	3,426.80	1.90	1.90
Pontiac	2,955	83	99	43.58	1,551.67	0.72	0.86
Portneuf	10,112	236	278	75.19	3,221.51	1.25	1.79
Quebec City	25,000	453	635	49.97	2,757.65	0.83	1.53
Quebec (county)	5,601	203	243	72.42	1,998.14	1.20	1.11
Richelieu	3,692	89	115	45.81	1,983.13	0.79	1.10
Richmond	7,288	229	250	101.26	3,222.78	1.68	1.79
Rimouski	2,977	125	140	47.69	1,137.87	0.79	0.63
Rouville	4,238	86	96	66.13	3,258.75	1.10	1.81
Saguenay	4,009	168	170	100.85	2,406.65	1.68	1.34
Shefford	3,917	101	119	41.21	1,598.25	0.68	0.89
Sherbrooke	11,682	337	394	112.85	3,912.00	1.87	2.17
Soulanges	2,145	67	79	69.90	2,237.87	1.16	1.24
Standstead	3,922	135	143	60.63	1,761.43	1.01	0.98
St-Hyacinthe	3,115	188	203	85.47	1,416.10	1.24	0.79
St-Jean	2,930	60	79	44.31	2,163.80	0.74	1.20
St-Maurice	8,262	262	287	96.60	3,046.35	1.60	1.69
Témiscamingue	4,421	124	131	49.69	1,771.59	0.83	0.98
Témiscouata	9,144	251	285	50.48	2,166.88	0.99	1.20
Terrebonne	3,847	123	152	38.09	1,191.32	0.63	0.66
Trois-Rivières (city)	2,865	94	132	44.13	1,345.01	0.73	0.75
Vaudreuil	1,917	63	69	57.25	1,742.09	0.95	0.97
Verchères	3,505	63	77	52.01	2,893.59	0.86	1.61
Westmount (county)	2,882	89	112	28.56	924.76	0.47	0.51
Wolfe	5,962	177	183	102.22	3,443.26	1.70	1.91
Yamaska	8,271	167	180	97.12	4,809.84	1.61	2.67
Quebec (province)	404,940	13,539	17,407	60.21	1,800.79	1.00	1.00

TABLE 6.10: APPENDIX B

Statistics used to analyze influenza, Quebec 1920

Counties	New cases of influenza	Deaths due to influenza	Deaths due to influenza, pneumonia, and bronchial pneumonia	Influenza per 1,000 inhabitants		SMR	SIR
				Mortality rate	Incidence rate		
Argenteuil	70	4	27	2.37	41.45	0.30	1.03
Arthabaska	16	17	47	6.95	6.55	0.87	0.16
Bagot	39	8	30	4.51	21.98	0.56	0.55
Beauce	0	24	66	6.05	0	0.76	0
Beauharnois	10	12	48	6.13	5.11	0.77	0.13
Bellechasse	0	20	41	9.32	0	1.17	0
Berthier	64	24	62	11.90	31.72	1.49	0.79
Bonaventure	69	41	68	14.33	24.11	1.79	0.60
Brome	176	7	17	5.32	133.71	0.67	3.32
Chambly	173	11	48	5.10	80.22	0.64	1.99
Champlain	12	49	145	9.19	2.25	1.15	0.06
Charlevoix	573	52	65	25.53	281.28	3.20	6.99
Châteauguay	71	8	25	6.00	53.24	0.75	1.32
Chicoutimi	0	16	41	4.33	0	0.54	0
Compton	173	17	49	7.51	76.38	0.94	1.90
Deux-Montagnes	17	12	26	8.53	12.08	1.07	0.30
Dorchester	23	25	60	9.49	8.73	1.19	0.22
Drummond	104	14	30	7.12	52.93	0.89	1.32
Frontenac	0	18	42	7.60	0	0.95	0
Gaspé	107	48	83	12.09	26.94	0.51	0.67
Hull (Ottawa)	85	34	108	6.28	15.70	0.79	0.39
Huntingdon	55	11	29	8.49	42.44	1.06	1.05
Iberville	10	5	21	5.47	10.39	0.68	0.27
Jacques-Cartier	28	32	137	5.24	4.58	0.66	0.11
Joliette	2	30	88	11.77	0.78	1.47	0.02
Kamouraska	0	12	32	5.54	0	0.69	0
Labelle	19	26	69	5.71	4.17	0.71	0.10
Lac St-Jean	196	25	47	7.15	56.06	0.90	1.39
Laprairie	0	10	24	8.42	0	1.05	0
L'Assomption	3	10	34	7.09	2.13	0.89	0.05
Laval	71	9	32	3.70	29.19	0.46	0.73
Lévis	15	31	73	9.46	4.58	1.18	0.11
L'Islet	20	17	44	9.68	11.38	1.21	0.28
Lotbinière	15	17	47	7.91	6.98	0.99	0.17
Maskinongé	0	11	29	6.88	0	0.86	0

▶

◄ TABLE 6.10: APPENDIX B

Counties	New cases of influenza	Deaths due to influenza	Deaths due to influenza, pneumonia, and bronchial pneumonia	Influenza per 1,000 inhabitants		SMR	SIR
				Mortality rate	Incidence rate		
Matane	62	32	69	8.96	17.36	1.12	0.43
Mégantic	3	16	55	4.84	0.91	0.61	0.02
Missisquoi	5	14	23	8.04	2.87	1.01	0.07
Montcalm	12	9	24	6.54	2.72	0.82	0.27
Montmagny	127	30	83	13.86	58.69	1.74	1.46
Montmorency	40	9	16	6.53	29.03	0.82	0.72
Montreal (city)	4,364	490	2,032	8.05	71.70	1.01	1.78
Napierville	0	6	20	7.63	0	0.96	0
Nicolet	7	20	42	6.85	2.40	0.86	0.06
Pontiac	20	20	37	10.17	10.17	1.27	0.25
Portneuf	5	35	81	10.79	1.54	1.35	0.04
Quebec City	1,564	61	248	6.51	167.01	0.82	4.15
Quebec (county)	30	21	50	7.25	10.36	0.91	0.26
Richelieu	45	25	45	13.00	23.40	1.63	0.58
Richmond	3	7	40	3.00	1.28	0.38	0.03
Rimouski	184	37	72	13.67	67.97	1.71	1.69
Rouville	7	3	15	2.23	5.21	0.28	0.13
Saguenay	0	6	13	2.49	0	0.44	0
Shefford	37	19	60	5.51	14.62	0.94	0.36
Sherbrooke	50	23	81	7.46	16.21	0.93	0.40
Soulanges	63	10	16	10.10	63.63	1.26	1.58
Standstead	2	13	33	5.65	0.87	0.71	0.02
St-Hyacinthe	95	18	50	7.92	41.81	0.99	1.04
St-Jean	136	10	26	7.15	97.23	0.90	2.42
St-Maurice	7	19	72	8.78	2.50	0.85	0.06
Témiscamingue	8	21	37	8.15	3.10	1.02	0.08
Témiscouata	0	74	124	16.98	0	2.13	0
Terrebonne	91	35	103	10.49	27.28	1.31	0.68
Trois-Rivières (city)	10	12	82	5.45	4.54	0.68	0.11
Vaudreuil	14	13	18	11.44	12.32	1.43	0.31
Verchères	49	13	38	10.39	39.16	1.30	0.97
Westmount (county)	78	8	41	2.49	24.23	0.31	0.60
Wolfe	11	13	41	7.27	6.15	0.91	0.15
Yamaska	1	6	25	3.38	0.56	0.42	0.01
Quebec (province)	9,346	1,855	5,646	7.99	40.24	1.00	1.00

PART 3

Influenza and the Limits of Modernity

7

Flu Stories: Engaging with Disease, Death, and Modernity in British Columbia, 1918-19

MARY-ELLEN KELM

M y family has a flu story. My maternal grandmother, born in 1902, had five sisters and one brother, Donald. In the fall of 1918, the whole family was relieved that he had been spared the ordeal of the trenches. He was nineteen that year and surely would have been sent to Europe had the war not ended in November. But their relief was short-lived. Before the end of the year, Donald contracted the flu and died. The story concludes at the graveside with my great-grandmother observing that she had now joined the substantial ranks of those who knew the pain of burying a child.

My mother told this story to illustrate two interrelated points. The first was that relief could be fleeting – a son saved from war could be taken by disease. The second also had to do with a sense of reprieve withdrawn. In my great-grandmother's era, losing a child was all too common. This flu story was a way to say that one of the greatest gifts of modernity was the reduction in childhood mortality. But that promise was not to be fulfilled, at least not for my mother's grandmother. The 1918-19 flu demonstrated the limits of modernity, for there was little in modern medicine to stem its tide or save its victims. In the end, my family's story seemed to say, modernity would prevail but not before the flu had taken its terrible toll.

For much of the twentieth century, the broader tale of the 1918-19 flu epidemic lay untold. Alfred Crosby called it America's forgotten pandemic and suggested that the collective amnesia regarding it had to do with its universality and its lack of impact on institutions and organizations. Still, like my grandmother, people remembered the flu vividly.[1] Alan Swedlund, in a recent paper, explains this odd contradiction by arguing that the confidence in modernity made people see their losses as personal, and so they did not weave them into the larger optimism of Progressive Era America.[2] More recently, emerging infectious diseases such as SARS, Avian flu, and AIDS have prompted people to look again at the 1918-19 flu.[3] This resurgence of interest provides all the more reason to re-examine how people who experienced the flu made meaning out of the event.

In this chapter, I examine the surviving flu stories in British Columbia. I begin with contemporary newspaper accounts from six regions of the province. Two of the newspapers, the *Victoria Daily Times* and the *Vancouver Daily Sun,* were strong supporters of the Liberal Party, and a third, the *Vancouver Daily World,* was founded by J.J. McLagan, another Liberal supporter. These connections to the Liberal Party may account for the similarity of their coverage of the flu, but there was remarkable unanimity within the press, whatever its political party affiliations, on the effects of the flu and on its reportage. It becomes clear that newspapers carried two different flu stories simultaneously. There were official accounts that balanced fear of the disease with faith in medical modernity. Such articles tracked the geographic spread of the epidemic, then brought home the good work of public health authorities and volunteers to contain it, and finally pointed to other populations that suffered more from the illness. Usually, the press portrayed these populations – Aboriginal people, Mennonite farmers, and Chinese labourers – as insufficiently modern. Alongside this dominant narrative were individual accounts of sorrow and loss, published in lengthy obituaries and in the "about town" sections of small-town papers.

After surveying the newspapers, I delve into the flu stories that emerged from a series of interviews conducted with elderly Vancouver residents in the 1970s. Mostly from the immigrant, working-class neighbourhood of Strathcona, they experienced the flu in intensely personal ways. For them, community, rather than medicine, helped them survive the incredible debilitation of the disease. Modernity had a limited impact on their understandings of it.

Finally, I study the stories that one of these "other" populations told about the flu. Of the published BC accounts from this era, only First Nations writers emphasize the flu and its impact on their communities. Although this emphasis reflects the devastation that the virus inflicted on First Nations, who died at rates seven times that of the provincial average, I argue that talking about influenza was also a way of revealing the limits

of modernity and perhaps of incorporating the flu into other epistemologies of disease.[4]

Charles Rosenberg writes that epidemics are dramaturgic in form. They
have an identifiable beginning, proceed through a course of events that
are limited in space and time, mount in intensity toward personal and
collective crises, and are followed by denouement and closure.[5] The press
coverage of the flu in British Columbia follows this pattern, with some
revealing tendencies. The main story presented by all the newspapers is
one of anticipation and subsequent containment. The alarm is raised as
the flu is tracked in coverage picked up from Eastern Canada and the
United States. Then the wise and self-sacrificing labour of public health
officials, the action of government, and the efforts of volunteers take centre
stage as these actors work to contain the disease and its impact. Finally,
the drama comes to an end as life returns to normal, bans on public meetings are lifted, and an assessment is made of the effects of the flu. But the
enormous human cost cannot be ignored, and here another story emerges
simultaneously. Obituaries express the losses felt by individual families
and their communities. Press reports of the devastation in Aboriginal,
Doukhobor, Mennonite, or Chinese communities, who appear to have
slipped the bounds of containment, underscore the broader message of
the triumph of modern medicine over epidemic disease. There are slight
regional variations in these press narratives. Vancouver resisted a full ban
of public meetings for much of the epidemic, setting its chief medical
officer, Dr. Frederick Underhill, in opposition to provincial authorities
and other city health officers. Some small southern Interior towns, only
lightly affected, gave in to the rhetoric of boosterism, attributing their
escape to the benefits of the salubrious climate in British Columbia's still
sparsely settled dry belt. Writers in Prince Rupert, Fort George, and Grand
Forks paid more attention to what was happening in nearby settlements
and reserves, and so the contrast between their own experience of the flu
and those of their often less fortunate neighbours is a more prominent
feature of their reporting. But overall, the message of the press was one of
containment, where the wisdom of modern medicine and the work of
interventionist health authorities were successful in limiting the
devastation.

The story began, to follow that dramaturgic metaphor, offstage. BC newspapers started to run articles about the epidemic in Eastern Canada and in the United States in late September 1918. With headlines such as "Spanish Influenza Is Ravaging Camps" and "Alarm in US over Influenza," they emphasized anxiety and tragedy.[6] Vancouver papers stressed the flu's imminence, reporting on deaths at the Bremerton Naval Yard or the University of Washington in nearby Seattle. Recommendations for preventatives, including reports of "the power of cinnamon for cutting short the invasion of influenza poison," accompanied coverage of the flu's spread.[7] But though newspapers might run advertisements for "Week's Break-Up-A-Cold tablets," they expressed more considerable faith in the prudent action of public health authorities who in Quebec, Ontario, and nearby Seattle were closing shops, banning public meetings, and recruiting volunteers into apparently state-coordinated responses to the epidemic.[8]

As British Columbians braced for the flu, news stories praised the readiness of public health officials. Fred Underhill, Vancouver's first city health officer, sought to calm fears early in October by saying that there was only one case under observation in the city, but he cautioned the public not to underestimate the virus. In an article that was picked up by other BC newspapers, Underhill emphasized that everyone had a duty to stay well and, if ill with the flu, not to pass it on to others. He then issued a thirteen-point list of "dos and don'ts," arguing that if the work of health authorities were to be effective, the public must take precautions.[9] The headline, "Vancouver Ready to Fight Epidemic of Spanish Grippe," said it all.[10]

The provincial government weighed in, too. On 5 October, Cabinet passed an order-in-council to allow municipalities to close all places of public assembly. The *Vancouver Daily World* assured its readers that "there need be no panic. The health authorities are prepared, before the disease becomes epidemic to close all schools and public assembly places and do everything possible to curtail its spread."[11] Within days, the paper wrote that Victoria and surrounding municipalities had closed poolrooms, theatres, and other places of public assembly as the first cases of flu arrived at hospital; soon after that, Victoria closed its schools.[12] But Vancouver's city health officer, Underhill, did not agree with closure. He thought closing schools just put children on the street infecting each other, and he saw no point in curtailing business or the work of industry by a full-scale closure. In response to such strong leadership, Vancouver's press wrote, "When Spanish influenza came to Vancouver it did not have any easy walkover. It was met with a barrage of disinfectants; official regulations and advice; intelligent conferences on best methods of combating it; and a public at least partially informed on how to avoid and treat it. It was about last Friday that the first cases were definitely identified. Since then the disease has not secured by any means a strangle hold. It has not frightened the city as yet into closing any of its public institutions."[13] The press expressed its confidence in modern approaches to the management of epidemics.

Medical authorities offered a variety of solutions. Some, such as the use of masks, signalled the widespread acceptance of germ theory. Colonel C.E. Doherty of the Canadian Expeditionary Force ordered two thousand masks from the Red Cross to be used by medical workers "to prevent them inhaling the germs."[14] Not all medical authorities accepted that masks would prevent the spread of the virus. Victoria's medical health officer, Arthur G. Price, scoffed at their use; indeed, he thought them unsafe for the general public as they would "collect germs that otherwise would be escaped."[15] Others disagreed heartily, including a prominent member of the Imperial Order Daughters of the Empire, who claimed that people who would not use masks were not taking the flu seriously. Dr. M.T. MacEachern, superintendent of Vancouver General Hospital, similarly endorsed the use of masks, saying that they prevented the "germ-laden moisture of another's breath" from reaching the face. He also stressed that fingers as much as breath carried the disease and that masks would prevent people from touching their nose and mouth.[16] Discussing prevention in terms of shielding the public from germs gave the impression that medical men and prominent social leaders were working together to apply the knowledge of modern medicine, particularly germ theory, to the threat of influenza. Hope placed in modern scientific medicine went so far as to include shipping the monkeys from Vancouver's zoo to the University of Toronto for experimental work on influenza.[17]

But what constituted modern medicine was very much still in formation. Modernity in medicine was not so much occasioned by a massive paradigm shift as by an enfolding of older ideas into emergent ones. Older configurationist approaches that situated disease in the "interactive, contextual and often environmental" vied and sometimes merged with those emphasizing contamination, in which disease is spread by "the transmission of some morbid material from one individual to another."[18] Thus, Fred Underhill could upbraid women whose clothing made them vulnerable to flu, saying, "If women would wear longer skirts and higher blouses and so keep themselves warm, they would do a great deal to render themselves immune from influenza," at the same time as he issued very detailed instructions to prevent the contagious spread of the disease through careless spitting or shared handkerchiefs, food, or candy.[19] Similarly, Victoria's health officer, Arthur G. Price, questioned the use of chemical disinfectants and claimed that the best disinfectant was sunshine.[20] As the numbers of sick continued to rise, Price blamed the constant rain, since "germs thrive better in the damp atmosphere," but, he continued, there was cause for hope, since the city's mild climate was not conducive to the most virulent form of the disease.[21] By contrast, Underhill credited the rain for a short downturn in new cases during the same week of 12 October.[22] Interior cities, affected by the flu in early November, were optimistic that they would be spared the more serious varieties because of the "exceptional climatic conditions in the Okanagan."[23] Indeed, the small Okanagan town of Oyama could not resist using the language of boosterism as it appeared unscathed by the flu.[24] Though confident that modern medicine could understand and control the virus, health officers combined configurationist and contaminationist ways of thinking about disease and advocated measures, such as quarantine and the use of warm clothing, that were social and personal in their orientation.[25]

The promise of modernity – that human intervention could change the world in a positive way – extended beyond the work of public health officials; ordinary British Columbians had a role to play, too. So the press paid attention to the importance of sacrifice, particularly of volunteer time, in ending the epidemic. In a sense, the battle against the flu was an extension of the war in Europe, and not surprisingly, the language of war pervaded press coverage. Volunteers who helped keep a local pharmacy open during the pandemic were said to be "stepping into the breach," and one volunteer in Vancouver marked the crest of the epidemic there by saying that "we have gone over the top now."[26] Just as in the war, optimism was a duty. The press reported on the new temporary and emergency hospitals that were opening to meet the crisis and lauded the work of nurses and volunteers. The message was the same in every city and town in British Columbia: those who were suffering were not alone, there was no cause for panic, each city's citizens were doing all they could to care for the sick.

The military and local businesses donated space for emergency hospitals, and the press first called for and then praised the work of volunteers, particularly women.[27] In Prince Rupert, women were asked to give their time and any spare beds they might have at home to help with patients coming in from outlying districts.[28] Vancouver's superintendent of relief, G.D. Ireland, used the language of wartime, calling flu victims "casualties" and describing those who cared for them as offering "worthy service."[29]

Authorities used pre-existing networks of volunteerism, heightened during the war, to appeal to public-spirited women.[30] Newspapers praised women volunteers, in particular. The *Prince George Citizen* put it thus: "A roll of honor should be inscribed with the names of the self-sacrificing women of Prince George and vicinity, who are helping to care for the afflicted in the local hospitals. A number of men are also doing a noble part in the work. In the case of the women particular honor is due, as they have laid aside their own household duties to assist in the greater duty of caring for the afflicted ones."[31] The *Citizen* published the names of volunteers on 15 November 1918, a practice shared by other small-town newspapers such as the *Kamloops Telegram*.[32] In this way, the press coverage focused attention on the saving interventions of humans against the chaos of disease.[33]

But it was not possible to transform all press reports into good news stories about how the flu was being contained. Around the edges of newspaper coverage, other stories emerged in the obituaries, the lists of dead, and in accounts of the flu's ravages in other communities. The extent to which the dead included the prominent as well as the obscure ensured that all deaths became news.[34] Since many of the dead were in the prime of life, their obituaries were heartbreaking as they left young families, bereaved spouses, and sometimes parents, too. The *Prince George Citizen* reported the death of one well-known woman:

> The deceased lady had been one of the first to volunteer for nursing service when the outbreak of influenza occurred and when stricken with the disease her strength was not equal to a successful fight with the malady. The case is doubly sad owing to the death about ten days ago of her little daughter and only child aged four years. The death of the little one had been kept from the mother's knowledge until her strength was equal to the blow. Besides her husband, who is overseas with the Canadian forces, the parents, Mr. and Mrs. Otto King of Fort George are bereaved.[35]

In many cases, the dead had been contributing members of their communities, and the loss, especially in small towns, was keenly felt. The *Kamloops Telegram* expressed it best when, in announcing the death of Chamber of Commerce member William T. Summers (aged thirty-two), it wrote, "On every hand, one hears among citizens expressions of the deepest regret that the late Mr. Summers was cut off in the prime of his young manhood – regret from a personal viewpoint and regret that Kamloops should lose so splendid a citizen, a young man who was an enthusiastic believer in the future of the city and an indefatigable worker in its up building ... Friends attribute his illness to exposure through hospital work in the emergency caused by the outbreak of influenza."[36]

The flu took community leaders and their families, city councillors (J.D. Smith in Prince Rupert, nursing volunteer Marjorie Moberley, daughter of Major Moberley of the military board of pensions), the wives of prominent professionals (Katherine Grant, the wife of well-known Vancouver lawyer Pollard Grant), newspapermen (William Fraser, formerly of the *Kamloops Telegram*), school principals (Ross F. Coldwell of Livingston Public School in Vernon), doctors (Dr. Harvey of Kamloops, Dr. Swenerton of Vancouver), and priests (Father McNeil of St. Paul's Hospital). Even Fred Underhill himself came down with the flu, though he recovered.[37]

Those who were strangers perished as well, their lonely deaths underscoring the atomization of transient workers in British Columbia's resource-based economy and the plight of those without family.[38] Vancouver General Hospital reported its deaths on 22 October 1918, including "Mr. Rose [who] is without friends in the city ... The other deaths [that day included] an Italian named Constani, and a Japanese named Iwatsuru."[39] The *Victoria Daily Times* reported on the death of boiler-maker Dan Morton, the "most pathetic victim of influenza," who died having spent at least a week alone, without food or blankets.[40] Near Kamloops, the dead body of a Chinese worker was found in an outbuilding; he had died alone three weeks earlier.[41] Readers of the BC newspapers would have agreed with Alfred Crosby's assertion that the flu respected neither class barriers, gender, nor racialized categories. A single column of obituaries in the *Victoria Daily Colonist*, for example, reported the deaths of Chong Lin, born in China, married and employed as a cook, Private Harry Johnston, Lena Grant, wife of physician James F. Grant, and Nora Pellow, a widow with seven grown children, including four sons on active service.[42] And on the same *Prince Rupert Daily News* page that announced the death of Alderman J.D. Smith, the paper reported that city council had granted permission to ten Sikh workers in that town to cremate their co-worker Harry Singh on a funeral pyre at the local cemetery.[43] Evidently, the flu respected no social boundaries, and for those who read the papers, it must have seemed universal.

But was it? Accounts of high mortality in certain communities permitted the press to express fears about the disease and the spectre of disorder it raised by talking about populations that were considered foreign, outsiders, or "others." In such cases, the devastation was safely at a distance, in remote mining and logging camps, on Indian reserves, or in urban

ethnic enclaves such as Chinatown. Here, it was hinted, devastation occurred precisely because their inhabitants were not fully modern. Their
lack of modernity constituted a threat to the rest of British Columbia
because they might act as reservoirs of disease ready to reinfect convalescents or those who had escaped the flu in the fall. So, amid the many
triumphalist articles published in newspapers is a sub-genre of narratives
that allowed the press to talk about death and disease, safely cordoned off
from settler and urban British Columbians. Early reports of the flu stressed
the "foreignness" of those infected. One paper described the situation in
Prince Rupert like this: "The disease appears especially severe among the
Indians and foreigners, though citizens also feel the effect."[44]

In urban and suburban areas of the province, the press reported on the
particular propensity of the virus to attack ethnic enclaves or nearby reserves. In Vancouver, when several deaths occurred in the Japanese district
along Powell Street, Underhill reminded readers that eight cases had occurred in one house.[45] In Victoria, the Chinese community was subject to
specific scrutiny.[46] Though it had been declared "safe" early in the epidemic,
by 30 October, the *Victoria Daily Colonist* was reporting suspicions about
the Chinese, writing, "It is stated that the conditions in Chinatown are
not as satisfactory as was at first believed. There seems to be a tendency
among some Chinese to hide all evidence of the epidemic in their district
from the health authorities. The police, however, are cooperating with
the Health Department in an effort to see that the Chinese carry out the
regulations in this respect."[47] In North Vancouver, the focus was on the
local reserves, as it was in Nanaimo on Vancouver Island.[48]

As the initial fall epidemic started to wind down, it became apparent
that some sectors of the population had been more seriously affected.
Especially in small-town papers, stories told of the epidemic's devastation
among First Nations. The *Kamloops Telegram* reported that there were a
number of Aboriginal victims in the Douglas Lake region and on the Chu
Chua reserve that abutted the CPR line.[49] As early as 1 November, the
Prince George Citizen reported that the Dakelh village of Stoney Creek
(Sai'k'uz) had been badly hit, with nearly 100 percent morbidity.[50] Within
the week, the *Citizen* published the gruesome tale of a local Lhedli-tenne
family succumbing to the disease at a campsite along the Fraser.[51] The
Kamloops Telegram reported a similarly grisly find by British Columbia
Provincial Police chief constable Aitken in the Big Bar area, in which an
Aboriginal woman lay dead in bed for five days because her family was
too ill to bury her.[52] Similar conditions prevailed among the Secwepemc,

where Chief Inspector Edens found families starving because they were too weak to get food for themselves.[53] In December, the *Prince George Citizen* announced that the official death tally among the Indians of British Columbia was set at 714.[54] Similarly, the predominance of the foreign-born among the dead was commented on in a number of papers. When, on 28 November, the *Chilliwack Progress* tallied the death toll in its region of the Fraser Valley, it reported four deaths among whites, one among the Japanese, two among the Chinese, and five among Aboriginals.[55] Similarly, the *Grand Forks Gazette* stated that Kelowna had experienced only ten flu deaths – nine Chinese and one South Asian.[56]

Newspapers rarely speculated on why racialized others succumbed to the flu, but what they did say is revealing. The *Vernon News,* writing of the situation in Keremeos, reported no deaths among white settlers, but two in Chinatown acquainted the local population with some "funny Chinese customs" relating to death, though the *News* made no connections between adherence to such customs and mortality.[57] The *Prince George Citizen* was much less reticent in attributing blame when it came to the deaths among a Mennonite group that was waiting to take up a pre-emption, a move that was exceedingly unpopular in the region. The *Citizen* stated that the Mennonites had been living in conditions "almost regardless of sanitary laws," and as a result many had become sick and some had died.[58] The *Citizen* had similarly clear views on the reasons for mortality among Dakelh people, who died at a rate over three times as high as their non-Native neighbours: "Mortality among the Indians was exceedingly heavy and may be attributed to lack of care consequent on their nomadic tendencies, coupled with a native stoicism when finally prostrated."[59] In the Kootenays, suspicion was cast on the Doukhobor communities. The *Grand Forks Gazette* reported that Doukhobor leaders were trying to hide the extent to which the flu had affected their colony and later blamed them for a resurgence of cases after the ban on public meetings was lifted on 6 December 1918. Popular perceptions of the Doukhobors, like those of the Mennonites, were of an insufficiently modern community, eschewing contact with secular society and, in the case of the Doukhobors, allegedly rejecting medical intervention.[60] Like First Nations who adhered to pre-modern modes of existence and the Chinese who retained their funny customs, these populations bore the brunt of the flu, the newspapers told readers, because they remained aloof from the life-saving interventions of medical modernity and, indeed, might have no roles to play in a developing, modern British Columbia.

MEMORIES OF FLU: STRATHCONA

If the promise of modern medicine was the theme of media stories about the pandemic, what dominated the memories of those who suffered from the disease? In the 1970s and 1980s, BC Archives funded a series of oral history projects capturing the province's past by recording the memories of Aboriginal people and settlers of all ethnicities, ultimately publishing them in forty volumes.[61] Though flu stories came up in more than one of these projects, only the Strathcona Project specifically asked participants to recall the flu. Strathcona in 1918-19 was a vibrant, bustling working-class neighbourhood and a major node of settlement for immigrants to Vancouver. It contained Chinatown and was home to the city's Italian, Eastern European, and African American communities. Representing as they do people who seldom left written records of their lives, the Strathcona oral histories, then, grant us access to experiences that evade documentary evidence. Intensely personal, speaking to the lived experience of suffering from influenza, they differ from the newspaper accounts. They remember the suddenness of its onset and the debilitation of its victims. Young adults and middle-aged healthy people were particularly affected; as one woman said, "It seemed the stronger they were, the harder they fell."[62] Though people had clearly assimilated ideas of contagion and acted on their fears by shunning the sick and by wearing gauze face masks infused with camphor, most received no help from the medical authorities the press was praising at the time. In the Strathcona stories, the community – neighbours and family – the traditional pre-modern loci of medical care, intervened to save lives. These accounts, though not anti-modern, reveal the limits of medical modernity.

As survivors, the Strathcona seniors provide an inside look at the flu. They, too, follow Rosenberg's dramaturgic path, but their focal point is narrow. The disease is experienced as embodied, personal, and familial. All remember with clarity the swiftness of onset. Violette Benedetti was at the Viaduct drugstore on Main Street, in the heart of Strathcona, when she became extremely dizzy. By the time she reached her family's apartment, she had to crawl up the stairs, "like a drunk," she said. Soon her whole family had the flu.[63] Adelaide Treasure could pinpoint the exact moment she got sick. She felt "as if some sharp thing had hit my back ... and instantly I knew I had the flu. And I just kept getting so weak and weak that I just had to go to bed and lie down."[64] The debilitation that followed was extreme. She could do nothing for herself or her husband,

Pete, who had contracted the disease as well. As she recalled, "I couldn't help Pete, you see. I knew he was dying but I couldn't help him. I couldn't do a thing. We were just lying in bed, waiting for death. That's really what we were doing."[65] The unusual pattern, in which the virus targeted the fit and healthy, also lingered in survivors' memories. They recalled that many strong men and mothers of young children died. As Elisa Negrin remembered, "It seemed to be the strongest, the heaviest people who went down, the ones that looked the healthiest and strongest, more than anyone else, who went down with it."[66] Or as Nora Hendrix put it, "Plenty people was dying, dying like flies. Oh the big, healthy people was just dying like nobody's business."[67] The number of deaths overwhelmed local funeral facilities: Violette Benedetti recalled looking into Hogan's Alley and seeing bodies piled high like cordwood, waiting to be dealt with by Edwards's undertaking parlour.[68]

Few interviewees credited modern medicine for the fact that they had survived the flu. Only Violette Benedetti's family was visited by a doctor, and it also received the ministrations of the Victorian Order of Nurses, of whom she said, "If it wasn't for them, we would have all been dead."[69] No others saw any health professionals.[70] The information about how to prevent the flu had clearly made the rounds, but what people understood about germ theory is harder to determine. Benedetti remembered that "everytime the doctor went on a call, he had a drink of brandy. You know ... so they wouldn't get the germ."[71] Nora Hendrix's husband, afraid he would catch the flu from the members of the golf club where he worked, cautioned Nora against going out in the rain and used mustard plasters and goose grease on the children to fend off the disease.[72] Others used camphorated masks sold by local department stores, whose efficacy, as we have seen, was open to debate among health officers.[73] Some remembered folk remedies. Mary Veljacic told interviewers that parents hung garlic around their children's necks to ward off the virus.[74] Chow Yin Wong reported that Chinese medicine was effective against the flu.[75] Though it is not clear that people feared germs specifically, many recalled that family members and neighbours stayed as far as possible from the afflicted.[76]

That said, survivors' strongest memories involved neighbours who risked infection to help the sick. Adelaide Treasure remembered the care she received from her neighbours, two young sisters who worked in the city. When she was too ill to help herself, she banged on the wall that connected their two flats. The older of the two women, probably no more than twenty-five, came to her aid, taking care of Treasure's three-year-old son Dick and even bathing her husband, Pete.[77] Neighbours brought food to five-year-old Gilbert Haines, who was coping on his own, and it was the niece of a friend who checked in on the Benedetti family and who may have arranged for those visits by the doctor and nurses. Flu survivors in Strathcona were indebted for their lives to their community, their families and friends, not to medical modernity. The Strathcona seniors offered no criticism of city officials or medical authorities in their recollections. Though some commented on the absence of medical care, none said that they had expected any. Perhaps the flu, when set within the larger context of long lives within the same community, simply diminished in importance, and so the absence of the very mechanisms the press boasted would contain it simply was not worthy of comment. The flu stories that emerge from Strathcona, then, deal extensively with the experience of the disease and the great numbers of deaths, but they speak very little of the modernity that so deeply inscribed the newspaper accounts.

First Nations Flu Stories

In the early 1990s, when I interviewed First Nations elders about their experiences of health and healing, only two were old enough to remember the 1918-19 flu epidemic. Mary Englund, St'at'imc, born at Port Douglas at the head of Harrison Lake, was a young girl in St. Mary's Residential School in 1918:

> We got it. We just stayed right in bed; every girl that was in the convent was in bed. I was so sick then. I tried to fight it, you know, and the nun kept saying, "You'd better go to bed," she'd say. So finally, I went to bed and she came upstairs and took my temperature. My temperature wasn't too bad, so I went to bed and I just covered up and I stayed right in bed. I'd cover my head and all and just stayed right there. Every once in a while the nun would come by and she'd say, "Are you still alive?"[78]

Margaret Gagnon, of the Dakelh reserve at Shelley, near Prince George, was at home when the flu struck. She contracted it during late fall and was unable to get out of bed before the spring. As she walked with her Granny through the village, she was astonished by the number of empty houses that bore silent witness to those who had died. As a result of the devastation to her own family, Gagnon was sent to Lejac Residential School the following fall.[79] Like the interviews with Strathcona seniors, the recollections of these elders were personal accounts of disease and death.

Epidemics also appear in histories published by First Nations writers, and the flu is no exception. This chapter now turns to five accounts from Aboriginal histories in British Columbia. The earliest is that of the Okanagan writer Christine Quintasket, or Mourning Dove, written in January 1919. Titled "The Red Cross and the Okanogans," it is reprinted in Jay Miller's edited version of Quintasket's autobiography, *Mourning Dove: A Salishan Autobiography*.[80] The next is a prose-poem by Secwepemc elder Augusta Tappage, recorded during the late 1960s or early 1970s by Cariboo writer Jean E. Speare and first published in 1973.[81] Two more come from Dakelh territory. The first appears in *Stoney Creek Woman/Sai'k'uz Ts'eke: The Story of Mary John,* written collaboratively by Bridget Moran and Sai'k'uz elder Mary John, and published in 1988.[82] The second appears in the self-published history by Nak'azdli writer Lizette Hall, called *The Carrier, My People,* which appeared in 1992.[83] The last flu story to be discussed here was also published in 1992 as part of a book project instigated by the Xeni Gwet'in in their fight to save their Nemiah Valley as an Aboriginal wilderness preserve. The book is called *Nemiah: The Unconquered Country,* and its influenza story, "The Big Flu," was told by Tsilquot'in elder Eugene Williams, published in English for the first time.[84] Set within their own community histories, these stories shed light on how First Nations writers have ascribed meaning to the events of the fall of 1918. Certain themes emerge. Almost all the stories link the flu with past epidemic events. Unlike the press, who situated the flu as a discrete disease episode, First Nations writers see it as part of a longer history, in which contact with non-Natives, manifest through global movements of people and goods, is pathogenic. And yet, modernity is not incompatible with non-Western thought and in these narratives is combined with indigenous epistemologies of disease, death, and survival. As in the Strathcona stories, the dramaturgic pattern of the epidemic narrative is much narrower than that of the newspapers; however, in these accounts, community rather than personal survival is at centre stage.

Quintasket's story, the only contemporary account, is a transborder comparison of responses to the flu among the Okanogan people in which she contrasts the heroic efforts of American officials and settlers with the "war weary and exhausted," "powerless and inert" reaction in Canada.[85] Quintasket reports that the Okanogan people connected the flu to previously devastating smallpox epidemics ("the Flu put fear into the Indians as much as did the dreaded smallpox") and referred to it, at least initially, as "whiteman's sorethroat disease."[86] Quintasket's story is played out on the stage of community, and so she names the sick and dying, and tells their stories both to build pathos and to counter dominant images of Aboriginal people, a project to which much of her writing was devoted. She gives an account of Chief Antoine Nachumchin, lying ill with flu while his brother suffered nearby from tuberculosis. Their younger sister nursed them both until she collapsed and died. Quintasket uses this narrative to comment on the valour of Aboriginal women, concluding, "The patience of the Indian woman endures without murmur or complaint even unto death. Can greater love and fidelity be found in any race?"[87] This narrative was intended to present a positive, and explicitly gendered, image of Aboriginal people to a non-Native reading audience.

But like the newspaper journalists, Quintasket could also be critical of the Okanogan responses to disease. She appears to have shared the prevailing faith in medical modernity. Only in the presence of doctors, nurses, and on hospital wards staffed by nuns could the flu's devastating impact be mitigated. South of the border, she asserts, Aboriginal people were "wholly unable to cope with the strange malady." They readily gave in to the entreaties of authorities to go to hospital, all except those whose adherence to pre-modern beliefs rendered them inert: "In some cases the aged and superstitious could not be induced to leave their squallid [sic] homes, but remained to fight fate with that stoic indifference to death for which our race is renowned."[88] On the Canadian side of the border, Aboriginal conviviality, according to Quintasket, had to be contained by Indian police because "the custom of indiscriminate visiting of the sick among the Indians is prolific of fatalities."[89] So, like that of the press, Quintasket's faith seems centred on medical modernity and the rational humanitarianism of individual volunteers rather than Okanogan responses.

And yet, for Quintasket, modernity was not the only solution. She attributes the survival of Inkameep residents to the use of a tea made with Okanogan sage.[90] Moreover, she speaks with trepidation about the health impacts of an inadequate transition to modernity. Like some agency physicians of the day, she seems to believe that Okanogan adaptation to modern housing had been too fast, without adequate supervision, and hence was unhealthy. She writes, "The casting aside of the tepee and the adoption of modern houses has had an evil effect on our race beyond calculation ... Owing to his former mode of life – in the open and well-ventilated tepee – the Indian does not understand how the air can become polluted and deadly."[91] Combining older configurationist views of disease etiology with a critique of government policy on housing, Quintasket expresses an ambivalence toward modernity that some medical commentators shared.[92] Her story ends with a plea that more Canadians and

Americans should be like the white settlers who helped the people at Colville Reservation in Washington State. Thus, it concludes not with the resolution of one epidemic but with the ongoing relationship between Natives and non-Natives of the Columbia Plateau.

Augusta Tappage's flu story is embedded in a larger narrative about a smallpox outbreak that struck her grandmother's village during the 1860s. In it, she contrasts her own experience with that of her grandmother. One day, a white miner passed through the village and camped nearby. In return for the food and hospitality they offered, he gave the villagers a Hudson's Bay blanket. Though he had shown no signs of smallpox, the whole village was soon sick and dying, and the people concluded that the blanket carried the disease. Tappage's grandmother survived because she was living in a pithouse outside the village.[93] While she was separated from them, everyone in the village died of smallpox, and she had to bury the dead. In some cases, she interred them in the pithouses where the disease had struck them, but she carried her brother's body up out of a pithouse, a difficult task for a young woman, prompting Tappage to conclude that "I guess she was strong in those days." The grandmother raised a flag over the place, warning people that what had once been a village was now a graveyard.

Tappage contrasts her grandmother's vitality with her own weakness during the 1918 flu. White men – "the soldier boys ... coming home" – brought this disease, too. The grandmother, now an old woman, was too weak to fight it, and Tappage herself was too sick with flu to help her. Whereas her grandmother had attended to her brother's corpse, Tappage could not do the same: "I was sick with the 'flu. I couldn't get up and help nobody! I couldn't help granny. I raised up in bed after they told me and I looked out the window. I saw my granny's coffin. It was bouncing around in the back of the rig. They were hauling her down to the graveyard to bury her. About a mile down the hill. I couldn't go. But I saw her go. I saw my granny go."[94]

This flu story has a narrower field of vision than Quintasket's. Outsiders, whether a white miner or soldiers, bring the disease, but they play no part in the ensuing drama. Family and obligations to the dead are at centre stage here. Though the devastation of smallpox was significant (killing off an entire village), for Tappage's family, the grandmother's escape and her ability to attend to the dead ensured cultural survival. By weakening Tappage so significantly, the flu rendered her unable to care for her grandmother either in life or death, a significant rupture in the cultural fabric.[95] Though the narrative brings the flu story into position with the past, the disease exerts a modernizing influence by challenging, through its over-whelming physical presence, the funerary customs that ensured commun-ity survival.

Mary John's flu story begins with her own experience of the illness, but the narrative scope quickly widens to her family and the community. She writes, "I may not have known what the 1918 flu was, but I knew that it made me very sick. Sick as I was, I was aware that many things, some good and some very sad, were happening on the reserve."[96] Like Tappage, she situates her story in the context of the flu as a family event. While she was lying ill, her mother gave birth to a baby boy, aided by a Dakelh midwife known here only as Agnes George's mother. This joyous occasion, however, is immediately overshadowed by the deaths on reserve, including that of the midwife herself. John writes that the practice of ringing the church bell with each death audibly brought home the magnitude of the epidemic, even as she was too sick to leave her bed. Like Quintasket, she reports that the local physician, Dr. Stone, ignored the Dakelh and treated the non-Native population instead. In contrast, the Catholic priest resident on the reserve, Father Coccola, worked tirelessly. Like the Strathcona seniors, John recalled that predicting who would die was difficult, as "some of the weakest survived and some of the strongest found their way to the village cemetery."[97] Those who were buried in a mass grave at the cemetery ultimately concerned John.[98] Years later, she and her children were clear-ing the cemetery of brush and crumbled gravemarkers when she discov-ered that the mass grave had sunk significantly. This physical remainder of the tragedy prompted her to tell her children about the flu and its impact on the Dakelh. But her account ends with the auditory image of the church bell silenced again as life returned to normal in the wake of the epidemic.

Like Tappage's story, John's is relatively short, but it contains key ele-ments. It notes the failure of the doctor, representative of medical modern-ity, to intervene, but the Catholic priest renders good service to both the sick and dying. John and her children are horrified by the care for the dead, or lack of it, and it is this aspect of the epidemic that leaves a vis-ible reminder, the uneven spot in the graveyard, that must be explained, forcing the story of the flu to the surface. Otherwise, birth and the return to normalcy contain this drama as it ends with the words "Life was good again."[99]

In *The Carrier, My People,* Lizette Hall tells the flu story from another Dakelh village, less than a hundred kilometres from John's Sai'k'uz village.

Hall's book is a very good example of the genre of writing Mary Louise Pratt calls "autoethnography."[100] Defined in opposition to colonialist study of the other, autoethnography fuses cultural and personal revelation. Hall's book ranges from discussions of the language, the clan structure, and the role of feasting in Dakelh society, to the place of the Hudson's Bay Company and Catholic missionaries, to a short biography of her father and a description of contemporary Dakelh villages. A section is devoted to epidemics. As with Tappage, it begins with smallpox and the role of Europeans in spreading it. Hall writes, "There were some epidemics that wiped out quite a few of the native people. One of which was the small-pox epidemic when the whites first came into the country. I will not go into details of how this happened. I am sure some people know the rea-son."[101] Here, she refers to the persistent belief among many BC First Nations that smallpox was intentionally spread via infected blankets.[102] Hall then turns to the 1918 flu, which struck Nak'azdli (Fort St. James) just as people from all around Stuart Lake were gathering for All Saints Day. Contact with the non-Dakelh world and mobility are key features of the narrative. The first to die in Nak'azdli was a man from Nadleh (Fort Fraser) who had accompanied a Hudson's Bay Company employee travel-ling with supplies. Others contracted the virus at the Aleza Lake sawmill, had been moved to hospital in Prince George, returning to nearby Vanderhoof by train and then by horse and wagon to Nak'azdli. Hall's account begins with a geography of transmission that ultimately links the Dakelh with disease through modern modes of labour, medicine, and transportation.

The care of the dead also stands out in Hall's flu story. After the first death, the church bell rang, but soon the priest asked that it be stopped as deaths came more frequently. Teams of horse and wagon carried coffins to the cemetery every day. Mass graves became necessary. Families who died on their traplines were eaten by their dogs. And when the epidemic was over and the Christmas season began, grief overwhelmed the com-munity. Hall recalls that at Midnight Mass, Father Coccola offered a black robe to a woman who, having lost no one to the flu, was wearing festive clothes. Hall's own family experienced the capriciousness of the disease since her mother, who nursed many ill and dying people, never developed symptoms. Hall situates and names all the dead and those who offered care, embedding the flu and its impacts within the community.

Her story has much in common with those of Augusta Tappage and Mary John. The infection comes from outside, specifically via contact with non-Native people, and in one case at a site of waged labour – the sawmill at Aleza Lake. In this respect, modernity is implicated in its origin and spread. As in the stories of Tappage and John, the flu is culturally disruptive in that customs involving the care of the dead cannot be maintained. Earlier in her autoethnography, Hall described the beliefs and rituals around death, including the ritual required when "too many deaths" occur.[103] In the larger context of her narrative, her depiction of the hasty and perfunctory funerals conducted during the epidemic clearly signifies cultural dislocation. In a book whose tone is largely triumphalist in that it documents the ongoing strength of the Dakelh, the story of the flu stands out as tragedy.

The most complex flu story to be considered here comes from the Xeni Gwet'in territory of Nemiah Valley on the Chilcotin Plateau. It is told by elder Eugene Williams as he heard it from Eagle Lake Henry, who experienced the flu first-hand. On their way home from a hunting trip, Eagle Lake Henry and his wife encountered a man named Bob Graham while camping at Tatla Lake. Graham reported that Eagle Lake was in the midst of a flu epidemic and offered rum and Lysol as preventatives, the rum to be taken in small, regular doses. Henry and his wife returned to their village, where they discovered the truth of Graham's words. The people had moved into camps on higher ground and were dying there. Henry's own parents were dead. So he and his wife cleaned their home with Lysol, draping the walls with rags soaked in the strong-smelling disinfectant. Finding the elder Nezulhtsis in his pithouse, near death, Henry bathed him in Lysol-steeped hot water, and Nezulhtsis said that he saw the disease crawling up the steam. He was saved from death.

Henry then considered the origins of the flu and implicated two Tsilquot'in men in its spread from Williams Lake. The first, a man named John, went to Williams Lake for a load of lumber to rebuild a local dance hall in time for Christmas and brought the virus to the reserve at Stone. The second, named Tsicone, brought the flu with the wood from Stone to the Nemiah Valley, though he had been warned to avoid the reserve because of the disease. Tsicone's guilt prompted him to use the purchased wood to build coffins.

Williams recounts two additional anecdotes related to influenza. In the first, his father, Sammy Williams, dreamt of the flu while staying at Tsuniah, distant from the communities it was affecting. He dreamt that "some soldiers came over to Nemiah and shot this disease with all kinds of colours going through the sky." Because of the dream, he stayed away from the Nemiah Valley. In the second anecdote, the people of Nemiah urged a medicine man, named Abiyan, to come and "sing with their sick people," and though his spirit helper was strong, he could not cure them of the disease. Williams concludes with the somewhat jarring statement that "this disease came from the Chilcotin War."[104] Here again, this First Nations narrative situates the flu in the longer history of Aboriginal-white contact. The Chilcotin War, the only armed uprising against settler interests staged by a BC First Nation, occurred in 1864. For Tsilquot'in people, it has become emblematic of their own attempts to resist colonization and the duplicity of the colonizers, who offered safe negotiation with Tsilquot'in leader Klatsassin only to arrest him and his followers, trying them in English and hanging them in Williams Lake as murderers. To the Tsilquot'in, the Chilcotin War was not just about territorial incursion; it was also about smallpox and depopulation. In their account of smallpox, which appears just a few pages before Eugene Williams's flu story, Henry Solomon tells how a Hudson's Bay Company employee spread the disease to the Tsilquot'in by trading blankets taken from smallpox casualties among the Nuxalk. In *Nemiah: The Unconquered Country*, the flu and smallpox narratives are juxtaposed in such a way that they become linked, just as they are in the works by Quintasket, Tappage, and Hall. Like the others, its flu story expresses ambivalence toward modernity. The desire for an improved dance hall sets in motion a chain of events that brings the virus with a load of sawn lumber. But commodities, such as rum and Lysol, can also be medicine. And Tsilquot'in prophesy remains effective even if its strongest healers do not, so that tradition itself is not counterposed to the flu. The Tsilquot'in influenza narrative is one of hybrids, in which the past soaks through the porous surface of the present, giving deeper meaning to the already dramatic events of the fall of 1918.[105]

CONCLUSION

What role does modernity play in the production of flu stories? As Alan Swedlund suggests, modernity may have placed certain limits on what would be told and what would be remembered. Certainly, the contemporary press asserted the triumph of medical modernity over the flu. Though it reported the link between the disease's reach and modern forms of transportation, particularly the railways, it nonetheless displayed a faith that humans, acting with knowledge and reason, would ultimately contain and then defeat the flu. Just as the virus travelled the PGE line up from Squamish, for example, so, too, could medical aid come by train. Indeed, where death and devastation dominated the press coverage, it was in discussions of populations not deemed modern enough. Only there, among Doukhobors, Mennonites, and First Nations, did the press speculate that the flu might find itself a reservoir. Surely, extending modernity's reach even among these groups, the newspapers seemed to suggest, would wipe out future disease threats.

Obituaries, with their profound expressions of grief and loss, could not be contained by the conventions that appear to have shaped the press coverage. But the tendency to run obituaries of ordinary people alongside reports on prominent members of society worked to present the flu as a universal phenomenon not bound by gendered, classed, or racialized social categories. In the flu stories from working-class Strathcona, modernity plays little part. The virus strikes with sudden randomness, and lives are preserved only through the intercession of community, not medicine. Among First Nations, community is also highlighted as the promise of medical modernity, so often recited by Indian agents, missionaries, and residential schoolteachers, is not fulfilled. Moreover, the modern world is grounded in the past, and in First Nations writing about the flu, history plays an important role. By invoking the memories of smallpox, First Nations situate the flu in the story of contact, of which modernity is but one chapter. Rather than silencing First Nations flu histories, modernity becomes part of the story. Whereas Quintasket, writing shortly after the epidemic, is uncertain that the Okanagon people can become modern, Lizette Hall and Eugene Williams, writing years later, can look back and see that the community did find ways of responding to the flu, and to modernity itself, that mitigated its impact. Like their non-Native neighbours, First Nations did not reject modernity; rather, their responses to the flu show that they employed it to craft hybrids.

ACKNOWLEDGMENTS

Special thanks go to Jen Hatton, research assistant extraordinaire, who made sense of the death certificates and travelled across the province in the middle of winter to collect newspaper sources. The Social Science and Humanities Research Council paid for the research.

NOTES

1   Alfred W. Crosby, *America's Forgotten Pandemic: The Influenza of 1918,* 2nd ed. (Cambridge: Cambridge University Press, 2003), 323-25.

2 Alan Swedlund, "Everyday Mortality in the Time of Plague: Ordinary People under Extraordinary Circumstances in Massachusetts before and during the 1918 Flu Epidemic" (paper presented to the 138th symposium of the Wenner Gren Foundation, Tucson, 18 September 2007).

3 Esyllt W. Jones, *Influenza 1918: Disease, Death, and Struggle in Winnipeg* (Toronto: University of Toronto Press, 2007), 5.

4 Mary-Ellen Kelm, "British Columbia First Nations and the Influenza Pandemic of 1918-1919," *BC Studies* 122 (Summer 1999): 23-48.

5 Charles Rosenberg, *Explaining Epidemics and Other Studies in the History of Medicine* (Cambridge: Cambridge University Press, 1992), 279.

6 "Spanish Influenza Is Ravaging Camps," *Prince Rupert Daily News*, 26 September 1918, 2; and "Alarm in US over Influenza," *Kamloops Telegram*, 26 September 1918, 4.

7 "Prevention and Cure of Influenza," *Victoria Daily Times*, 4 October 1918, 1; "Cure for Spanish 'Flu,'" *Vernon News*, 17 October 1918, 4; and advertisement, *Kamloops Telegram*, 10 October 1918, 9.

8 "Theatres and Churches Are Closing in the East," *Victoria Daily Times*, 4 October 1918, 1; and "Seattle Tries to Curb Grippe," *Vancouver Daily World*, 5 October 1918, 1.

9 "Provincial Health Department Has Issued Bulletin on the New Disease," *Vernon News*, 10 October 1918, 1; and "Don't Kiss; Don't Get Your Feet Wet, Says Dr. Underhill," *Vancouver Daily World*, 7 October 1918, 1.

10 "Vancouver Ready to Fight Epidemic of Spanish Grippe," *Victoria Daily Times*, 7 October 1918, 1.

11 "The World Power of Influenza," *Vancouver Daily World*, 8 October 1918, 1.

12 "Victoria Is Quiet as on Sundays," *Vancouver Daily World*, 9 October 1918, 1; and "Close Victoria Schools," *Vancouver Daily World*, 8 October 1918, 4.

13 "Seventeen New Cases of Spanish Influenza Reported Yesterday," *Vancouver Daily Sun*, 9 October 1918, 1.

14 "Some 'Flu' Cases in New Westminster," *Vancouver Daily Sun*, 9 October 1918, 2.

15 "City to Secure 'Flu' Hospital," *Victoria Daily Colonist*, 26 October 1918, 1.

16 "Other Cities Enforce Use of 'Flu' Masks; Serums Are Found to Prevent Infection," *Vancouver Daily Sun*, 4 November 1918, 3.

17 "Fourteen New Cases of 'Flu,'" *Vancouver Daily World*, 10 October 1918, 1.

18 Rosenberg, *Explaining Epidemics*, 295.

19 "Short Skirts and Open Blouses Invite 'Flu,'" *Vancouver Daily World*, 8 October 1918, 1. Underhill's tactics reveal yet another shift away from the broader social approach of the sanitarians and toward more individual indexes of risk and contamination. Paul Starr, *The Social Transformation of American Medicine: The Rise of a Sovereign Profession and the Making of a Vast Industry* (New York: Basic Books, 1982), 189-91; and Mary Poovey, *Making a Social Body: British Cultural Formation* (Chicago: University of Chicago Press, 1995).

20 "Fourteen New Cases of 'Flu,'" 1.

21 "Number of Cases Still Increasing," *Victoria Daily Times*, 11 October 1918, 1; "Dry Weather Will Halt the Epidemic," *Victoria Daily Colonist*, 12 October 1918, 1; "Decrease Shown in Influenza Cases," *Victoria Daily Times*, 12 October 1918, 1; and "Epidemic Shows Signs of Waning," *Victoria Daily Colonist*, 13 October 1918, 1.

22 "Third Death in City from 'Flu,'" *Vancouver Daily World*, 12 October 1918, 1.

23 "Influenza Seems to Be Subsiding," *Vernon News*, 7 November 1918, 1; and "The Influenza," *Vernon News*, 21 November 1918, 4.

24 "Happenings throughout the District: Oyama," *Vernon News,* 28 1918, 4.
25 The closing of public venues was the subject of considerable debate. Almost everywhere across the province, this was the preferred method of containment. By instituting public closures under the authority of the province, municipalities demonstrated that they were doing everything possible to prevent the spread of the disease. Victoria closed schools shortly after the virus arrived in the city. Prince Rupert closed its poolrooms, theatres, and cabarets by the middle of October. North Vancouver closed all schools and public meetings on 15 October, New Westminster followed suit on 17 October, and Kamloops did the same on 18 October. At the same time, Fred Underhill repeatedly defended his decision to keep the city open by saying that this afforded the best way to survey the situation. Called in to deal with the "war on flu" in Vancouver, the provincial medical health officer, Henry Esson Young, closed the city through an order-in-council on 18 October, having expressed dissatisfaction with Underhill's interpretation of prevention. Margaret Andrews, "Epidemic and Public Health: Vancouver 1918-19," *BC Studies* 34 (Summer 1977): 21-44.
26 "Drug Store Staff Has Been Depleted," *Prince Rupert Daily News,* 26 October 1918, 1; and "Local 'Flu' Cases Show Decrease in Known New Cases," *Vancouver Daily Sun,* 27 October 1918, 1.
27 "Nurses Required to Deal with Influenza Cases," *Victoria Daily Times,* 10 October 1918, 1.
28 "Volunteers Asked to Aid in Coping with Influenza," *Prince Rupert Daily News,* 19 October 1918, 1.
29 "Influenza Said to Be on Decline," *Vancouver Daily Sun,* 2 November 1918, 1.
30 "Kingston Street Fire Hall Is Opened as Emergency Hospital," *Victoria Daily Times,* 22 October 1918, 3; and "Drop In Number of Cases of Flu Still Continues," *Vancouver Daily Sun,* 5 November 1918, 1.
31 "Little Improvement Shown in Local Influenza Situation," *Prince George Citizen,* 1 November 1918, 2.
32 "Helped to Attend Influenza Patients," *Prince George Citizen,* 15 November 1918, 4; "Women and Girls Are Assisting at Hospitals," *Kamloops Telegram,* 7 November 1918, 3; "Items of Local Interest," *Kamloops Telegram,* 14 November 1918, 6; and "Board Thanks All Who Served," *Kamloops Telegram,* 12 December 1918, 5.
33 The conclusions here contrast with those of Debra Blakely for American newspaper coverage of the 1918-19 flu. See her *Mass Mediated Disease: A Case Study Analysis of Three Flu Pandemics and Public Health Policy* (Lanham, MD: Lexington Books, 2006), 21-66.
34 The first flu deaths in Vancouver and Victoria received specific newspaper coverage. In each case, medical authorities stressed that the dead had recently travelled outside the community. "Sgt.-Major Smallwood Dies of Influenza," *Victoria Daily Colonist,* 9 October 1918, 4; "Two Deaths, Seventy Cases," *Vancouver Daily World,* 11 October 1918, 4; "Miss Wylie Seriously Ill," *Kamloops Telegram,* 17 October 1918, 4; and "Talented Kamloops Girl Suddenly Carried Away," *Kamloops Telegram,* 24 October 1918, 1.
35 "Obituary," [no name given] *Prince George Citizen,* 29 October 1918, 4.
36 "Is Great Loss to Community," *Kamloops Telegram,* 15 November 1918, 4.
37 "Well Known Stockman Is Victim of Pneumonia," *Kamloops Telegram,* 24 October 1918, 1; "Lionel Stobart Passes Away," *Kamloops Telegram,* 21 November 1918, 1; "Flu Deaths Are Lower than for Many Days Past," *Vancouver Daily Sun,* 29 October 1918, 2; "Wife Dies; Husband Ill," *Vancouver Daily Sun,* 31 October 1918, 3; "Prominent Citizen Is Victim of Pneumonia," *Kamloops Telegram,* 31 October 1918, 4; "Number of 'Flu' Cases Increases," *Vancouver Daily Sun,* 1 November 1918, 1; "Late Kamloops Newspaper Man Dies of

Influenza," *Kamloops Telegram,* 7 November 1918, 3; "Ross F. Coldwell Claimed by Death," *Vernon News,* 7 November 1918, 3; and "Believe Influenza Epidemic Is Now on the Decline," *Prince George Citizen,* 29 October 1918, 1.

38 For example, the *Vancouver Daily Sun* reported the death of a "hindu whose name is un-known." "Flu Situation Still Improving," *Vancouver Daily Sun,* 10 November 1918, 1.

39 "Four Deaths at General Hospital," *Vancouver Daily Sun,* 22 October 1918, 1.

40 "Lonely End for Disease's Victim," *Victoria Daily Times,* 21 October 1918, 4.

41 "Body of Chinese Victim of 'Flu' Found," *Kamloops Telegram,* 28 November 1918, 4.

42 "Obituary Notices," *Victoria Daily Colonist,* 23 October 1918, 4.

43 "Unusual Ceremony of Cremation," *Prince Rupert Daily News,* 23 October 1918, 1; see also "Alderman Is a Victim of the Epidemic," *Prince Rupert Daily News,* 23 October 1918, 1.

44 "Two Deaths Took Place in Hospital," *Prince Rupert Daily News,* 15 October 1918, 1; "Indians Are Having Hard Time from Flu," *Prince Rupert Daily News,* 17 October 1918 4; and "Three Men Dead from Pneumonia Attacks," *Prince Rupert Daily News,* 18 October 1918, 1. Other newspaper accounts that stress the outsider status of the infected early in the epidemic are "Flu Deaths," *Grand Forks Gazette,* 6 November 1918, 1; and "Disease Spreads with Rapidity," *Victoria Daily Colonist,* 19 October 1918, 1. The *Prince George Citizen* made a similar point, stating that of the twenty-one known dead in Prince George as of 26 October, no more than six were local to the city. All the rest had come from outlying regions. "Believe Influenza Epidemic Is Now on the Decline," 1; "Picture Shows Are Closed Up in Fernie," *Vancouver Daily Sun,* 26 October 1918, 4; and "Outlying Sections in Grip of Epidemic," *Victoria Daily Colonist,* 26 October 1918, 1.

45 "Third Death in City from 'Flu,'" 1.

46 "Influenza Continues to Claim Sufferers," *Victoria Daily Times,* 14 October 1918, 1; and "Chinatown Safe," *Victoria Daily Colonist,* 29 October 1918, 4.

47 "Epidemic Still Has Strong Grip," *Victoria Daily Colonist,* 30 October 1918, 1.

48 "Most Increase in Cases Is South of the City: 100 Cases on North Shore," *Vancouver Daily Sun,* 20 October 1918, 1; "Another Drop in Number of 'Flu' Patients," *Vancouver Daily Sun,* 26 October 1918, 1; and "Nurses Fall Victims," *Vancouver Daily Sun,* 29 October 1918, 1.

49 "Items of Local Interest," *Kamloops Telegram,* 21 November 1918, 4.

50 "Little Improvement Shown in Local Influenza Situation," *Prince George Citizen,* 1 November 1918, 2.

51 "Influenza Epidemic Rapidly Subsiding," *Prince George Citizen,* 5 November 1918, 2; and "Many Indians Die of Spanish Influenza," *Prince George Citizen,* 15 November 1918, 5.

52 "'Flu' Conditions around Clinton," *Kamloops Telegram,* 14 November 1918, 4.

53 "Say Conditions Are Appalling," *Kamloops Telegram,* 14 November 1918, 8.

54 Untitled article, *Prince George Citizen,* 10 December 1918, 5.

55 Untitled article, *Chilliwack Progress,* 28 November 1918, 2

56 Untitled article, *Grand Forks Gazette,* 29 November 1918, 2.

57 Untitled article, *Vernon News,* 28 November 1918, 8.

58 "Mennonites Suffer from Influenza," *Prince George Citizen,* 23 November 1918, 2.

59 "Eighteen Hundred Cases of Influenza in Northern BC," *Prince George Citizen,* 14 January 1919, 2. Settlers in the Prince George area had a mortality rate of 22.5 per 1,000 people, whereas the death rate for Dakelh on reserves in the vicinity was 79.0 per 1,000. See British Columbia, Vital Statistics, Death Registrations, vols. 003, 995, British Columbia Archives (BCA), Victoria.

60 "Spanish Influenza among the Doukhobors," *Grand Forks Gazette,* 6 December 1918, 13 December 1918, 6

61 Saeko Usukawa et al., eds., *Sound Heritage: Voices from British Columbia* (Vancouver: Douglas and McIntyre, 1984).

62 Phyllis Culos, interview by Daphne Marlatt and Carole Itter, 16 May 1977, BCA, Strathcona Project, T2742:1, tape only.

63 Violette Benedetti, interview by Daphne Marlatt, 1 April 1977, BCA, Strathcona Project, T2679:1, transcript.

64 Adelaide Treasure, interview by Rich Mole, 9 September 1979, BCA, Christmas in British Columbia Project, acc. no. 3552-1-1-2, transcript.

65 Ibid.

66 America Bianco, Elisa Negrin, and Dora Trono, interview by Daphne Marlatt, 9 May 1977, BCA, Strathcona Project, T3181:0001.

67 Nora Hendrix, interview by Daphne Marlatt, 14 July 1977, BCA, Strathcona Project, T2727:3, transcript.

68 Benedetti interview, Strathcona Project.

69 Ibid.

70 Adelaide Treasure stated emphatically, "We couldn't get a doctor. You couldn't get a nurse." Treasure interview, Christmas in British Columbia Project. Mary Veljacic spoke fondly of a Dr. Tompsett who worked in the neighbourhood, but when asked if he was around during the flu, she did not recall seeing him; perhaps he was away in the war, she wondered. Mary Trocell Veljacic, interview by Carole Itter and Daphne Marlatt, 2 June 1977, BCA, Strathcona Project, T2699:0003, tape only.

71 Benedetti interview, Strathcona Project.

72 Hendrix interview, Strathcona Project.

73 Culos interview, Strathcona Project; Benedetti interview, Strathcona Project.

74 Veljacic interview, Strathcona Project; Culos interview, Strathcona Project.

75 Chow Yin Wong, interview by Carole Itter and Daphne Marlatt, 13 January 1977, BCA, Strathcona Project, T3174:00011, transcript.

76 Treasure interview, Christmas in British Columbia Project; Benedetti interview, Strathcona Project; Gilbert Martin Haines, interview by Michael Taft, 13 July 1982, BCA, Tall Tales of British Columbia collection, T3973:0013.

77 Treasure interview, Christmas in British Columbia Project.

78 Mary Englund, interview by author, 15 May 1993, Lillooet, BC (audiotape in author's possession).

79 Margaret Gagnon, interview by author, 25 September 1994, Prince George (audiotape in author's possession).

80 Jay Miller, ed., *Mourning Dove: A Salishan Autobiography* (Lincoln: University of Nebraska Press, 1990), 189-92. Alanna Brown disputes Quintasket's authorship of this piece, attributing it to a collaborator, but her reasons for doing so are not clear. See Alanna Kathleen Brown, "The Evolution of Mourning Dove's *Coyote Stories,*" *Studies in American Indian Literatures,* 2nd ser., 4,2-3 (Summer-Fall 1992): 172, 180, http://oncampus.richmond.edu/. "Okanogan" is the American spelling.

81 Jean E. Speare, ed., *The Days of Augusta* (1973; repr., Vancouver: Douglas and McIntyre, 1992), 30-32.

82 Bridget Moran, *Stoney Creek Woman/Sai'k'uz Ts'eke: The Story of Mary John* (Vancouver: Tillicum Library, 1988), 24-25.

83 Lizette Hall, *The Carrier, My People* (Cloverdale, BC: privately printed, 1992), 19-21.

84 Terry Glavin and the People of Nemiah Valley, *Nemiah: The Unconquered Country* (Vancouver: New Star, 1992), 89-103.

85 Miller, *Mourning Dove,* 191.

86 Ibid., 192.

87 Ibid., 191.

88 Ibid., 190.

89 Ibid., 191.

90 Ibid.

91 Ibid., 192.

92 Mary-Ellen Kelm, "Diagnosing the Discursive Indian: Medicine, Gender, and the 'Dying Race,'" *Ethnohistory* 52 (Spring 2005): 371-406.

93 Tappage does not explain why her grandmother was living in a pithouse on her own, but she may have been experiencing either puberty or menstruation seclusion. See Mary C. Wright, "The Woman's Lodge: Constructing Gender on the Nineteenth Century Pacific Northwest Plateau," in *In the Days of Our Grandmothers: A Reader in Aboriginal Women's History in Canada,* ed. Mary-Ellen Kelm and Lorna Townsend (Toronto: University of Toronto Press, 2006), 251-69.

94 Speare, *The Days of Augusta,* 31.

95 James Alexander Teit, *The Lillooet Indians,* vol. 2, pt. 5 of *The Jesup North Pacific Expedition* (New York: G.E. Stechert, 1906), 270.

96 Moran, *Stoney Creek Woman,* 24.

97 Ibid., 25.

98 Ibid.

99 Ibid.

100 Mary Louise Pratt, *Imperial Eyes: Studies in Travel Writing and Transculturation* (London: Routledge, 1992), 7.

101 Hall, *The Carrier, My People,* 19.

102 Michael Harkin, *The Heiltsuks: Dialogues of Culture and History on the Northwest Coast* (Lincoln: University of Nebraska Press, 1997), 78.

103 Hall, *The Carrier, My People,* 8.

104 Glavin and People of Nemiah Valley, *Nemiah: The Unconquered Country,* 91.

105 Ibid., 88-90.

8

Spectral Influenza: Winnipeg's Hamilton Family, Interwar Spiritualism, and Pandemic Disease

ESYLLT JONES

The matching baby books of twin brothers Arthur Lamont and James Drummond, the sons of Lillian and Thomas Glendinning Hamilton of Winnipeg, give brief records of their developmental milestones – when they laughed, sat up, walked, and talked – and gentle observations on their personalities. Arthur's baby book includes his mother's bittersweet remembrance of the night he became seriously ill with the pandemic influenza from which he would die on 27 January 1919. Arthur was the smaller and less robust of the brothers, the second of the twins to be born. His mother noted that Arthur had crawled with one foot tucked under and did not learn to walk as quickly as James. At age three, beginning to show a love of music, he was also "rather nervous and high strung, given to scolding," and he spoke with a lisp. "The night he was taken ill he said the following little rhyme ... with the most adorable little lisp and chuckle," Lillian wrote. His "Aunt Billy" soothed Arthur with her gentle teasing, "Where's the Hamilton twins?" Arthur responded, "Thems us. Mamma I kith Aunt Billy wiff mithletoe."[1] Arthur's death not long afterward reconfigured the familial and spiritual practices of the Hamilton household. In the coming years, Lillian, Thomas, and the family would continue a poignant engagement with their adored Arthur, communicating with him beyond death, in an afterlife they believed existed. As the Hamiltons grew to public prominence in Canada's interwar spiritualist movement, they maintained their bond with Arthur in seances "akin to a family reunion" (see Figure 8.1).[2]

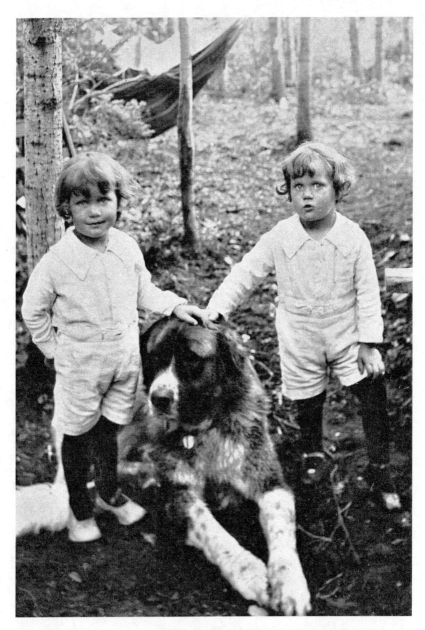

FIGURE 8.1   Arthur Lamont and James Drummond Hamilton, twins, circa 1918.
Source: University of Manitoba Archives and Special Collections, Hamilton family fonds, UM_pc272_A10-001_001_0001_008_0001

The Hamilton family history allows us to connect the private manifesta-
tions of influenza grief to a broader cultural moment: the appeal of spiritualist exploration and practices, especially communing with the dead, in
a grieving interwar society. This research contributes to an emerging focus
among historians on the impact of the disease on ideologies and mental-
ities, popular culture, and memory and mourning in the interwar period.[3]
With Mary-Ellen Kelm's essay in this collection, it interrogates the ways
in which the influenza pandemic confounds the modern/not modern bi-
furcation of early-twentieth-century cultural history. The flu pandemic,
like its spiritual response, read as fundamentally not modern. Journalists
at the time compared it to the Black Death; Winnipeg during the pandemic seemed medieval to them. However, in its blending of traditional
and modern means of managing death and grief, influenza suggested
continuities in human experience, emblematic of modernity's capacity
to incorporate multivalent identities and beliefs. Thomas and Lillian
Hamilton were medical professionals (Thomas a physician, Lillian a trained
nurse), and they lived an active Protestant Christian faith; yet they sought
to find in the spiritualist ethos an affirmation of human survival beyond
death. Although they were previously intrigued by telepathy, table lifting,
and other occult incidences, their interest in psychic phenomena deepened
following their son Arthur's unexpected death from influenza. Thomas
Hamilton would go on to establish an international reputation as a spiritualist, largely based on his photographs of spirit ectoplasm. Publicly framed
as scientific psychic research into evidence that life persisted after death,
the Hamilton seances were at the same time a domesticated ritual central
to sustaining family and friendship, in a context of grief and loss, and
shaped by gender, ethnicity, and class.

INFLUENZA IN THE HAMILTONS' NEIGHBOURHOOD

The fall 1918 wave of pandemic influenza arrived in the city of Winnipeg
during the closing days of September 1918, carried by both military and
civilian vectors. In a city of approximately 180,000, over 1,200 lost their
lives to the disease. Infection rates, of course, were much higher than this
mortality suggests. At the epidemic's peak toward mid-November, several
hundred new cases were being reported each day, and many more were
probably never reported to health officials. The city's health authorities
(under the powers granted them by the provincial board of health and the

Public Health Act) took measures to contain the disease, which were quite similar to those of other major urban centres across North America. Incoming trains were inspected, and if necessary affected passengers were quarantined. A ban was placed on large public gatherings, and schools, universities, and places of entertainment (theatres, billiard parlours, concert halls) were closed. A public information campaign began, informing residents of appropriate precautions and urging them to report the disease and seek medical care if they or a family member became ill. The city's pathologist, William Boyd, travelled to the Mayo Clinic in Minnesota to obtain a vaccine, thousands of doses of which were then manufactured by the provincial laboratory under the direction of Gordon Bell. The vaccine was offered free of charge at stations across town. After these measures failed to stop the spread of the disease through October 1918, the City issued a quarantine order at the end of that month, although it lacked the will or the human resources to enforce it.[4]

Health authorities were openly concerned about the increasing number of influenza cases in the working-class and immigrant districts in the north end of town, and believed that once the disease took hold there, they could do little to control it. In the early days of the epidemic, most cases occurred in the south and centre of the city, which gave health officials some optimism that they could contain the disease. By early November, however, the locus of the disease shifted to the district surrounding the railway tracks and northward, including Elmwood, where the Hamiltons lived and where Thomas Hamilton practised medicine. Elmwood was a predominantly Anglo-Canadian working-class neighbourhood, across the Red River from the north end, also an area of immigrants and workers. In 1918, Elmwood's population was 11,500. Originally a district of market gardens and wooded swampy land, its urbanization and industrialization occurred, as elsewhere in the city, after the building of the railway, which traversed Elmwood. By the time of the First World War, pedestrian and streetcar links, as well as the Redwood and Louise Bridges, connected it to the city on the west side of the river. Businesses and residents were attracted to Elmwood because land and taxes were cheaper there than across the river. For workers, it offered job opportunities in local industries such as the meat-packing plant, a large wooden box and barrel factory, the Dominion Foundry, Western Iron and Steel, several coal and fuel firms, a millworks, and a farm implement manufacturer. As Winnipeg historian Jim Park states, "It was considered a tough, labouring class neighbourhood, polluted by all the industry along the tracks."[5]

The social geography of Elmwood had been clearly laid out by the Great War era. On the west was the large Elmwood Cemetery, where Arthur Lamont Hamilton was buried. The main thoroughfare, Kelvin Street (now Henderson Highway), had a variety of local merchants; this was where Thomas Hamilton's office and home were located. Kelvin Street formed a kind of social boundary line in Elmwood: middle-class and more stately homes lay to the west of it, in the heavily wooded area between Kelvin and the river; working-class housing was located on its east side. To the east and south, the homes of working families ended at the industrial area and railway tracks, and eventually Elmwood itself gave way to the growing worker suburb, Transcona.

Like other districts of the city where many families lived in relative poverty and in poor housing, Elmwood was hard hit by influenza. Its residents suffered a high death rate, as high as that across the Red River in the north end. Rates were 6.3 per 1,000 population in the North End and 6.4 in Elmwood, compared with 4.0 in the more wealthy area south of the Assiniboine River.[6] Elmwood was underserviced, with limited health care infrastructure. It had no hospital. Some of its flu victims were isolated and received treatment at the LaSalle Hotel, at the foot of the Louise Bridge, which had been converted into an emergency hospital by public health authorities.

Experiences with influenza in Winnipeg were highly mediated by class and ethnicity. Working-class and immigrant districts had the highest death rates, and poorer citizens faced many material challenges in confronting the disease. This is not to suggest that the financially secure did not contract influenza or die from it; no sector of society was immune. Many prominent Winnipeg families lost loved ones. Nevertheless, the dominant social response to the pandemic cast middle-class and elite Winnipeggers (men and women) as leaders in the fight against the disease, as fully engaged in the struggle in a way that workers and the poor were not. Health officials and the press tended to portray working-class immigrants as passive victims, relying on the charity and skills of their social betters to rescue them. In one sense, then, physicians and health authorities employed their social power during the pandemic. Yet ironically, many physicians experienced influenza as a highly disempowering disease, because medical treatment was largely ineffectual and failed to save so many of the ill.

A leader in the local medical profession, Thomas Hamilton would perhaps have shared such a contradictory and at times frustrating encounter with the pandemic, although he left no account of his experiences. As a general practitioner in Elmwood during a time when physicians were in short supply due to military service, Hamilton would have cared for many influenza sufferers in their homes and at the Winnipeg General Hospital, where he had admitting privileges. Health professionals were particularly vulnerable to the flu because of their proximity to the infected, and Hamilton himself may have brought it into his household. The Hamilton twins became very ill with influenza in January 1919, as the pandemic reached the end of its fall-winter wave. Perhaps the family had believed it had escaped the worst, but instead all became infected.[7] In Winnipeg, flu mortality typically targeted adults, who died in the largest numbers, with 60 percent of all deaths occurring among those aged twenty to thirty-nine, about evenly distributed between men and women. It was relatively rare for children of Arthur's age (three years) to die from influenza; in fact, according to public health department statistics, three- to four-year-olds were much less likely to die than infants under age two. This makes sense given what we now know regarding the risk of influenza complications such as pneumonia for children under twenty-four months of age. James Hamilton's symptoms were so severe that he lost an eardrum.[8] Arthur, who perished on 27 January, was one of only thirty-three children in his age cohort to die of the flu in Winnipeg between the beginning of October 1918 and the end of January 1919.[9]

Because the pandemic was most lethal for adults, few historians have noted the impact of childhood deaths from the disease; this sets historical treatments of influenza apart from those for the more ubiquitous infectious illnesses of this era, such as diphtheria and scarlet fever. Yet, children did die, especially the very young. The impact of the disease on family life was deep and varied, as families had to reconfigure themselves in a wide variety of ways after the deaths of mothers, fathers, children, and siblings. According to Arthur's older brother, Glen, and his sister, Margaret, much later in life, the loss of the little boy was traumatic for Thomas Hamilton, resulting in deep sadness and grief. He may have believed, as a "strict Calvinist Presbyterian," that the death of a beloved child was a punishment from God.[10] His daughter, Margaret, who was nine when Arthur died, recalls her father weeping inconsolably: "I can remember crawling into his bed and putting my arms around him and patting him and saying 'Well, dad, you've got the rest of us, don't cry so hard. We love you too.' But that was a very small comfort because nothing could replace the loss of a beloved child." Glen recalled, "He felt here he had lost a beautiful little boy. Where had the soul gone?"[11] In both of these sibling recollections, the impact of Arthur's death was still powerfully evident sixty-eight years later when they were interviewed by researchers. Glen, who was seven in 1919, recalled seeing his brother lying dead: "My mother and father took me into the bedroom where he was lying in his crib. He looked just like a little wax doll."[12] Beside him were an oxygen tank and eucalyptus oil in a basin of boiling water, a combination of orthodox medical treatment and popular remedies, neither of which saved his life.[13]

The influenza pandemic, then, affected Thomas and Lillian Hamilton as health professionals and as parents – in their "public" and "private" lives. As leaders of a spiritualist revival in the city, the Hamiltons afford us insight into how the epidemic shaped both private and public expressions of grief and loss.

SPIRITUALISM AND ITS CONTEXTS

Although few histories discuss the spiritual impact of the influenza pandemic, several historians have argued that it posed a particular challenge to established religious frameworks. In Africa, David Simmons has recently suggested, the epidemic resulted in a "crisis in faith." Non-Christian Africans saw it as "a plague sent by the ancestors ... or ... the result of witchcraft."[14] Other scholars have perceived influenza as contributing to innovative forms of spirituality, generating a "new spiritual idiom."[15] In response to its devastating impact, Pentecostal spiritual movements arose all over southern Africa, in black, white, and coloured communities, many of them led by black African prophets who viewed the pandemic as both a punishment and a spiritual opportunity. These included the spirit churches of Zimbabwe, the Aladura Church of Nigeria, the Kimbanguist Church of Zaire, and the South African followers of Xhosa prophetess Nontetha Nkwenkwe.[16] Nontetha had survived influenza but lost a child during the pandemic. She began proselytizing after experiencing a series of prophetic dreams during its aftermath.

The possibility of an intimate relationship with the spirits of influenza's dead informed the American Mormon covenant "Vision of the Redemption of the Dead," authored by Joseph F. Smith in October 1918. "Death had surrounded him throughout his life," one scholar notes, and he was personally familiar with grief, but the context of both the Great War and the flu pandemic led him to write this text. Smith saw in 1918 "vast concourses of the dead." His vision saw missionization continuing beyond the grave, with the "work of salvation among the dead."[17] Like spiritualism, Mormonism responded to the loss, grief, and metaphysical questioning of the era by positing a world of the dead with whom the living might commune.

Spiritualism, a broad category encompassing several historical moments and diverse in its practices and practitioners, has been defined as "the belief that the spirits of dead people can communicate with people who are still alive (especially via a medium)."[18] In North America, the foundational event in the history of spiritualism was the "rappings" heard by the young Fox sisters in upstate New York in 1848, which over the next few decades led to spiritualist circles emerging all over North America and across the Atlantic, in which participants communicated with the dead through mediums, automatic writing, table levitation, and other forms of spirit communication. Spiritualism has often been studied as a Victorian or antebellum movement. However, recent studies by Jenny Hazelgrove on Britain, and Stan McMullin on Canada, demonstrate that it experienced a revival of sorts during the period between the world wars in the early twentieth century.[19] Some fascinating parallels exist between the social and cultural contexts within which spiritualism flourished during the nineteenth and twentieth centuries. Both were eras of war, revolution, rebellion, and reform – and epidemics.[20] During the mid-nineteenth century, the American Civil War and devastating epidemics of cholera shook the social order.[21] In both eras, spiritualist movements emerged out of particular historical moments, shaping and being shaped by experiences of mass death and grief, but also co-existent with social movements of a diverse variety, including feminism, anti-racism, labour struggle, middle-class reformism, and religious revivalism.[22] These parallels suggest that spiritualism can usefully be linked with a particular kind of social transformation and mass mourning.

Although there were many paths to spiritualist belief, and not all participants were drawn to it by experiences of grief, many leaders of spiritualist movements had experienced personal loss, often of children, parents, or siblings. Ann Braude begins her study of spiritualism and women's rights in the United States with the story of socialist feminist Annie Denton Cridge, whose first child died in infancy in 1857. Cridge was comforted in her grief by witnessing the spirits of her own dead parents caring for her child's spirit body.[23] Another commonly cited example is that of Sir Oliver Lodge, a physicist and core member of the British Society for Psychical Research, who lost his youngest son, Raymond, aged twenty-six, at Ypres in 1915.[24] In 1916, Lodge published *Raymond,* an explication of the family's spiritualist searches for evidence of Raymond's afterlife. This book went through a dozen printings between 1916 and 1919. The Lodge family's experience has helped to establish the standard historical narrative of twentieth-century spiritualism, which links the growth in spiritualist practice to war death and mourning. The interwar spiritualist revival is generally described in social and cultural histories of the era without reference to the influenza pandemic, as a "powerful means by which the living 'saw' the dead of the Great War."[25] Many influential spiritualists themselves privileged the role of the war in their texts. The Great War's importance in shaping interwar cultural patterns of loss, faith, and memory in North America and Britain has thereby significantly overshadowed the significance of the pandemic.[26]

This dominant narrative can be misleading. However powerful the vocabulary of wartime sacrifice and military commemoration, not all tragedy in these years took place in the theatre of war. Consider the experience of Sir Arthur Conan Doyle and his wife, Jean. Several members of their extended family, including two brothers-in-law and two nephews, died in battle. But Doyle's son from his first marriage, Kingsley, died during the influenza pandemic while caring for patients as a medical intern. Because Kingsley had been injured at the Somme, his death is commonly described as war-related.[27] He recovered from his war wounds, however, only to die in London at the end of October 1918 from complications of influenza. Four months later, Doyle's younger brother, Innes, to whom he had long been close, died of pneumonia following influenza.[28] Although Doyle had been interested in spiritualism, it was after these events that he became an active proponent, lecturing and touring internationally on the subject.[29] In his 1926 novel *The Land of Mist,* the protagonist, Professor Challenger, is converted to spiritualism after his wife dies "suddenly from virulent pneumonia following influenza," after which "the man staggered and went down."[30]

The Doyles sought often to communicate with their dead son. On 7 September 1919, with the help of a medium, Welsh spiritualist Evan Powell, the couple spoke with Kingsley. Doyle described this experience:

> Then came to me what was the supreme moment of my spiritual experience. It is almost too sacred for full description, and yet I feel that God sends such gifts that we may share them with others. There came a voice in the darkness, a whispered voice, saying "Jean, it is I." My wife felt a hand upon her head, and cried, "It is Kingsley." I heard the word "Father." I said "Dear boy, is that you?" I had then a sense of a face very near my own, and of breathing ... A strong hand then rested upon my head, it was gently bent forward, and I felt and heard a kiss just above my brow. "Tell me, dear, are

you happy?" I cried. There was silence, and I feared he was gone. Then on a sighing note came the words, "yes I am so happy."[31]

The Lodges and the Doyles were famous voices in a broader transatlantic spiritualist movement. Many Canadians, like their counterparts in Britain, the United States, and elsewhere, responded to the loss of life characteristic of the 1914-20 era – deaths caused not only by war but also by pandemic disease – by reshaping their religious and spiritual practices. One of the expressions of this phenomenon, albeit by no means the only one, was a revival of interest in spiritualism. During this period, attempts to commune with the deceased beyond the grave increased dramatically in number. The curious and the committed gathered to investigate psychical phenomena and founded spiritualist circles and churches across Canada.[32] In July 1923, Arthur Conan Doyle came to proselytize the "proofs of immortality" in Winnipeg. Nearly two thousand people came to hear him speak at the Walker Theatre.[33] Doyle found a vibrant spiritualist community in the city, of which he wrote in his memoir, *Our Second American Adventure*.[34] He and Jean Doyle formed a long-lasting friendship with the Hamilton family. Like the Doyles, with whom they shared the experience of losing a child to the flu pandemic, Thomas and Lillian Hamilton sought solace in their emergent spiritualist practice and belief. The spiritualist practices of the Hamilton circle demonstrate the private and familial connections between the pandemic – which broke the boundaries between civilian and soldier – and a flourishing interwar spiritualism in Canada.[35]

The Hamiltons in Social Context

Although some cultural historians have focused on nineteenth-century spiritualism as being an oppositional movement, embraced by feminists and radicals of a wide variety, scholars have also pointed to its diversity and broad appeal over time and across social boundaries. Literary scholar Helen Sword has argued that "its widespread appeal seems to have depended, above all, on its elastic capacity to offer something for everyone, the empowered as well as the powerless."[36] Spiritualism attracted religious reformers, seeking "a less hierarchical, more personal context with God," as well as scientists "who hoped to reveal material explanations for what they considered to be very real and plausible psychic phenomena."[37] Stan McMullin has argued that spiritualism, particularly for Protestants, was an attempt to integrate tensions between science and faith, a rejection of the sometimes crude materialism of science, a "scientific religion."[38]

In Canada, spiritualism attracted the well educated and professionals, many of them, like Thomas Hamilton, physicians. Medicine, however, was not always welcoming or sympathetic to spiritualist pursuit. In the late nineteenth century, as other scientists showed curiosity about the claims of spiritualism, physicians remained largely opposed to it. In fact, as a number of scholars have shown, orthodox physicians pathologized and sought to medicalize spirit mediumship, developing diagnoses such as "credo-mania" and "mediomania," the latter associated with the dysfunction of the female reproductive organs.[39] For some medical men, spiritualism was a disease that should be studied and treated: neurologists attributed it to altered blood flow to the brain during excitement; psychological medicine tended to argue that it was caused by neuroses; or perhaps it was a hereditary defect.[40] The less hostile advocated objective empirical research and observation. S.E.D. Shortt has suggested that by the late nineteenth century, medicine, with its professionalizing claims to scientific objectivity, had disavowed religion and metaphysics, and become a secular science.[41] Diseases, including epidemics such as cholera, were to be understood not through the lenses of faith or managed through religious practices such as fasting and prayer, but by public health ordinances and hygiene.[42]

There is much in the Hamilton story that suggests a less firm boundary between medicine and faith than the secularization thesis of medical history suggests. Nonetheless, it is clear why Thomas Hamilton the physician preferred to describe himself as a psychical researcher, not a spiritualist. He wished to be publicly perceived as a scientist attempting to document the existence of psychic phenomena. In this essay, spiritualism is employed as a label in part because, despite his claims of scientific objectivity, Hamilton was not an impartial observer of his mediums and experiments. At the same time, whatever the protestations of adherents that they were interested only in rational, skeptical, scientific observation, some role must be given to unconscious desire.[43] Hamilton and his family, like many other practising spiritualists in interwar Canada and elsewhere, were drawn to spiritualism for complex reasons, many of them deeply emotional, psychological, and metaphysical.

The Hamiltons were a respectable, aspiring middle-class Protestant Winnipeg couple, both of them ethnically Scottish Canadian and Presbyterian. Thomas was born on 27 November 1873 in Agincourt, Ontario, and moved with his family to homestead in Saskatchewan in

1883. They built their home on the bank of the North Saskatchewan River in what is now Saskatoon. After the death of his father and sister, Thomas moved with his mother and four of his five brothers to Winnipeg in 1891. He trained as a teacher at Manitoba College and taught classes to raise funds to attend medical school. He graduated from the Manitoba Medical College in 1903, and in 1905, he began his private practice in Elmwood, where he lived and worked throughout his medical career. Hamilton has been described as "Elmwood's first doctor."[44]

In 1906, when he was thirty-three years old, Hamilton married Lillian May Forrester. She was born in Emerson, Manitoba, into a family of Scots ancestry. She trained as a nurse at the Winnipeg General Hospital nursing school, graduating in 1905 and winning the medal for "Highest General Proficiency" among her class. After graduation, she was briefly employed as a staff nurse at the Winnipeg General Hospital. Like other women of her era, she did not continue to work professionally (at least in a hospital setting) after her marriage. She was active in a number of women's and church organizations, including the Woman's Missionary Society, the Medical Faculty Women's Club of the University of Manitoba, and the Women's Musical Club.[45] Together, the Hamiltons had four children, two of them twin boys, James Drummond and Arthur Lamont, born on 27 September 1915.

Like many other early-twentieth-century spiritualists in Canada, Thomas Hamilton was a liberal Protestant social reformer. He was active in medical professional organizations: "In 1921 he was elected President of the newly formed University of Manitoba Alumni Association and President of the Manitoba Medical Association. As well, he published the first edition of the Manitoba Medical Association Bulletin. In 1923 he was appointed one of Manitoba's two representatives to the Executive of the Canadian Medical Association – a position he held until 1933."[46] The Hamiltons were active congregants of the Presbyterian King Memorial Church. In fact, their first experiments with telepathy were conducted with its minister, Dr. Daniel McLachlan, in 1918, before the influenza pandemic. Hamilton would write down his thoughts and attempt to transmit them telepathically to McLachlan, in the next room.

Had Hamilton never become famous for his psychical research, he would have been known for his role in the Liberal government of T.C. Norris (1915-20), which instituted a high number of reformist initiatives, including the enfranchisement of women (the first province to do so in 1916), a Minimum Wage Act, a Mothers' Allowance Act that provided for widows' pensions, amendments to the Public Health Act, a Pharmaceutical

Act to restrict the sale of cocaine and morphine, electoral reforms, and a Workmen's Compensation Act. After having served as a school trustee for Ward 7 from 1906, Hamilton was elected as a member of the legislature in 1915, where he served until 1920, when he was defeated by a labour candidate. Although not a member of Norris's Cabinet, Hamilton served on and chaired a number of standing committees and helped to guide the passage of legislation that made the Manitoba Medical College part of the University of Manitoba, in keeping with the recommendations for university-based medical training made by the Flexner report.[47]

Hamilton was also the first chairperson of the Winnipeg committee of the Mothers' Allowance Commission. In 1916, Manitoba had introduced Canada's first social security program for single mothers (widows and those whose husbands were in prison, insane asylums, or sanitaria). Applications were processed and benefits administered under the auspices of local boards, which were made up of community members (not professional social workers). Although not created for this purpose, the Mothers' Allowance program became essential for the financial stability of about 120 female-led Manitoba households after the deaths of their husbands from influenza. After exhausting their existing resources (indeed, the program required them to spend their savings before applying), influenza widows with two or more children under the age of sixteen were entitled to benefits in support of costs such as rent, food, and clothing. The program was not financially generous, but it allowed the wives of flu victims to keep their families together.[48] As Winnipeg committee chair, Hamilton would have learned about the lives of the dozens of influenza widows, most of them working class, who applied in desperation to the program after the pandemic.

GRIEF AND THE TURN TO SPIRITUALISM

According to her daughter, Margaret, Lillian Hamilton immediately turned to notions of the afterlife as consolation after Arthur died. She read and "studied" Frederick Myers's *Human Personality and Its Survival of Bodily Death,* first published in 1906. A Cambridge-trained poet and essayist, Myers was one of turn-of-the-century Britain's most prominent spiritualist investigators and a co-founder of the Society for Psychical Research. Lillian's grief was "assuaged" by his arguments and the level of his personal belief in the afterlife.[49] However, her husband's interest in life after death was very real in the immediate aftermath of influenza, as was that of his closest friend, clergyman Daniel McLachlan. The two shared the experience of witnessing their children suffer from the flu. All three of McLachlan's children contracted it, and as he nursed them through a long night, he had a psychic experience. Years later, Margaret Hamilton recalled his description of the event: "He entered his study and he saw, seated at his desk, the living figure of a living woman at midnight ... And he told my father about this and he said 'As God is my witness I saw the living figure of my dead sister, Margaret.'"[50] The figure was "dressed in a white garment, brown hair falling over her shoulders, and who looked at him in a perfectly calm and composed manner. He noted the light – which came from the hall – shining on her hair, on her beautifully moulded arms, and saw that she was indeed a living woman."[51] Margaret Hamilton believed that McLachlan's experience had an influence on her father, particularly because he felt the same anguish at the illness of his children during the epidemic and could comprehend McLachlan's belief that he had seen his sister "from the other side."

From this point on, led initially by Lillian, the Hamiltons explored in much greater depth the possibility of life after death and communication with the deceased through the spiritual realm. Like the Doyles, whose governess had been the first household member to manifest automatic writing during the war, the Hamiltons began their experimentation within the domestic realm of the family. Elizabeth Poole (later known as the medium Elizabeth M.) was a working-class Scottish immigrant living in Elmwood. She was intimately familiar not only with the Hamiltons, but also with their recent bereavement. Thomas Hamilton knew her from her work as a practical nurse. Before and during the pandemic, she was employed in the Hamilton household. She was close to the children and continued to care for them into the 1920s. Elizabeth Poole thus represents a crucial link between the Hamilton family's experience of death and grief, and its incipient spiritualist belief. Margaret said of Elizabeth, "She was our second mother, and a dearly loved friend and nurse, our nurse during influenza [in] 1919. We owe her so much."[52] Lillian Hamilton described her as "uneducated, illiterate, but loved by all who knew her well, for her sunny gaiety, her warm kindliness, her loving and childlike heart." "Elizabeth's gifts," she wrote, "were both physical and mental."[53]

In 1920, Lillian convinced her husband to attend one of her meetings with "Elizabeth M.," as Poole became known, during which a table rose off the floor (see Figure 8.2). In the early years of the Hamiltons' experimentation with psychic forces, Elizabeth M. was the medium in nearly four hundred seances. These were attended by the Hamilton circle, which included several prominent physicians, professionals, and Protestant clergy

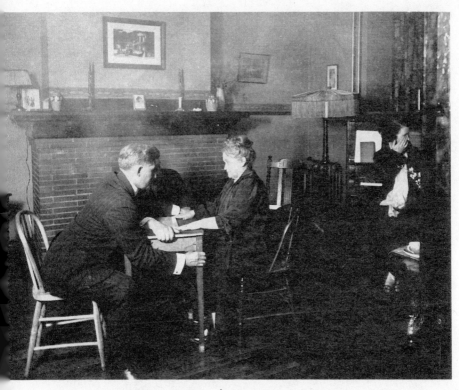

FIGURE 8.2   Telekinesis #1 – first experiment. Home of Dr. Thomas Glendenning
Hamilton, 26 March 1923. Pictured are Dr. Hamilton, Mrs. Poole (Elizabeth M.), and
D.B. MacDonald. *Source:* University of Manitoba Archives and Special Collections,
Hamilton family fonds, UM_pc012_A79-041_009 _0001_001_0001

and theologians, including Isaac Pitblado (an eminent city lawyer), Dr.
Bruce Chown (son of Dr. Gordon Chown and later a key researcher in
the discovery and management of Rhesus disease in newborns), and Dr.
Ross Mitchell. Elizabeth Poole believed herself to have the gift of second
sight, or what Lillian Hamilton referred to as "pre-vision." Poole said her
mother had called her a "witch."[54] She manifested an array of psychic
abilities over the years of her mediumship in the Hamilton group, including telekinesis (table tipping), rapping, precognition, clairvoyance, automatic writings, and deep trance visions and speech.[55] She was also a key
intermediary in the later mediumship of Mary M., which produced the
Hamilton circle's spectacular ectoplasm photographs.
    While in her trance, Elizabeth M. received communications from
luminaries such as Robert Louis Stevenson, missionary David Livingstone,

and Camille Flammarion, a French astronomer.[56] Many of her spirit communications came from W.T. Stead, the Victorian British journalist, author
of *The Maiden Tribute of Modern Babylon* (1885). After achieving public
prominence in the English spiritualist movement, Stead focused on jour-
nalism and politics until 1909, when his eldest son, Willie, died suddenly
at the age of thirty-three. For Stead, this was the true test of his commitment to spiritualism:

> I had always said I would never make my final pronouncement on the truths
> of Spiritualism until someone near and dear in my own family passed into
> the great beyond. Then I should know whether Spiritualism stood the test
> of a great bereavement, bringing life and immortality to light. And I am
> here to tell you that the reality of my son's continued existence, and of his
> tender care for me, have annulled the bitterness of death ... When my boy
> was here, our offices were connected by telephone, and it is much the same
> now. He writes to me through several mediums, he shows himself to my
> friends. I myself have seen his materialised face. One friend has seen him
> at least three times fully materialised, as was our Lord after His resurrection.
> He is here to-night beside me. I am as sure of that as I am of the fact that
> I am speaking to you. When I realise the difference it makes to have this
> knowledge, and to be without it, I feel I must testify to you as to the reality
> of the unseen world around us.[57]

Stead, who died in 1912, often came through and communicated with the
Hamilton circle. A chapter is devoted to these communications in Thomas
Hamilton's posthumously published study of psychic phenomena, *Intention
and Survival.*[58]

The child Arthur Lamont Hamilton's manifestation during the deep
trances of Elizabeth M. first appears in the written records of the Hamilton
seances in 1923, then again in 1927. There is no evidence at this stage of
sustained regular contact with him. He appeared to Elizabeth M. in a
vision on 27 January 1929, the tenth anniversary of his death.[59] In April
of that year, Lillian Hamilton's recently deceased father and dead brother
also appeared to Elizabeth M. The 1920s were years of gradual development
in Elizabeth M.'s psychic abilities, when the Hamilton family's level of
engagement with psychic research escalated. In this process, a struggle of
sorts occurred in Thomas Hamilton and in the family itself, as its members
sought to come to terms with the significance of their psychic experimentation and the tension between private beliefs and public revelations of
their spiritualist practice. Publicly, both Hamiltons were silent on the role

Arthur's death played in their beliefs. They never made any public confession, similar to those of Stead, Lodge, or Doyle, that grief had motivated the desire to communicate with the dead.

Although scholars have suggested that nineteenth-century spiritualism was subversive in its granting of mediumship and power to women, Hazelgrove has recently argued that twentieth-century spiritualists drew on traditional images of "transcendent femininity."[60] The Hamiltons certainly approached their spiritualist practices in very gendered ways. Of the two Hamilton adults, it was Lillian who connected their seances more openly and directly, albeit privately, with their grief and mourning of Arthur's death. She wrote of her commitment to a belief in survival in an unpublished synopsis of this early period:

> Especially was I enthralled by his [Myers's] great epilogue – a summing up of his studies of mental phenomena written from the standpoint of the scientist, the classical scholar, the poet, and the deeply religious thinker. Without stressing this discovery to anyone – not even T.G. [Thomas] – for me the problem was settled: religious faith in survival no longer walked alone but went hand in hand with evidence of a scientific nature. A new world had opened up – a world of belief that helped me part with Arthur without tears and with an inner joy that one of my beloveds was safely over and ready for other-world evolutionary endeavors.[61]

In this personal narrative, Lillian's motherhood moves her to explore the possibility of communicating with her child, and her femininity makes her a "natural" participant in spiritualism, although never a spirit medium herself. She seeks out, helps to develop, and facilitates the deployment of the spiritualist gifts of the working-class Scot, Elizabeth Poole, a medium with whom she shares a bond and an experience of grief, but over whom she is nevertheless assured of her class superiority.

Thomas Hamilton's stance was guided by his commitment to science, manly stoicism, and perhaps by a sense of personal reserve; he made every attempt to frame the seances as scientific experiments that would prove the veracity of psychic phenomena rather than the survival of his young son. His records of psychic experimentation are filled with graphs and diagrams, such as Figure 8.3, which rigorously maps the characteristics of deep trance. For the first five years of experimentation in paranormal activity, Hamilton kept his views entirely private. Over time, he began to speak and write publicly, although he remained cautious. Hamilton the public figure, politically active and a leader in his profession, had his reputation

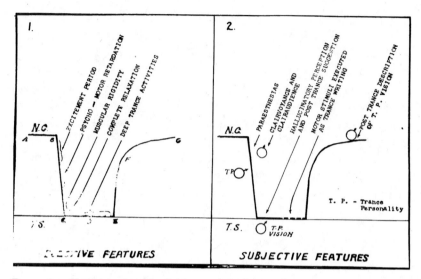

FIGURE 8.3   Trance #41 – graph of objective and subjective features of trance condition. *Source:* University of Manitoba Archives and Special Collections, Hamilton family fonds, UM_pc012_A79-041_009 _0002_041_0002

to consider. Worried that his own personal grief would call his scientific credibility and objectivity into question, he made it clear that his research was not based in "sentiment."[62] In *Intention and Survival,* his emphasis remains firmly on experimentation and scientific proof of ectoplasm and continuing life force after death. The book contains very little that is personal or reflective.

Nonetheless, the Hamiltons were privately utilizing spiritualist practice to maintain their connection to their dead loved ones. During the late 1920s and early 1930s, in two separate sets of seances, a breakthrough occurred in their search for confirmation of Arthur's survival. Mary Marshall (known as Mary M.) had joined the Hamilton circle as a medium in 1928, and through her mediumship the group began to focus on teleplasm, or ectoplasm, as scientific evidence for life after death (see Figure 8.4). Like Elizabeth Poole, who introduced her to the Hamiltons, Mary Marshall was born in Scotland.[63] In a short autobiography she wrote for Lillian Hamilton, no doubt to verify her lack of education or any background that would allow her to fraudulently recreate the works of Stevenson and others through her mediumship, Mary told a story rich in pathos. Born to poor working-class parents in Glasgow, she lost her mother at age three. For a time, she and her older brother lived with her grandmother in

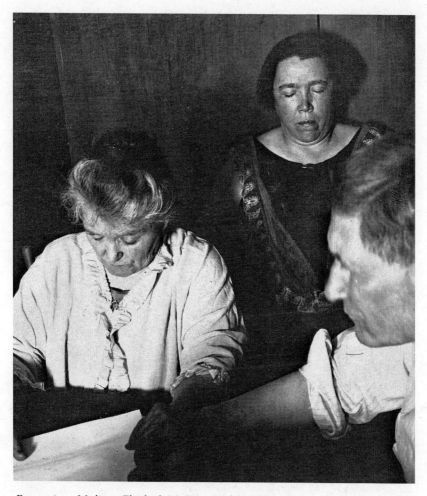

FIGURE 8.4   Mediums Elizabeth M. (Mrs. Poole) and Mary Marshall, in a deep trance state prior to the materialization of the spirit at a seance at the home of Dr. Thomas Glendenning Hamilton on 10 March 1930. Dr. Hamilton is holding the arm of Mrs. Poole. *Source:* University of Manitoba Archives and Special Collections, Hamilton family fonds, UM_pc012_A79-041_009 _0009_028_0001

Ireland, who died and left them in the care of two unmarried aunts, who supported themselves as millworkers. After the sisters quarrelled, the father took the children back, and at age six, Mary was put to work keeping house for him. She ran away, back to Ireland, where her aunt sent her to an orphanage. Secure and cared for, Mary noted that this was "the happiest time of my life." However, the orphanage arranged for her to do domestic work in the household of an English Presbyterian clergyman and his wife, where she was treated kindly. Mary could not adjust to her improved circumstances: "I felt like a fish out of water I had never had the love of a woman nor a kiss from anyone." She moved in and out of domestic service, kept house for her father and brother, and then married. She and her husband emigrated to Canada.[64]

Mary M. demonstrated psychic powers beyond those of Elizabeth M., most particularly the ability to generate ectoplasm, which was believed to be a physical manifestation of a spirit: a gauzy, cloudy substance, it demonstrated a spirit's material presence. It was excreted through the orifices (mouth, nose, and in some cases vagina) of the spirit medium. The term "ectoplasm" was coined by French physician Charles Richet (winner of the 1913 Nobel Prize in Physiology/Medicine for his role in the discovery of anaphylaxis), who had a long-standing interest and involvement in psychical research. The Hamilton group used photography in an attempt to prove the presence of ectoplasm, and the family archive contains numerous fascinating shots taken by Thomas Hamilton with the help of other members of the circle, which show ectoplasm emerging from the body of Mary M. In some of these photos, the ectoplasm congealed to reveal the faces of the spirits whose communications Mary was transmitting.

Arthur's survival was suggested by the appearance of his face in ectoplasm, which was photographed during a 25 November 1928 seance at the Hamilton home (see Figure 8.5). At the seance were W.B. Cooper (who worked in the insurance sector), a Mrs. Alder, the transportation engineer Hugh Reed, Ada Turner (a university-educated English teacher), Harry Green, fellow Scot and CPR lawyer, and Dr. James A. Hamilton, Thomas's brother. At this sitting, both Elizabeth M. and Mary M. were acting as mediums, working together as they often did in this period. The spirit control known as Walter, who through Mary (and Elizabeth) often communicated between the living and the dead, instructed Thomas Hamilton regarding when and how to photograph the ectoplasm: "Walter: Ready? Ready? One! ... Do you know about the signals? Dr. T.G. [Hamilton]: Yes, I'm to fire 2 seconds after your three." While the medium relayed Walter's commands, the others held hands and sang, the medium violently beating her elbows on a table in time to the music. Harry Green is described as experiencing "acute spasms." After two rounds of photographs, with four different cameras, Walter expressed his exhaustion and frustration: "O-o-h! No more tonight. There's one of them that's not right, one of the cameras. You didn't get it, the way you want it. It's not as good as I thought it would

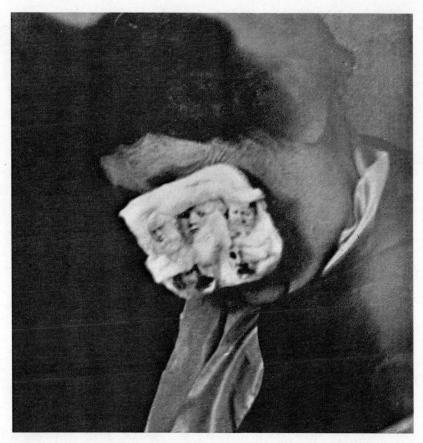

FIGURE 8.5   Teleplasmic mass attached to the face of the medium, Mary Marshall. Top left, Grandfather W. Centre, Arthur Lamont Hamilton. Top right, unrecognized. Lower left, Robert Louis Stevenson. Lower right, David Livingstone. Seance at the home of Thomas Glendenning Hamilton, 25 November 1928. University of Manitoba Archives and Special Collections, Hamilton family fonds, UM_pc012_A79-041_009 _0004_009_0003

be ... There are two you won't be able to recognize, there's too much ecto-plasm. The conditions are not as good as I would like them to be: there is too much attention; you are too tense." As Walter had stated, Arthur appears in the picture, as a baby, younger even than he was when he died.

Toward the end of the sitting, Ada Turner spoke to Walter, asking him, "Walter, when I get so weary, are you using me or am I just sleepy?" Walter replied, "I use every body, even the little fellow." The transcription of the seance then stated, "Here general laughter follows when little Jim is discovered in the corner. Up to this point he has been as quiet as a mouse."[65] Little Jim was the youngest of the surviving Hamilton children, Arthur's twin, who would have been just fourteen when this event took place. Despite their youth, it was not uncommon for the Hamilton children to be involved in the circle's psychic experimentation, although Glen was much less often mentioned. His relationship with the family and its spiritualism appears to have been troubled at times. Correspondence between Lillian Hamilton and Elizabeth Poole (who continued to work for the family as child care provider and nurse) suggests that James and Glen had a conflicted relationship during the early 1920s. Glen was teased at school about the family's reputation, and in interviews, he recalled children chalking "This is the Ghost House" on his home. This "ribbing" prevented him from publicly discussing the Hamilton research; it also seems to have contributed to his own partial withdrawal from the family's preoccupation with spiritualism.[66]

The seances occupied a central role in Hamilton family life during the 1920s and early 1930s. This period saw weekly sessions with a larger group and an additional weekly seance with a smaller, more intimate group limited to family; the latter ran from 1920 until 1935, when Thomas Hamilton died suddenly of a heart attack. Again, useful comparisons can be drawn with the Doyle household. Historian Ruth Brandon has described the Doyle home circle as "an intense, emotional, and highly motivated affair."[67] The same can be said of the Hamilton small circle. Their intensity was particularly demonstrated by Lillian and her daughter, Margaret, who attended most family sittings (Margaret recorded the sessions). James occasionally participated, and Glen did so infrequently. The mediums in the larger Hamilton circle were almost all women. However, in its more private spiritualism, the family began to work with a male medium, John (Jay) MacDonald, who spoke messages from the deceased. In these seances, Arthur came through regularly, as did better-known figures such as Claude Debussy (known as Sterge), Robert Louis Stevenson, Harry Houdini, and Frederick Myers.[68] During the early 1930s, Arthur communicated regularly. In February 1933, Lillian, Thomas, and Margaret gathered for a seance with MacDonald, Margaret recording. Through the medium, "Arthur purported to speak. He greeted the sitters, remarked that his father was present at this time and after about 2 or 3 minutes conversation left, giving place to Sterge [Debussy]. Sterge: 'That was a gift to you (meaning Arthur's presence). The old man [Thomas] was so dumb that he didn't know it! We have to use your boy to help us and we are letting him practise. He knows where you are (to T.G.H.).'" In the 1933 sittings of the small circle, Arthur comes through as a young man, kind and playful. James, his twin, began to attend sessions regularly in May 1933.

There was often gentle teasing and laughter between the family and Arthur. The written record shows that this everyday banter, particularly between Lillian and the children, became quite relaxed over time. In June 1933, Arthur "reminisce[d] about the lake and holidays, and says he comes with us from year to year." In September, he reminded Lillian and Margaret of his impending birthday. In March 1934, Glen Hamilton attended, an unusual occurrence. Arthur's spirit was excited by the presence of all the family, called his father "Pop," and told "Glen that he will be used in his work as an instrument through his own motivation, but with the help of unseen friends." Later that year, just before Margaret was to be married, he teased her about preparations for the wedding, joking that "if they [the Hamilton family] do this for the departure of a daughter, what more will they do for the return of a son?" Lillian and Arthur together imagined his prodigal return, "Arthur seeing himself clad in armor, like King Arthur. We chat together, and Arthur leaves very quietly, with no apparent effect on the medium," Margaret records.[69] Thomas Hamilton was absent from this seance.

Even in death, Arthur was trying to perform for the family, to show his eagerness to contribute to its psychic researches. Many of his messages to his family were not explicitly of comfort or longing but rather of usefulness. On 9 March 1933, at a sitting with Lillian, Margaret, and the medium, Arthur explained his spirit role:

Hello mother! Hello Margaret! Your atmosphere is awfully good tonight, quite calm, no noise or bustle. It's so quiet and restful that even the mice won't wake up! That's as long as I can stay; my message is more personal than vital. I hope my message will be vital someday. It is hard for me to give evidence that could be used with others. It is a big question, that's why I am not trying to be a witness but simply a communicator; but I hope someday to be a control worthy of the family. Give my love to all that are away – my brothers and my father and good night and God bless you.[70]

A week later, after greeting his family and joking about making better puns than his twin brother, James, Arthur gave a long speech about his hopes for building his own spirit control capacities:

I'm getting through better. There, that's better now! I'm becoming quite good at it. I can come fluently. You see, we put Walter through first and then I come through to clean up. I'm a street cleaner, just a wiper ... Sit back, Dad, you'll wear yourself out listening like that. There, that's better. Save yourself.

I think the foremost and best thing I do is to work for you. I have nothing to tell you until I have served and worked ... You see, I've been over here a comparatively long time but there is much I want to know. I am going to make a study of communication ... But tonight I was with you when you were dining. I stood there thinking of communication of the strangeness and of the miracle of it. And I thought of mediums, that is, controls to you. We have an instrument which is sometimes good, sometimes poor.

Over the course of this seance, the medium became very tense, his breathing snarling, "heavy and rough," and he grasped Thomas by the throat, as if to strangle him. He then dropped back into his chair, and Arthur appeared, as a gentle and healing spirit attempting to diffuse the impact of the angry spirit who preceded him. He explained, "It's so much easier for me to smooth things because I'm less earthly. My emanations are not earthy, they are more emanations of the spirit, since my emotional development on earth, and the things that go with it, has been so little. My emotions are more pure. Therefore I am more tranquilly. I flow through and when I have flown through I leave nothing for another control to combat. I not only clean up but I clear up."[71] Arthur continued to perform this emotionally calming and nurturing role throughout the small circle seances in 1933. On one occasion, he promised to look after a "poor soul" who had died a violent or painful death and who appeared through John MacDonald as a man named Woods.[72] Sterge referred to this and other cases as Arthur's "rescue" work.[73]

After Thomas Hamilton's death in 1935, Lillian became increasingly open about her interest in the afterlife, revealing a more popular strand of spiritualism in the group's experiments.[74] Before her husband's death, she had published few writings about spiritualism, but her 1940s and 1950s articles in spiritualist journals such as *Light* offer a slightly modified history of the couple's earliest encounters with the spirit world. According to Lillian, some of their first research was done with a ten-year-old girl identified as Lucy, the daughter of a local clergyman, who demonstrated "astonishing gifts" while playing with a Ouija board. Using the Ouija board, Lucy correctly identified words that Thomas Hamilton conveyed telepathically. In the same article, Lillian referred to communication between a

Margaret M. and her son, who died of war injuries in 1917.[75] During the mid-1940s, Lillian received messages via Mary M. from her dead husband. He reassured Lillian that he was among friends and fellow spiritualists on the other side. This narrative, of a circle of friends experimenting with Ouija boards in the presence of children and communicating with their deceased loved ones, was a domesticated, if not feminized image of psychic research that Thomas Hamilton was careful to publicly avoid. By the 1950s, Lillian was less constricted by concerns about potential damage to her husband's credibility or professional status and was willing to reveal a more domestic and emotional side of the family's earliest attempts to demonstrate the truth of psychic phenomena than was evident in her husband's copious publications on the subject.

CONCLUSION

It has not been my intention to demonstrate that interwar spiritualism was attributable solely to the impact of the influenza pandemic. Rather, I provide an example of a prominent spiritualist family whose pursuit of evidence of the afterlife was shaped by its personal experience of the pandemic. As Helen Sword has noted, "Young men who have died in battle hold no monopoly on inducing parental grief."[76] Parents, husbands, wives, siblings, and even animal lovers have sought to establish ongoing relationships with their loved ones. The grief of the Hamilton family was expressed through its desire to believe in Arthur's survival of death and was "rooted in primal sorrow."[77] The Hamiltons were among the many who sought to find solace in the wake of a catastrophic and unanticipated global pandemic, coming at the end of a brutal war, in a hybrid blend of science and faith. As their experience attests, spiritualism's hybridity may have been shaped within the confines of gender and class relations, but it was flexible enough to allow for meaningful reparations of grief, however complex and diverse.

In the history of the influenza pandemic and cultural responses to it lies a creative tension between modernity and science, on the one hand, and more traditional venues for the expression and management of loss and grief, such as Christian faith in the afterlife. The Hamiltons demonstrate how these interpretive frameworks could be bridged in the lived experience of the family. Those psychic researchers who, like Thomas Hamilton, attempted to distance themselves from any sentimentality and "hysteria" in popular spiritualism must be understood as simultaneously driven by a familial and personal desire to ascertain the truth of life beyond death and to maintain contact with their loved ones. Their spiritualist practice makes the fullest sense only within the context of their grief and that of their community, which had survived a crucible of loss.

NOTES

1 Baby book of Arthur Lamont Hamilton, University of Manitoba Archives and Special Collections (UMASC), Hamilton Family fonds, A10-01, Winnipeg.
2 Stan McMullin, *Anatomy of a Seance: A History of Spirit Communication in Central Canada* (Montreal and Kingston: McGill-Queen's University Press, 2004), xiv.
3 "Given the cultural turn in current historiography," Guy Beiner wrote recently in the journal *Cultural and Social History,* "it is beyond belief that no cultural history of the pandemic has been written to date." Guy Beiner, "Out in the Cold and Back: New-Found Interest in the Great Flu," *Cultural and Social History* 3,4 (October 2006): 496.
4 Esyllt W. Jones, *Influenza 1918: Disease, Death, and Struggle in Winnipeg* (Toronto: University of Toronto Press, 2007), Chapter 3.
5 Jim Park, *On the East of the River: A History of the East Kildonan-Transcona Community* (Winnipeg: City of Winnipeg Community Parks and Recreation, 2002), 99.
6 "14,029 Persons Are Attacked by 'Flu' in Winnipeg between October 5 and End of January," *Winnipeg Tribune,* 12 March 1919, 3. See also Jones, *Influenza 1918,* 59.
7 According to a 1987 interview with Glen F. Hamilton, Thomas Hamilton's son, quoted in James Nickels, "Psychic Research in a Winnipeg Family: Reminiscences of Dr. Glen F. Hamilton," *Manitoba History* 55 (June 2007): 53.
8 Janice Hamilton, pers. comm., 11 May 2010 (correspondence in author's possession).
9 "14,029 Persons Are Attacked by 'Flu,'" 3.
10 Nickels, "Psychic Research," 53.
11 Quoted in ibid.
12 Ibid.
13 Nickels, "Psychic Research," 53.
14 David Simmons, "Religion and Medicine at the Crossroads: A Re-Examination of the Southern Rhodesian Influenza Epidemic of 1918," *Journal of Southern African Studies* 35,1 (2009): 30.
15 Terence Ranger, "The Influenza Pandemic in Southern Rhodesia: A Crisis of Comprehension," in *Imperial Medicine and Indigenous Societies,* ed. David Arnold (Delhi: Oxford University Press, 1989), 183.
16 Ibid., 184-85; Robert Edgar and Hilary Sapire, *African Apocalypse: The Story of Nontetha Nkwenkwe, a Twentieth-Century South African Prophet* (Athens: Ohio University Center for International Studies, 1999), xx, 10. See also Howard Phillips, *Black October: the Impact of the Spanish Influenza Epidemic of 1918 on South Africa* (Pretoria: Government Printer, 1990), Chapter 8. For the Nigerian Aladura Church, see Deidre Helen Crumbley, "On Being First: Dogma, Disease and Domination in the Rise of an African Church," *Religion* 30 (2000): 169-84.
17 George S. Tate, "'The Great World of the Spirits of the Dead': Death, the Great War, and the 1918 Influenza Pandemic as Context for Doctrine and Covenants 138," *BYU Studies* 46,1 (2007): 12, 34-36.

18 "Spiritualism," WordNet: A Lexical Database for English, http://wordnetweb.princeton.edu/.

19 Jenny Hazelgrove, *Spiritualism and British Society between the Wars* (Manchester: Manchester University Press, 2000); and McMullin, *Anatomy of a Seance.*

20 Molly McGarry, *Ghost of Futures Past: Spiritualism and the Cultural Politics of Nineteenth-Century America* (Berkeley: University of California Press, 2008), 1.

21 For cholera in Canada, see Geoffrey Bilson, *A Darkened House: Cholera in Nineteenth-Century Canada* (Toronto: University of Toronto Press, 1980). For the USA, see Charles Rosenberg, *The Cholera Years: The United States in 1832, 1849 and 1866* (Chicago: University of Chicago Press, 1962). For Europe, see François Delaporte, *Disease and Civilization: The Cholera in Paris, 1832* (Cambridge, MA: MIT Press, 1986); and Richard J. Evans, *Death in Hamburg: Society and Politics in the Cholera Years, 1830-1910* (London: Penguin Books, 1987). For Britain, consult R.J. Morris, *Cholera 1832: The Social Response to an Epidemic* (London: Croom Helm, 1976). For a discussion of some of the relationships between social change and epidemic disease, see the collection edited by Terence Ranger and Paul Slack, *Epidemics and Ideas: Essays on the Historical Perception of Pestilence* (Cambridge: Cambridge University Press, 1992).

22 For Canada, see Ramsay Cook, "Spiritualism, Science of the Earthly Paradise," *Canadian Historical Review* 65 (March 1984): 4-27. For Britain, see Logie Barrow, *Independent Spirits: Spiritualism and English Plebeians 1850-1910* (London: Routledge and Kegan Paul, 1986); and Alex Owen, *The Darkened Room: Women, Power, and Spiritualism in Late Victorian England* (London: Virago, 1989). For the USA, see Hans Baer, *The Black Spiritual Movement: A Religious Response to Racism* (Knoxville: University of Tennessee Press, 1984); and Ann Braude, *Radical Spirits: Spiritualism and Women's Rights in Nineteenth Century America* (Boston: Beacon, 1989).

23 Ibid., 1.

24 Helen Sword, *Ghostwriting Modernism* (Ithaca: Cornell University Press, 2002), 47.

25 Jay Winter, *Sites of Memory, Sites of Mourning: The Great War in European Cultural History* (Cambridge: Cambridge University Press, 1995), 54.

26 See, for example, Ruth Brandon, *The Spiritualists: The Passion for the Occult in the Nineteenth and Twentieth Centuries* (New York: Alfred A. Knopf, 1983), Chapter 6; Hazelgrove, *Spiritualism and British Society;* Sword, *Ghostwriting Modernism;* and Winter, *Sites of Memory,* Chapter 3.

27 While discussing twentieth-century spiritualism as a response to the war, Jay Winter states that Kingsley "was wounded while serving at the Somme and died of pneumonia in London in 1918." Ibid., 58.

28 Dinah Birch, "The Ghosts of Sir Arthur Conan Doyle," *Times Literary Supplement,* 7 November 2007, http://entertainment.timesonline.co.uk/.

29 For an alternative opinion that downplays the relevance of Doyle's emotional experience, see Alex Owen, "'Borderland Forms': Arthur Conan Doyle, Albion's Daughters, and the Politics of the Cottingley Fairies," *History Workshop Journal* 38 (1994): 67.

30 Arthur Conan Doyle, *The Land of Mist* (London: Hutchinson, 1926), 11.

31 Quoted in Kelvin I. Jones, *Conan Doyle and the Spirits: The Spiritualist Career of Sir Arthur Conan Doyle* (Wellingborough, UK: Aquarian Press, 1989), 136.

32 McMullin, *Anatomy of a Seance,* xvii. See also Walter Meyer zu Erpen and Joy Lowe, "The Canadian Spiritualist Movement and Sources for Its Study," *Archivaria* 30 (Summer 1990): 77.

33 "Crowded House Hears Conan Doyle Speak," *Manitoba Free Press* (Winnipeg), 4 July 1923, 9. See Michael W. Homer, "Arthur Conan Doyle's Adventures in Winnipeg," *Manitoba History* 25 (Spring 1993), http://www.mhs.mb.ca/.

34 Arthur Conan Doyle, *Our Second American Adventure* (Boston: Little, Brown, 1924), 223-31.

35 McMullin, *Anatomy of a Seance,* 107.

36 Sword, *Ghostwriting Modernism,* 3. See also S.E.D. Shortt, "Physicians and Psychics: The Anglo-American Medical Response to Spiritualism, 1870-1890," *Journal of the History of Medicine and Allied Sciences* 39 (1984): 341.

37 Sword, *Ghostwriting Modernism,* 3-4.

38 McMullin, *Anatomy of a Seance,* 16.

39 Shortt, "Physicians and Psychics," 343; and Braude, *Radical Spirits,* 159.

40 Shortt, "Physicians and Psychics," 347.

41 Ibid., 351-52.

42 Rosenberg, *The Cholera Years,* 213-25.

43 Owen, "'Borderland Forms,'" 71.

44 "Elmwood's First Doctor," *Elmwood Herald,* 10 June 1954, 2.

45 "Mrs. T. Glen Hamilton Early Elmwood Resident Dies, Aged 75 Years," *Elmwood Herald,* 20 September 1956, 8.

46 "Biography of T.G. Hamilton," Manuscript Finding Aid, UMASC, Hamilton Family fonds, http://umanitoba.ca/.

47 "Biography of T.G. Hamilton," Manuscript Finding Aid, UMASC, Hamilton Family fonds.

48 Jones, *Influenza 1918,* Chapter 6.

49 "Interview with Margaret Hamilton Bach, November 26, 1980," 7, UMASC, Hamilton Family fonds.

50 Ibid.

51 Lillian Hamilton described this same event in her papers. Lillian Hamilton, "An Interval," UMASC, Hamilton Family fonds, MSS 14, box 15, folder 6.

52 Margaret Hamilton Bach, "Elizabeth Macdonald Wilson (Mrs. John Poole)," UMASC, Hamilton Family fonds, MSS 14, box 9, folder 15.

53 Mrs. Glen Hamilton, "'Elizabeth M': The Wonderful Story of Dr. Glen Hamilton's First Medium," *Light,* 18 June 1936, 385.

54 Ibid.

55 "The Various Psychic Phenomena Manifested by the Gifted Psychic Mrs. Elizabeth Poole, 1920-1927," UMASC, Hamilton Family fonds, MSS 14, box 9, folder 15.

56 T.G. Hamilton, *Intention and Survival: Psychical Research Studies and the Bearing of Intentional Actions by Trance Personalities on the Problem of Human Survival* (Toronto: Macmillan, 1942), 236.

57 Quoted in Estelle W. Stead, *My Father: Personal and Spiritual Reminiscences* (1913), 311-12, W.T. Stead Resource Site, http://www.attackingthedevil.co.uk/.

58 Hamilton, *Intention and Survival.*

59 Sittings, Group III: January – April 1929 – 'Amorphous Masses,' 27 January 1929, UMASC, Hamilton Family fonds, MSS 14, box 15, folder 14.

60 Hazelgrove, *Spiritualism and British Society,* 81.

61 Hamilton, "An Interval."

62 McMullin, *Anatomy of a Seance,* 202.

63 Nickels, "Psychic Research," 55.

64 Mary Marshall to Lillian Hamilton, July 1945, UMASC, Hamilton Family fonds, "Lillian Hamilton Correspondence Incoming 1901-1932," MSS 14, box 5, folder 5.

65 "Report of Sitting Held Sunday November 25, 1928," UMASC, Hamilton Family fonds, MSS 14, box 15, folder 13. For biographical information on the Hamilton circle, see McMullin, *Anatomy of a Seance,* 209-12.

66 Nickels, "Psychic Research," 58-59.

67 Brandon, *The Spiritualists,* 220.

68 McMullin, *Anatomy of a Seance,* 204.

69 Jay McDonald Scripts, 10 February 1933, 24 June 1933, 22 September 1933, 30 March 1934, 22 June 1934, UMASC, Hamilton Family fonds, MSS 14, box 14, folder 17.

70 Jay McDonald Scripts, 9 March 1933, UMASC, Hamilton Family fonds, MSS 14, box 14, folder 17.

71 Jay McDonald Scripts, 17 March 1933, UMASC, Hamilton Family fonds, MSS 14, box 14, folder 17.

72 Jay McDonald Scripts, 19 May 1933, UMASC, Hamilton Family fonds, MSS 14, box 14, folder 17.

73 Jay McDonald Scripts, 24 June 1933, UMASC, Hamilton Family fonds, MSS 14, box 14, folder 17.

74 McMullin, *Anatomy of a Seance,* 206.

75 Mrs. T. Glen Hamilton, "Telepathy Plus Spiritism in the Hamilton Researches in Winnipeg," *Light,* April 1951, 470-74, UMASC, Hamilton Family fonds, MSS 14, box 2, folder 7.

76 Sword, *Ghostwriting Modernism,* 47.

77 Ibid.

PART 4

Influenza and Public Health in
the Contemporary Context

9

Toronto's Health Department in Action: Influenza in 1918 and SARS in 2003

HEATHER MACDOUGALL

"Mommy, are you going to die?" This plaintive question from the young daughter of a Toronto nurse fighting infection with severe acute respiratory syndrome (SARS) in Mount Sinai Hospital in April 2003 exemplifies the fear and concern which outbreaks of infectious disease provoke in the families of front-line workers.[1] For historians, both the role of the media in highlighting the dangers of an epidemic outbreak and the response of health authorities recalled nineteenth- and twentieth-century reactions to cholera, typhus, yellow fever, smallpox, bubonic plague, and poliomyelitis rather than to HIV/AIDS.[2] But what part was Toronto's health department to play in an international health crisis? As the SARS outbreak once again demonstrated, local public health organizations are the foundation for concerted community efforts to manage disease and to control public panic.[3] By comparing and contrasting the way in which public health authorities in Toronto managed the 1918 influenza pandemic and SARS in 2003, we can see how a century of medical advances had conditioned the public and health care professionals to expect prompt control of communicable diseases, speedy development of a prophylactic vaccine, and effective exchange of information at the provincial, national, and international levels. But both outbreaks also demonstrated the power of negative ethnic and class stereotyping, the impact of the media in both educating and frightening the public, and the high cost in terms of human lives and devastation of the local and national economies.[4]

In 1918 and 1919, the worldwide influenza pandemic is estimated to have killed between 20 and 40 million people. For European and North American nations who were just coming to the end of the First World War, with its toll of 6 to 9 million dead and wounded, the flu seemed to be the fourth horseman of the apocalypse.[5] War, famine, pestilence, and death challenged Canadians, Americans, and their allies and foes to respond both to the immediate threat and to institute more formal national and international organizations to ensure that future pandemics were controlled before they could spread beyond their countries of origin. The great pandemic also gave a further impetus to biomedical research, which resulted in the discovery of the causative virus by British researchers in 1933.[6] As research continued, however, the complexity of influenza strains became apparent. But did public perceptions of the disease change? Was it seen as a killer or simply as an annual nuisance that appeared in North America every fall and winter after it had completed its attacks on the southern hemisphere and Australasia? In 2003, the question for many epidemiologists and health authorities was whether SARS was the feared new version of the 1918 strain or another type of disease.[7] Lack of a readily available diagnostic test or specific symptomatology significantly hampered the health authorities' response to the 2003 outbreak and prompted some officials to seek historical precedents for their containment efforts.

By their very nature, epidemics reveal the strengths and weaknesses of the societies in which they occur. Using Toronto as a case study to examine the reaction of citizens and their health departments to influenza in 1918 and SARS in 2003 provides an opportunity to probe into the changing role of local health departments and their staffs in two key crises. In 1918, Toronto was a bastion of white Anglo-Saxon Protestantism, with less than 10 percent of its population of neither Canadian nor British origin. The city had undergone a wave of physical expansion through amalgamation of newly developed suburbs prior to 1914 and was the focal point for industry and commerce in Ontario. As the provincial capital, it not only housed the legislature, the provincial board of health, the principal university, and the leading medical facilities, but also administered a budget equivalent to that of the provincial government. Overshadowing these characteristics was Toronto's fervent support of the war effort; it was the most imperialistic of Canadian cities in 1914, and for four long years, its 490,000 citizens provided volunteers for the Canadian Expeditionary Force (CEF), the Canadian Army Medical Corps (CAMC), and the field hospitals in France, Britain, and Canada. Civilians played their part and turned out munitions, food supplies, and clothing, bought war bonds, and planted victory gardens.[8] The arrival of a virulent strain of influenza with the returning soldiers added further stress to the final days of the conflict and challenged existing public health staff to organize to combat disease with limited numbers, limited medico-scientific knowledge, and limited resources.

By 2003, the former city of Toronto had been forcibly amalgamated with five surrounding municipalities to create a combined population totalling 2.5 million, nearly 50 percent of whom had not been born in Canada. From 1945 on, the city had been a magnet for successive waves of refugees and immigrants seeking a better life for their children. By the 1980s, Toronto was the dominant economic engine for the nation.[9] But as the federal and provincial governments adopted Thatcherite and Reaganite economic policies, the city lost much-needed funding for its aging infrastructure and services. This did not bode well for Toronto's Public Health Department (TPH), which relied on municipal taxes as well as provincial grants. Furthermore, in 1997, the province updated the mandatory programs which local health units were expected to provide and then changed the tax base to limit business taxes which Toronto had used to fund innovative health and education programs.[10] Was Toronto Health ready for a possible pandemic?

The arrival of SARS demonstrated the devastation that disease outbreaks impose as businesses and public facilities close in response to local, national, and international fears of disease transmission. Indeed, one of the most striking differences between the two outbreaks was the administrative complexity created by the presence of competing provincial and federal authorities in 2003.[11] In 1918, Canada did not have a federal health department, provincial health departments were very small, and no international health agency equivalent to the World Health Organization (WHO) existed.[12] By comparing and contrasting the abilities of the two local medical health officers – Drs. Charles Hastings and Sheela Basrur – to coordinate disease control efforts, develop and maintain sufficient capacity to respond to outbreaks, and to communicate effectively with fellow citizens, the media, and external authorities, we will be able to gauge the impact of their activities during these crises. The parallels and differences in the two outbreaks demonstrate how the lessons of the past need to be deeply ingrained in both collective memory and public policy if present and future challenges are to be met with courage and effectiveness.

INFLUENZA 1918-19: TORONTO'S EXPERIENCE

By October 1918, the nearly half a million Torontonians had endured four years of war in which seventy thousand of their sons, husbands, fathers, and co-workers had enlisted in the CEF and served overseas in the trenches on the Western Front.[13] Concern for the troops was matched by the growing recognition that social conditions at home demanded improvement if the sacrifices being made in Europe were to be meaningful. Under the dynamic direction of Dr. Charles J. Hastings, Toronto's medical officer of health (MOH) from 1910 to 1929, Ontario's capital became a showplace for modern methods of public health administration and preventive activity.[14] Between 1910 and 1917, Hastings spearheaded the introduction of pasteurized milk, well-baby clinics, municipal housekeepers, and health education by public health nurses, based on successful examples found in leading British and American cities.[15] He quickly became a spokesman for progressive public health activists, arguing that "one reason why advances in preventive medicine have been so slow is that prevention lacks dramatic interest" and that, as a result, appeals to humanitarianism had to be supported with economic arguments which demonstrated that spending on public health administration was an investment, not an expense.[16] Starting with a staff of three public health nurses in 1910, Hastings moved quickly to expand the health education component of his staff's work and in 1914 created a Division of Public Health Nurses. Based in district offices shared with either the police force or social agencies, the public health nurses quickly became "guides, philosophers and friends" for the women and children in their areas. Using a generalized system that stressed health education rather than curative services, Toronto's Department of Public Health (DPH) devoted great attention to forging links with more than two hundred local voluntary groups through the Neighborhood Worker's Association (NWA).[17] This reciprocal relationship intensified during the First World War as many families received coordinated assistance from the DPH and NWA as a greater emphasis on "scientific" social service developed.[18] Thus, the concept of teamwork was well understood and widely shared when warnings about a flu epidemic began to arise in the spring and summer of 1918.

The influenza outbreak is thought to have begun at Camp Funston in Kansas in March 1918 and to have accompanied American troops to France, where it spread to the combatant armies.[19] Canadian soldiers began to fall ill during the spring, and the return of some troops in the summer of 1918 triggered the epidemic in Canada. The federal government was responsible for military cases, but provincial medical officers and their municipal counterparts knew that they would be fighting the outbreak with limited resources since so many doctors, nurses, and inspectors were serving in the armed forces. On 19 September, the *Toronto World* reported cases in a military camp in Ontario. For Toronto's medical officer and its local board of health (LBH), this presented a challenge because influenza was not a reportable disease under the 1912 Ontario Public Health Act, and most doctors were hoping that the outbreak would be similar to the one in 1889-90, which had attacked primarily the elderly and apparently provided some immunity to those who survived.[20]

These hopes were soon dashed. Military doctors were well aware that the flu was killing soldiers between twenty and thirty-nine with great rapidity.[21] When the disease spread into the community, it devastated the workforce, made entire families ill, and left orphans and the elderly in its wake. But what could be done to stop it? Communicable disease control was one of the main functions of municipal and provincial health departments in Canada during the late nineteenth and early twentieth centuries, but in the past it had created opposition and imposed economic hardship on those who were quarantined in their homes or sent to municipal isolation hospitals.[22] Should these conventional tactics be used against the flu?

As English Canada's leading health department, Toronto had a well-established Division of Communicable Disease, a municipal laboratory for testing TB and diphtheria samples, an isolation hospital, and a division of vital statistics to provide the data needed for decision making.[23] But as Hastings was well aware, the usual approach to controlling the spread of infectious disease was proving ineffective against influenza. Articles in the October issue of the *American Journal of Public Health (AJPH)* and personal contact with health authorities in the United States made it clear to Hastings, who was president of the American Public Health Association (APHA) in 1918, and his provincial counterpart, Dr. John W.S. McCullough, Ontario's chief medical officer, that there was much disagreement about the benefits of these approaches.[24] Indeed, McCullough conducted a survey of provincial and state health officers on the merits of quarantine and isolation, and found that the majority had concluded that "these measures are impracticable."[25] But the mayor, Thomas L. Church, the press, and most of the public expected such actions, and in cities such as Milwaukee, they were apparently effective.[26] In Toronto, however, quarantine and isolation were not implemented since the disease toll escalated so quickly as to render them ineffective on a case-by-case basis.

In his capacity as president of the APHA, Hastings left Toronto from 5 to 8 October to travel to Boston, New York, and Washington to see the ravages of the epidemic first-hand.[27] Since flu was not a reportable disease, the statistics for its spread and virulence are suspect, but each of the communities which experienced an outbreak quickly recognized its propensity to overwhelm standard disease control measures and facilities. When the disease first appeared in Toronto, the MOH and military authorities appealed for calm, provided a detailed description of the symptoms, strongly recommended resting in bed, and exhorted the sick to call for medical assistance.[28] The first civilian casualty was a schoolgirl who died in Toronto General Hospital on 29 September 1918. In spite of growing public pressure for isolation and quarantine, Hastings did not issue the order, because the bulk of cases were military men in the base camp located in the city. But the child's death was a prelude to a typically rapid increase in cases and deaths; within a week, more than 10,000 students and staff out of the 66,000 students and 1,630 teachers were sick.[29] The impact on the city's hospitals was immediate and overwhelming. By 8 October, the Toronto Western Hospital was full, and half the nurses at the Grace Hospital were ill.[30] Toronto General, the city's newest and largest facility, had almost 50 percent of its 676 patients ill with the flu by mid-October, eighty nurses fell ill, and three died.[31] As a result, surgery was cancelled except for emergency operations. Similar problems beset the 350-bed St. Michael's Hospital, but the situation was further compounded by the absence of medical staff on duty overseas. The Sisters of St. Joseph used student nurses, their own teaching staff, and teaching Sisters from Loretto Abbey to keep the hospital functioning during the epidemic.[32]

With a population of roughly 490,000 and the fear that 40 percent or more of the population would become ill if the European and American experience was repeated in Toronto, the MOH and his provincial counterpart moved swiftly to create additional hospital accommodation and to train volunteers to care for the sick. Two hotels were commandeered and turned into emergency hospitals. To staff them, the province issued a call for an Ontario Emergency Volunteer Health Auxiliary, which provided training to create a volunteer group known as the Sisters of Service.[33] Women's groups, teachers, and other women whose jobs were eliminated when their workplaces were closed attended the three-lecture course on the care of the sick and the sickroom.[34] Willing volunteers were then assigned to one of the six health department district offices or to the temporary hospitals. But as the staff at Central Neighborhood House, a settlement in one of Toronto's slum areas, noted, few of the Sisters of Service were willing to serve in their part of the city.[35] This was especially problematic for the poor and non-English-speaking immigrants because "the assistance of neighbours, usually freely rendered during illness, was negligible owing to the contagious nature of malady," and this required settlement house workers to provide nursing, housekeeping, and child care during the epidemic.[36]

Nevertheless, volunteer work was vital as the public health nurses (PHN) were working "to the point of exhaustion" dealing with the rapid increase in sick families. Early in the outbreak, the MOH informed the *Globe* that the nurses were focusing their entire attention on assisting the sick and that various inspectors had been put on twenty-four-hour duty to provide food, fuel, and other necessities to stricken families.[37] According to the anonymous author of an in-house history of the Public Health Nursing Division, "As much hourly nursing care as could possibly be arranged was given, but it did not begin to cover the need. There were very few days that the nurses did not come into the district offices and relate some unbelievably harrowing stories."[38] As the epidemic progressed, Health Department staff also caught the disease, and by 23 October, 54 of 319 staff were ill, including 22 nurses and 4 doctors.[39] To deal with the growing demand for nursing care and for food, fuel, and "bedding, night clothing, towels and even pneumonia jackets," the DPH turned to the Neighborhood Worker's Association. Using Toronto's newspapers to publicize these needs, the NWA appealed to Torontonians' patriotism and civic spirit by informing readers that any and all donations of soup, money, or volunteer time would be gratefully received and that the former would be delivered to stricken homes by Boy Scouts.[40] Twenty-seven depots to receive these items were set up throughout the city as Torontonians rallied to care for the sick.

The same issue of the papers reported that approximately fifty people a day were dying of flu or broncho-pneumonia. The MOH had already ordered schools to close, and various organizations such as the Canadian and Empire Clubs as well as Masonic Lodges were cancelling their meetings. The LBH and Mayor Church were in agreement that other places should also close to help prevent the disease from spreading, so, on Saturday, 19 October, all theatres, moving picture shows, pool- and billiard rooms, and bowling alleys were closed for the duration.[41] Further precautions included prohibiting the circulation of public library books, while allowing the libraries to remain open, and persuading Toronto's churches to hold only a single service on Sundays – Mass for Catholics in the morning and evening services for the Protestants. The university was closed and fifth-year medical students were assigned to assist busy general practitioners in making home visits and to work in the newly opened temporary hospitals.[42] The Health Department also relied on the work of the Victorian Order of Nurses and the St. Elizabeth Visiting Nurses for bedside care of the sick.[43]

During the epidemic, the Health Department staff made 17,108 visits to stricken households, and its records indicate that there were approximately 1,750 deaths in 150,000 cases.[44] The latter is probably an underestimate given the extent to which the press of work prevented accurate reporting of cases and deaths.[45] As well, the military was compiling its own statistics in the base hospital located in the eastern part of the city and at the base camp at the Exhibition Grounds. Whether these were included in the city's tally is unclear. But the impact of the epidemic was profound. The newspapers contained short items noting the deaths of many specific individuals, advertisements apologizing for delays in delivering bread and milk, news stories describing board of health meetings and the actions which resulted from its deliberations, and hortatory calls for more volunteers. The *Toronto World* also printed an impassioned plea arguing the benefits of gauze masks and asking that "Everybody Wear A Mask To Work On Saturday Morning."[46] Neither Hastings nor McCullough felt that wearing masks in public was warranted, with the result that Ontarians were not required to use them as were their counterparts in Alberta and several American states.

The economic consequences of the epidemic were significant. Munitions plants and other war industries slowed as workers became ill. The municipal firefighters and policemen took sick as did trainmen and Bell Canada employees. The cold rainy weather added further stress to the epidemic when coal became difficult to obtain, and fuel supplies for the sick and for industry diminished.[47] In a society which lacked unemployment insurance, the task of responding to the needs of the sick and their families fell on a populace that had already donated its time, effort, and money to winning the war and buying Victory Bonds. Nevertheless, the Toronto Board of Trade created an Influenza Fund and worked with the NWA and other community groups to distribute the proceeds.[48]

By the beginning of November, the situation began to ease. The schools were supposed to open on 5 November, but the fuel shortage postponed the reopening for a week. Sporting events resumed, hospitals began to report empty beds, and on 11 November, the Armistice was signed.[49] The celebrations which this unleashed may have contributed to another wave of the flu, but for Charles Hastings, the 1918 epidemic revealed a crucial lesson: "We require the centralization of authority. Whether that be a public health service, a local government board, a department of health, a ministry of health or a secretary of health, it matters little, but all authority should be centralized under one department, if we are going to have efficient results. Every human body may be a battlefield against these invisible foes. Consequently, every individual must be trained a fighter, and though we march apart, we must fight together under one command."[50] To his Canadian counterparts, Hastings was clearly calling for the creation of a federal health department, and in March 1919, legislation to this effect was introduced. The ravages of the flu epidemic were cited as one of the factors justifying the extension of federal involvement in an area of exclusive provincial jurisdiction.[51]

But the real impact was at the provincial and municipal levels. In Toronto, Hastings and his staff had demonstrated the benefits of a well-organized department which had made links to other municipal services, local hospitals, and non-governmental organizations. Their experience enabled them to move quickly to take command in a crisis situation. The role of provincial authorities was somewhat more complex. As chief medical officer (MO), Lieutenant-Colonel John W.S. McCullough had responsibility for all parts of the province which lacked permanent public health staff, but he was also deeply involved with his military duties. The solution was to allow Hastings and his staff to demonstrate effective community engagement and then to use this model for the rest of the province.[52]

When standard disease control measures proved ineffective at stemming the rising numbers of cases, Hastings turned to prevention. He brought back a *B. influenzae*–based vaccine from his visit to the New York City Laboratory to start flu vaccine production in Toronto. Most civilian and military health officers pinned their hopes for controlling the epidemic on either a preventive or a prophylactic vaccine. In 1914, the Connaught Laboratories had opened in Toronto to produce diphtheria antitoxin, but it quickly became the main supplier of vaccines for the war effort.[53] During the flu epidemic, Dr. R.D. Defries, the acting director, undertook the production and testing of flu vaccine using eighteen strains of the New York source and additional ones from Canadian soldiers at the base hospital. Although he was impressed by the impact of the vaccine on "desperate cases," he was alert to growing evidence that the vaccine was ineffective since researchers were unable to demonstrate that the Pfeiffer bacillus was the cause of the disease and indeed had begun to argue that it was a filterable virus instead.[54] Defries later argued that "the preparation and trial of vaccine was fully warranted by the existent knowledge of the disease and its etiology," while Hastings commented in November 1919 that during the flu epidemic the medical profession was "severely censured for not having discovered a vaccine," indicating that the public, too, expected science to provide a preventive for the disease.[55] But as many reports published in Canadian and American medical journals indicated, there was little clinical evidence that preventive or prophylactic vaccination made a difference.[56]

And what about the citizens? One of the most striking features of the outbreak was the extent to which Torontonians of all social classes suffered and yet sought to help each other. The middle class and well-to-do volunteered themselves and their cars to take food, medical and nursing supplies, and doctors and visiting nurses to their patients.[57] Workers tried to maintain essential services while their customers faced a final round of privation prior to the end of the war. Teachers, homemakers, nursing, medical, and dental students volunteered their services in hospitals and in the community. Settlement workers noted that the poor were so severely affected that they were unable to provide assistance to their neighbours – a breach of customary practice. And various immigrant groups were presented with additional challenges as the information provided in pamphlets and local newspapers had to be translated into languages that they understood. As the anonymous scribe who wrote about public health nursing noted, "The epidemic lasted approximately two months and it was an unforgettable experience for us all."[58]

For the health authorities who had directed local and provincial or state efforts during the epidemic, the influenza outbreak provided a challenge to their authority and expertise that led figures such as Sir George Newman and Victor C. Vaughan to lament the inability of officials to either control or prevent the disease.[59] At the rescheduled annual APHA meeting in Chicago in December 1918, a committee was formed to prepare "A Working Program against Influenza," which was published in the January 1919 issue of the APHA journal. This comprehensive review of the strengths and weakness of the efforts to combat the disease justified its prescription for action by noting that health agencies "must act in light of present knowledge," even if that knowledge is limited or flawed.[60] But it is clear that there were many variables that affected the progress of the disease and that finding the cause and an effective vaccine were high on the medical community's agenda. For local health officers, however, the extent of public cooperation during attempts to prevent the spread of disease was paramount.[61] They were also concerned about relief measures and effective organization of existing staff and services.[62] Nearly all had discovered a significant lack of trained personnel and were hoping that the outbreak would spur the creation of additional positions in their organizations. Indeed, one of the results of the epidemic was the conversion of the Canadian Red Cross war effort into peacetime service, which included funding the development of public health nursing programs at Canadian universities and supporting nurses to attend them.[63]

In May 1919, the Canadian Public Health Association, the Ontario Health Officers Association, and the Ontario Medical Association all met together in the Physics Building at the University of Toronto. On 26 May in the morning, the delegates heard papers on the new federal department of health by Dr. Michael Steele, member of Parliament, and state health insurance by Dr. Charles Hastings, and then in the afternoon, there was a symposium on influenza that featured speakers such as Drs. Wade Hampton Frost of the United States Public Health Service, Augustus Wadsworth of the New York State Laboratory, and John McCullough.[64] Clearly, the flu epidemic had influenced both clinical and preventive medicine in terms of organizational structure, administrative process, and scientific research. But would the lessons of this outbreak continue to influence public health practice?

Ironically, the support which Toronto's Health Department had received in 1918 proved limited. As the city returned to "normalcy" in 1919, the mayor and Board of Control recommended budget cuts to municipal services, including the Health Department. The effective organizing and yeoman services that staff had performed during the flu epidemic were forgotten or ignored when a mild form of smallpox appeared in October 1919. Anti-vaccination groups organized rallies attended by some city councillors who objected to Hastings's dynamic leadership and his demand that mandatory vaccination be instituted. This well-established preventive measure was condemned as "German Born Compulsion" and rejected as antithetical to the principles of liberty and democracy for which the war had just been fought. Were the anti-vaccinationists reflecting concern at the inability of the medical profession to prevent the flu epidemic through immunization, or was their opposition to compulsory vaccination a postwar rejection of the social and moral authority of Progressive experts and their domination of the war effort?[65]

SARS 2003

From 1919 to 2003, municipal and provincial health departments continued to be legally responsible for control of communicable disease. But with the development of vaccines against childhood diseases, the eradication of smallpox, and the use of antibiotics to treat tuberculosis and sexually transmitted diseases, the war on disease appeared to be won. As attention and staff interest shifted to behaviour modification and encouraging community development, the financial resources and personnel devoted to disease surveillance, infection control, and isolation/quarantine diminished.[66] Instead of TB sanatoria, preventoria, and mass chest screening and tuberculin testing, for example, the Communicable Disease Control (CDC) unit in Toronto was using directly observed therapy against a resurgence of tuberculosis in the late 1990s.[67] But would this client-specific approach prove effective against a future pandemic? What role would municipal health departments be expected to play in the event of such outbreaks?

Experts and pundits began to warn about the possibility of a worldwide pandemic of influenza during the 1970s and 1980s in the wake of the 1957 and 1968-69 outbreaks. The appearance of legionnaires' disease, HIV/AIDS, Ebola, and drug-resistant strains of tuberculosis followed by human deaths from avian flu were coupled with growing concern about environmental degradation.[68] In Ontario, the 2000 pathogenic outbreak of E. coli as a result of water contamination in Walkerton demonstrated the price that communities paid for failing to maintain basic services. A commission chaired by Mr. Justice Frank O'Connor highlighted the effect of provincial government cuts to the Ministry of the Environment and noted that it had failed to share vital information with local and provincial health authorities.[69] During the Harris regime from 1995 to 2002, the provincial government pursued tax cuts and reorganization of provincial services that focused on downloading duties to municipalities and regional governments. Convinced that Toronto and its surrounding cities – Scarborough, North York, the Borough of York, East York, and Etobicoke – were duplicating services, the province compelled them to amalgamate in 1997. This meant that the Toronto Health Department had to incorporate staff from the other five municipalities, determine whether its programs and services were appropriate to the new city, and try to find economies that would assist the new city's budget committee in dealing with its declining revenues.[70] The new MOH, Dr. Sheela Basrur, was a graduate of the University of Toronto (MD 1982, MHSc 1987), who had been the MOH of the East

York Health Unit, which had approximately fifty employees. In 1998, she became the leader of over eighteen hundred staff serving a population that was significantly different from its historical roots.[71] In addition to expanding in terms of territory, the new city had a multi-ethnic population that included 14.7 percent East and Southeast Asians, 10.8 percent South Asians, 1.9 percent West Asians, 2.6 percent Africans, 6.0 percent Caribbeans, 19.0 percent North Americans, 27.4 percent British, and 1.0 percent Aboriginals.[72] Fortunately, Toronto Health had been hiring community workers from the various ethnic groups since the 1980s in recognition of the need to provide culturally sensitive approaches to health education and preventive services.

But would Toronto Public Health, as the new entity was known, be able to maintain its national and international reputation for innovative community-responsive public health services in the face of the province's Mandatory Programs and limited funding? The 1995 election of the Progressive Conservatives led by Mike Harris compounded the financial difficulties already facing Toronto Public Health as a result of the recession of the early 1990s. The Harris regime was committed to cutting government spending and staff, dismantling publicly owned utilities, remaking the public education system, downloading as many social service and welfare activities as possible, and privatizing certain environmental and health services. For TPH, staff cuts, program closures, and pressure to reorganize and redefine future goals meant focusing on children, families, and specific "high risk" groups such as HIV/AIDS victims and street people rather than expanding CDC activities.[73] In addition, the city's many acute care hospitals and long-term care facilities were struggling to maintain service levels because of funding shortfalls and declining numbers of staff. A widespread flu outbreak in the winter of 2002 had resulted in the deaths of several citizens who had not received prompt assistance in overcrowded emergency wards. As a result, the province introduced mass flu vaccination in the fall of 2002. The immunization program was offered free to citizens through public clinics or their family physicians. But would this voluntary program be sufficient to protect Torontonians from the feared pandemic? Health Canada had been attempting to develop a national flu pandemic program, but Ontario was not supportive, preferring to develop its own approach since the Harris Conservatives were engaged in an ongoing conflict with the Chrétien Liberals over which level of government had the authority to design programs and deliver services. As Mr. Justice Archie Campbell's 2004 interim report noted, "To put together a provincial pandemic plan a number of parts needed to come together, including public health, labs, hospitals branch, emergency response and emergency management ... Had a pandemic flu plan been in place before SARS, Ontario would have been much better prepared to deal with the outbreak."[74] Toronto was in fact developing its own flu pandemic management plan, but like most other Ontario health units was waiting for the Public Health Branch of the provincial ministry to provide a template for responding to such a calamity. And then, through a fluke of nature, Toronto became the North American centre of the SARS outbreak.

In mid-February 2003, a vacationing Torontonian, seventy-eight-year-old Mrs. Sui-chu Kwan, was waiting for the elevator on the ninth floor of the Metropole Hotel in Kowloon when another guest, a doctor from Guangdong province in China, began to cough vigorously. He was ill with the atypical pneumonia which had been raging since November 2002 but had not been reported to the World Health Organization until early February. After Mrs. Kwan flew back to Toronto on 23 February, her symptoms – a high fever, muscle aches, and a dry cough – worsened, and she went to her family doctor's office on 28 February. Unfortunately, her condition deteriorated and she died at home in Scarborough on 5 March. Her forty-four-year-old son, Chi Kwai Tse, went to Scarborough Grace Hospital on 7 March with "a high fever, a severe cough, and difficulty breathing. He shared the open observation ward of a busy emergency department for 18 to 20 hours while awaiting admission."[75] This would prove to be the index case for the first phase of the SARS epidemic in Toronto. Mr. Tse died on 13 March, having infected several family members, emergency staff, and fellow patients. The respirologist who had treated him in the ER had sent samples out to test for infectious tuberculosis and had called Toronto Public Health to alert it to this possible problem. By 13 March, however, the tuberculosis test was negative, more people were sick, and infection control experts at other Toronto hospitals were working with TPH to identify the new disease. On 12 March, the World Health Organization had issued a global alert announcing outbreaks of atypical pneumonia in Hong Kong and Hanoi, and this enabled TPH and Dr. Allison McGeer, an infectious disease specialist at Mount Sinai Hospital, to identify the mystery illness.[76]

TPH swung into action: "In consultation with provincial and federal health officials, TPH held a press conference on March 14, activated its emergency response plan, established a public information hotline and assigned staff full-time to the outbreak investigation."[77] This succinct statement fails to convey the sense of crisis that existed as all three levels of health authorities discovered the weakened state of communicable disease control measures. For more than fifty years, TPH had not imposed quarantine on its citizens, and although the provincial Health Promotion and Protection Act contained provisions to do so, TPH staff lacked recent experience. Even more challenging was lack of knowledge regarding the disease itself. What was its cause? How was it spread? Where was it most likely to be contracted? What was the incubation period? How should it be treated? Who should be responsible for informing the public, provincial and federal authorities, and the WHO about suspected and probable cases?

The SARS outbreak starkly revealed the lack of coordination between federal and provincial health officials, and this conflict added to the demands being placed on TPH staff when they found themselves providing the same information to two different sets of officials. Differences of opinion about the confidentiality of patient information further challenged TPH containment efforts since they needed names of contacts to determine who should undergo a ten-day quarantine.[78] In contrast to 1918, when there had been a united front against influenza, the SARS outbreak illustrated the gap between prevention at the community level and care in hospitals or other tertiary facilities. The situation was further complicated because of international air travel and the growing demand for preventive precautions at Pearson International Airport, which was located in Mississauga, outside the bounds of TPH's jurisdiction.

With virtually no scientific information to guide them at the start and confused lines of communication with senior governments, Basrur and up to seven hundred of her staff began to track cases, monitor contacts, provide infection control advice to long-term care facilities and hospitals with SARS patients, and respond to growing public concern about the extent and nature of the outbreak. In addition to its printed materials, the TPH website posted descriptions of the symptoms as well as guidelines on handwashing and quarantine procedures in fourteen languages. More than two hundred staff did daily double shifts from 8:00 a.m. to 11:00 p.m. on the SARS Hotline that received over 300,000 calls during the outbreak, 47,567 in a single day. Although staff worked diligently, they were aware that the fragmentary information that they provided early in the outbreak caused frustration for many callers. As Justice Archie Campbell commented, "The problem was not lack of dedication and effort, but the fact that it was impossible in the middle of a rapidly expanding crisis to create the necessary infrastructure."[79] Nevertheless, in recognition

of the ethnic diversity of the city and the origins of the outbreak, TPH
worked closely with the Chinese community, which had created a
Community Coalition Concerned about SARS. This group trained
Chinese, Mandarin, and Cantonese-speaking volunteers to staff a 6180
hotline (the numbers sound like the Chinese word for "I'm willing to help
you"), produced and distributed Chinese-language SARS material, did
promotional activities for hard-hit Chinese businesses, and raised research
money for SARS studies.[80]

During the course of the outbreak, TPH's Case Management Team
was involved in two thousand investigations which required consultation
with infectious disease specialists because the symptoms were atypical and
no diagnostic test was available even though the genetic sequence of the
corona virus was established by British Columbia's Michael Smith Genomic
Sciences Centre on 12 April.[81] The lack of clear diagnostic criteria complicated control procedures because TPH staff and their clinical colleagues
were aware of the stigma attached to the disease and of the danger of
missing a case. To compound their difficulties, technology failed at this
critical moment. When the outbreak started, the only available disease-
reporting system was a fourteen-year-old DOS-based one known as RDIS
(Reportable Disease Information System). It was quickly apparent that
this disease-specific program would not work, and TPH turned to paper
files with Post-it Notes to keep track of cases and their contacts. Within
two weeks, Excel spreadsheets were also in use, but at no point was the
technology sufficiently flexible to provide the type of information and
analysis that would have enabled a clearer picture to emerge.[82] The challenge of contact tracing and quarantine supervision was immense as over
23,300 people were identified as contacts in each of the two waves of the
disease, and 13,374 spent ten days isolated in their homes. While they were
in quarantine, staff from TPH phoned once or twice a day to see if they
had any symptoms and to find out if emergency food supplies from the
Salvation Army or Canadian Red Cross were required. In spite of frustration caused by having to review their situation with each TPH staff member
who contacted them, very few Torontonians refused to comply with
voluntary quarantine procedures. Only twenty-seven isolation orders were
issued during the outbreak.[83] In a post-outbreak survey of health care
workers and the general population who had been isolated, an American
organization discovered that respondents cited "protecting others" as their
main motivation for undergoing quarantine. This strong sense of personal
and collective responsibility for community welfare mirrors the dedication
of visiting nurses and volunteers during the 1918 flu epidemic.

In part, the good behaviour by the general public may have stemmed from the growing recognition that SARS was apparently a nosocomial infection.[84] The outbreak was confined mainly to hospital staff, patients, visitors, and family members who had close contact with the index cases.[85] But in response to growing concern about SARS spreading more widely, the Ontario government declared a state of emergency on 26 March 2003 and ordered all of Toronto's hospitals to move to Code Orange emergency procedures. As in 1918, this resulted in the cancellation of all surgical procedures, limited emergency access, and the cancellation of appointments and elective procedures. All visitors were banned, including families seeking to care for dying relatives. Four days later, this draconian measure was applied to the province in general to protect health care workers and to prevent the spread of SARS into the general population.[86]

By the middle of April, the number of new cases was declining, and health authorities began to think that the worst was over.[87] Provincial officials and hospital spokespeople had issued daily reports on the number of actual, probable, and suspected cases, and provided the media with information to calm public anxieties over the Easter and Passover holidays. As in 1918, religious groups were asked to use common sense and to avoid shaking hands, kissing, sharing common communion cups, and organizing large gatherings, including funerals. But as post-outbreak studies indicated, the mixed messages which the daily briefings provided did not convince external observers that the situation was under control.[88] Imagine their surprise and shock when the WHO imposed a travel advisory on Toronto on 23 April.[89] This unwelcome decision required Dr. Barbara Yaffe, Toronto's director of communicable disease control, to travel to Geneva with federal officials, the Ontario minister of health and long-term care, and the province's chief medical officer to meet with World Health Organization officials to reassure them about the success of containment measures.[90] On 30 April, the ban was lifted but the international publicity and the continuing cancellation of conferences and conventions meant that Toronto's economy was suffering greatly.[91] The loss of jobs in the tourism and hospitality industries added to the stress, and the civic and provincial governments turned to marketing campaigns in an effort to reassure Torontonians and visitors that the city was safe to visit.

During late April and early May, staff from North York General Hospital sought advice from TPH regarding possible SARS cases in the psychiatric ward and among elderly post-operative orthopaedic patients. Since none of these people could be linked epidemiologically to previous cases, the situation remained in flux until an ICU nurse from North York General was admitted to the Toronto Western Hospital with SARS. In the interim, possible SARS patients had been transferred to St. John's Rehabilitation Hospital and the Baycrest Centre for Geriatric Care.[92] The province announced publicly that a second wave of the disease had appeared on 23 May, and the criticisms of all the flaws and failures that external critics had been making about the city's inability to control the disease increased in volume. Prime Minister Jean Chrétien had already appointed a national commission led by Dr. David Naylor, then dean of medicine at the University of Toronto, to investigate the outbreak, and now the Ontario minister of health, Tony Clement, announced the creation of an expert panel on SARS and infectious disease chaired by Dr. David Walker, dean of medicine at Queen's University in Kingston. And finally, on 10 June, Ontario's then premier, Ernie Eves, named Mr. Justice Archie Campbell to head a judicial commission to take testimony from patients, families, health care workers, and their representatives. These reviews made SARS one of the most intensively studied disease outbreaks in Canadian history, and the Naylor, Walker, and Campbell reports have all stressed the lack of coordination, capacity, and communication that bedeviled federal/ provincial/municipal relations in Ontario during the crisis.

On 30 June, the first nurse to die in the outbreak perished. Her death was followed by that of a colleague on 19 July and by that of a family physician on 13 August. Out of the national total of 438 cases, Toronto had 224, with 44 deaths.[93] Twenty-nine nurses, 14 doctors, and 30 other health care workers including respiratory therapists, radiology and ECG technicians, paramedics, registered assistants, housekeepers, clerical staff, and security personnel suffered from SARS, and many are still trying to recover.[94] In comparison to the morbidity and mortality of the 1918 flu, these numbers may seem small, but a century of medical progress had conditioned the public and health care workers themselves to expect medical professionals to provide prompt diagnoses and effective cures. The apparent speed with which SARS could spread and the lack of provincial laboratory support for diagnostic purposes left Toronto Health reliant on volunteers from other health units in Ontario and medical researchers based in the city's hospitals for the information that it needed to determine whether individuals were at risk of contracting or spreading the disease. When experts like Allison McGeer became ill with SARS, not only was there concern for her, but the experts with whom she had been consulting had to undertake ten days of quarantine during the height of phase one.[95] The colleagues who cared for them as well as the public health staff who supervised quarantine activities for their families will never forget the stress which this outbreak brought.

LESSONS FROM EXPERIENCE?

What does reviewing the history of disease outbreaks and epidemics have to contribute to improving our understanding of disease transmission and control? What does this type of analysis tell us about how society reacts to disease threats? And how can the lessons of these traumatic experiences be integrated into future planning? In comparing and contrasting the Toronto Health Department's response to pandemic influenza in 1918 and SARS in 2003, three main areas of comparison emerge: coordination, capacity, and communication. In 1918, Charles Hastings was indisputably in charge of the city's efforts to stem the flu because there were no senior agencies to provide direction from either Ottawa or Geneva. Ninety years later, Sheela Basrur had a similar role and responsibilities under the Health Protection and Promotion Act, but she was not recognized as the dominant leader because the disease had national and international implications, and therefore Health Canada, the Ontario Ministry of Health and Long-Term Care, and the province's emergency measures and public safety unit all participated in determining how the outbreak would be handled. As the Naylor, Walker, and Campbell reports make clear, Basrur and her staff worked twenty-hour days to contain SARS. They were assisted by volunteers from other Ontario health departments, other provinces, and the United States but found that in contrast to the close, collegial links which Hastings and his staff had with Toronto hospitals and provincial authorities, there was conflict and confusion over activities and authority.[96] Gradually, informal links with nearby health units emerged as SARS spread beyond Toronto and York County into Peel and Durham regions, but the shared sense of camaraderie that marked 1918 did not materialize because there had not been the type of sustained contact and trust-building that had occurred in Toronto from 1914 to 1918.

Both outbreaks demonstrated the logistical and political challenge which contagious diseases pose to local public health administrators. In 1918, Hastings and McCullough knew that their plans would be overset by lack of personnel. But they also knew that they could call on willing volunteers for support and that the mayor and local board of health backed them. Almost a century later, Toronto Public Health had 250 to 300 people working in its communicable disease control section, but they were dealing with an unknown disease that quickly uncovered the gaps in existing procedures for infection control in public institutions. Although TPH staff had worked with the seventy-eight long-term care facilities in the city to ensure that their infection control practices were effective, they had not provided the same level of service to acute care hospitals because of budget cuts and because there were supposed to be infection control officers and committees in place.[97] As a result, the trust which enabled Hastings and McCullough to rely on their academic and hospital-based colleagues for curative services did not exist, and TPH moved to create effective relationships with Toronto hospitals by establishing a communicable diseases hospital liaison unit. This was fully funded by the province from June 2003 to March 2004 with a commitment for 50 percent funding thereafter. But as the *Toronto Star* reported, city bureaucrats think that unless the province pays for the entire cost that the city should scrap the unit. Not surprisingly, TPH has argued that this unit is a critical part of future disease control efforts if a seamless transition from preventive to curative services is to be provided.[98]

In both outbreaks, communication was a vital part of the MOH's role. In October 1918, Hastings responded promptly to press queries, relying on his well-established ties with various newspapers to ensure that a message of calmness and fortitude was presented. The extent of the epidemic meant that many reporters, typesetters, and delivery boys were among the ill, with the result that the official view was rarely questioned. As well, stories about the final days of the First World War occupied many readers' attention. In 2003, the local press was initially very supportive and provided excellent summaries of existing knowledge regarding symptoms and where to seek help.[99] The nightly news included the daily press conferences attended by senior provincial officials, local infectious disease specialists, and Dr. Basrur. Her calmness throughout the crisis had an impact, according to one Toronto hospital's administrative assistant: "When the medical officer of health gets on TV and says everything is ok, we believe her."[100] Unfortunately, the information provided by hospital-based specialists and provincial authorities seemed to contradict the MOH's steady confidence in her staff and their activities.[101] As the Naylor, Walker, and Campbell reports suggest, this approach was ultimately perceived as indicating a lack of leadership and a possible attempt at covering up the extent of the outbreak. In retrospect, a single spokesperson would have been advisable, but there was little that any of the officials could do to overcome the voracious appetite of the media for information.

The information and misinformation that was broadcast internationally undoubtedly contributed to the WHO travel advisory and to the decline in tourism and convention business.[102] As a result, politicians at the provincial and federal levels tried to demonstrate their faith in the disease control efforts by TPH and its supporters by having widely publicized meals in Chinese restaurants. Gallant as these attempts to jump-start Toronto's economy and to promote solidarity with potential voters were, they did not mask the underlying tension between the two levels of government. TPH was caught in the middle because it was the body which had to help people qualify for federal employment insurance, provide food and other necessities while they were in quarantine, and respond to all the calls for information that flooded the hotline. Perhaps the most difficult ones to deal with were those asking for assistance in avoiding ethnic stigmatization. With its origins in China, SARS provided critics of Canadian immigration policy with a platform from which to vent their concerns. But the April outbreak among a charismatic Filipino religious group meant that it too was treated with hostility and fear.[103] As previously noted, nineteenth- and twentieth-century epidemics were replete with racist critiques directed against the presumed human vectors of diseases such as cholera, typhus, and plague. Even AIDS prompted a similar response because of the high morbidity rate within the Haitian community.[104] But one of the striking features of the SARS outbreak was the uniform condemnation of racist epithets by politicians, reporters, and concerned members of the public.

And when it became clear that SARS was predominantly hospital-based, health care workers also found themselves socially isolated. Each of the official reports commented on the sense of "fear, anger, guilt and confusion" that health care professionals felt as they tried to protect themselves and their families from the disease and from the fear evinced by their fellow citizens. Even more perturbing was the rift that appeared when provincial public health experts suggested that some of the in-hospital transmission occurred because of lack of handwashing, lack of proper use of N95 masks, and lack of common sense about staying home if symptomatic.[105] A team from the Centers for Disease Control and Prevention in Atlanta was invited to Toronto to adjudicate this dispute, but well after the outbreak was over, it was revealed that very few of the N95 masks had been properly fitted. Little wonder that hospital-based nurses who appeared before each of the commissions of inquiry were vehement in their criticism of the way that the outbreak was handled.[106] For these front-line workers, the SARS outbreak demonstrated once again the gap between theory and practice in clinical settings and the continuing hierarchy which privileged medical rather than nursing and other staff. A century of evolution in professional identities and status expectations was laid bare by SARS.

In 1918, flu was a known disease whose virulence seemed unaccountably to have mutated to the point that it became lethal. SARS was an unknown virus whose incubation period, degree of virulence, symptomatology, treatment, and sequelae were determined through experience and monitoring events in Hong Kong, Singapore, Hanoi, and other stricken centres.[107] In both instances, local public health agencies were the principal agents of the state because they provided the organization and staff to conduct case-finding home visits, arrange contact tracing and quarantine measures, and to organize hospital accommodations for the seriously ill. These standard disease control measures were overwhelmed by the magnitude of the 1918 epidemic, but the volunteer efforts of many citizens meant that the supportive care needed to prevent flu sufferers from succumbing to pneumonia and other sequelae was available. In 2003, the unity of purpose which had linked Toronto's Health Department, city hospitals, and the Neighbourhood Workers Association no longer existed. The hospital sector dominated much of the press coverage, and the cleavage between provincial officials and nurses' unions became widely known as a result.[108] "Name, blame, shame" replaced the deference to authority which had marked early-twentieth-century news reports. Nevertheless, the work of TPH staff was recognized by international experts, and on 12 July 2004, Mayor David Miller presented Dr. Barbara Yaffe, the acting MOH, and front-line staff with the Canadian Public Health Association Certificate of Merit Award for "their exceptional contribution in managing the SARS crisis" by "controlling the outbreak and implementing one of the largest quarantines in modern history."[109] Such recognition from peers and colleagues across the country is welcome confirmation that in spite of all the flaws and failures, Toronto Public Health fulfilled its obligations. And in his second interim report, Mr. Justice Archie Campbell argued for the primacy of local and provincial medical officers, stating that they "must have the lead role in public health emergency mitigation, management, recovery, coordination and risk communication."[110]

CONCLUSION

When the SARS outbreak began, reporters looked for parallels and historical models. The 1918 flu epidemic was cited by epidemiologists and historians as a possible parallel, largely, one suspects, because it has recently been the subject of renewed research and because it was worldwide.[111] But was there perhaps another reason? Were reporters and newscasters seeking reassurance that all would be well and that civilization would survive? In the Western media, attention was divided between the war in Iraq and the SARS outbreak. In the twenty-first century, death in combat seems somehow more comprehensible than death from disease. But as environmental degradation proceeds and species-jumping viruses and bacteria multiply, the certainties that pervaded twentieth-century Western medicine are beginning to fade. In their place is increasing respect for the ability of micro-organisms to mutate and a determination to use all available scientific tools to combat threats to human health. To date, three vaccines have been developed against SARS, the Sino-European project on SARS Diagnostics and Antivirals has reported that cinanserin, a drug for schizophrenia, is a useful therapy, and Dr. Josef Penninger's research team has demonstrated that the protein ACE2 can be used to combat the fluid buildup that killed SARS patients.[112] Clarifying the clinical picture and finding effective medications may remove the fear that epidemic diseases create, but as this review of disease control activities has demonstrated, however, age-old methods such as case identification, contact tracing, quarantine, and isolation are the first stage of containment and hopefully eradication. Toronto's experiences in 1918 and 2003 demonstrate "the power of public health" as the bedrock of disease control efforts.

But is it the historian's responsibility to point out the "lessons of the past"? If so, to whom should her observations be addressed? Policy-makers and public health administrators will be using the recommendations of the three reports as the foundation for change, and indeed, the federal government has already created a junior minister of state for public health, while Ontario under its new Liberal government has promised $41.7 million over the next three years to create the Ontario Health Protection and Promotion Agency. Dr. Sheela Basrur has been appointed the new chief medical officer of health, and the powers of the position have been expanded to enable future planning and better coordination.[113] Does this signal the senior governments' recognition of the crucial importance of prevention? Has the balance of power within the biomedical world shifted, or will the SARS outbreak fade from memory as quickly as the events of 1918? These questions will challenge future historians to explain the long-term impact of epidemic disease on society and to analyze the role of local health departments in the ever-expanding war on disease.

POSTSCRIPT: RECOLLECTING THE PAST?
SARS, PANDEMIC INFLUENZA, AND THE ROLE OF HISTORY

Both the influenza pandemic of 1918-20 and the SARS outbreak of 2003 garnered international attention and had a profound impact on Canada, resulting in the creation of the first federal health department in July 1919 and the opening of the Public Health Agency of Canada (PHAC) in September 2004. But was disease the cause or simply a catalyst for the establishment of these new government bodies? What role did history play in persuading policy-makers, politicians, and the public that an immediate response to epidemic disease was necessary to protect citizens' health and to maintain the national economy? As Jacalyn Duffin writes in her introduction to *SARS in Context: Memory, History, Policy,* historians found themselves being constantly queried by reporters seeking answers to questions about the nature of epidemics and their consequences for society in 2003.[114] But would they be consulted in its aftermath and as the world prepared for a potential avian flu epidemic? And if so, what did the media, policy-makers, scientific experts, and the public expect from them?

In *Historians on History,* John Tosh points out that historians and the public have a wide variety of expectations about the meaning and practice of the discipline. In general, the public views history as a means to create national identity or a shared sense of purpose and as the provider of insights or lessons from the past for current issues. This utilitarian view must be approached with caution, not merely because contemporary historiography in either its social history or postmodernist guise would repudiate it, but also because policy historians, like their peers, understand "that all social experience is historically constructed and therefore subject to change."[115] That renders simple analogies and predictions dangerous when planning for the future. But it does not absolve historians from contributing to the development of new institutions, policies, and programs.[116]

In May 2003, Dr. David Naylor was appointed to chair a national inquiry into the SARS incident, and when the report of his committee, *Learning from SARS: Renewal of Public Health in Canada,* was released in October, it gave a very critical recounting of events. It also used history to justify its call for a significant funding increase for public health activities and the creation of a new arm's-length agency whose role would include both pandemic/disease control planning and action and health promotion work to ensure continuing improvements in Canadians' health status.[117] But was the history on which the report was based window dressing or a genuine attempt to educate politicians, policy-makers, and the public about the vital role that prevention and environmental sanitation have played in controlling disease and improving the quality of life? As both a doctor and a medical historian, Naylor drew on the tradition among public health practitioners of using history to justify their calls for funding, new legislation, and public support.[118] But unlike in previous efforts, the shock of the SARS crisis resulted in political action.

In February 2004, the Jean Chrétien government appointed a junior minister of state for public health, Dr. Carolyn Bennett, MP for the St. Paul riding in Toronto, who met with stakeholders from around the country to discuss the structure and role of the new public health agency.[119] By September 2004, PHAC was based in Winnipeg and Ottawa, and Dr. David Butler-Jones had been appointed as the country's first chief medical officer.[120] The new agency was staffed by former employees of Health Canada's Population and Public Health Branch and given $165 million to pursue five priorities: "Emergency response capacity; disease surveillance; the creation of regional centres of excellence on communicable disease epidemiology; capital upgrades at the National Microbiology Laboratory in Winnipeg and the Laboratory for Foodborne Zoonoses in Guelph; and improving international collaboration."[121] That meant that one of the first tasks facing Minister Bennett and Butler-Jones was revising the national pandemic plan that had been publicized in February. Although SARS garnered worldwide attention and put Canada well ahead of other nations in terms of preparation, its reappearance in China during April 2004 re-animated fears about local, regional, and provincial/territorial abilities to control the spread of either SARS itself or the new challenge on the horizon, avian influenza.[122]

For policy historians, the development of a new national public health agency was paralleled by the media's interest in post-SARS endeavours to create a preventive vaccine. Sustained press coverage indicated that modern efforts bore an interesting resemblance to similar attempts during the 1918 influenza pandemic and seemed to have roughly the same result. Canadian experts, for example, stopped testing their versions of a SARS vaccine when serious side effects negated its effectiveness.[123] In contrast to European researchers during and after the Spanish flu pandemic, who questioned the validity of bacteriological science and who lost confidence in its applicability to influenza research, which Eugenia Tognotti has so clearly demonstrated, North American scientists post-SARS continued to probe the genetic structure of the 1918 flu virus in their efforts to aid other researchers in developing an effective vaccine.[124] In October 2004, an artificial flu virus similar to that of 1918 demonstrated its ability to kill mice, which died from symptoms similar to those suffered by humans in 1918-19.[125] A year later, Jeffrey Taubenberger announced that he and his team had sequenced the genome of one of the 1918 second-wave viruses and that it was an H1N1 virus, linked to avian influenza.[126] Informative as this discovery was, it did not aid public health professionals working to prepare their cities, regions, provinces, and territories for a possible flu pandemic. For, as researchers and health professionals worldwide understood, influenza viruses mutate through antigenic "drift" and "shift," which makes designing and producing an effective vaccine or preventive drug difficult since it has never been clear which strains are dominant. Thus, a human version of avian flu would be a new phenomenon.[127] If science could not provide a preventive, what could or should authorities do to implement the historical lessons derived from previous epidemics?

On 11 October 2005, the World Health Organization and the United States Department of Health and Human Services announced that an avian flu pandemic was likely; this raised even more public alarm than had occurred earlier, when various provincial and national pandemic plans had been presented.[128] Although the expert panels that had created these plans had clearly extrapolated potential morbidity and mortality from algorithms based on the 1918 pandemic death rates, had included sections dealing with the use of public facilities as temporary morgues, and had provided estimates of the numbers of caregivers required and the potential impact on the economy, they had neglected to compare the social structure of early-twenty-first-century Canada to its twentieth-century predecessor. Would urban Canadians rally to provide support for friends and neighbours?[129] Would they agree to quarantine and isolation? How much support could local health authorities and hospital staff anticipate? Did the women's groups that created soup kitchens and provided bedding, pneumonia jackets, and nursing support still exist? Had the lessons of the SARS outbreak been learned and applied in these plans?[130] Would twenty-first-century Canadians be as resilient as their forebears in the face of epidemic disease? As these questions demonstrate, there is a vital role for historians to play in aiding policy-makers, politicians, and the public in understanding the social dimensions of epidemics and their aftermath; and the essays in this collection demonstrate the range of issues that still require consideration in future program planning.

As historians published articles comparing the handling of SARS to that of the 1918 pandemic, health care professionals, political scientists, and policy-makers began to incorporate the social and political insights from this work into their calls for changes to public policy.[131] But in general, they did not grapple directly with issues of class, race, and gender since most public health law (and practice) still endeavours to deal with society as a collectivity in spite of ongoing evidence that social status, sexual preference, and ethnic origin are significant determinants of health.[132] Given the cracks that the SARS outbreak revealed in the acceptance of multiculturalism in Toronto and growing understanding that an avian flu pandemic was likely to originate in the Western Pacific region, shouldn't authorities have devoted more attention to the potential for a resurgence of racism and fear-based discrimination? Through the remainder of 2005 and into 2006, news stories highlighted the growing number of cases of bird-to-human and ultimately human-to-human transmission of avian flu in various Asian countries. Polemicist Andrew Nikiforuk provided a vivid picture of the 1918 pandemic juxtaposed with SARS and the 1997 avian flu eruption in Hong Kong in his *Pandemonium: Bird Flu, Mad Cow Disease, and Other Biological Plagues of the 21st Century.*[133] How did this use of history affect policy-makers and the public?

Clinicians Vincent Lam and Colin Lee took a more moderate approach to aid Canadians in preparing for the possibility of avian flu, in *The Flu Pandemic and You: A Canadian Guide.*[134] They not only discussed the history of previous pandemics while providing recommendations to enable individuals, families, and communities to cope with the outbreak but also described Asian farming practices and noted Western dependence on other nations for food supplies.[135] They underscored the impact that eliminating home-based poultry production would have on Asian people and their economies, and argued for more comprehensive efforts to compensate small farmers whose flocks were culled to contain the disease.[136] In doing so, they were echoing the work of the World Health Organization.

WHO had responded to the SARS episode by assuming a leadership role and afterward working with its member states to revise the International Health Regulations to make new and emerging disease threats reportable as soon as they arose.[137] Even with pandemic plans and stockpiling anti-virals, the medical experts at WHO and in most health ministries were well aware that less-developed countries could not afford to provide preventive drugs, vaccines, or hospital care to their citizens during a pandemic and that containing the disease before it spread was probably the most effective measure.[138] But containing disease depends on early reporting and prompt action to implement "social distancing" measures by local and national governments, and once again WHO had to challenge Chinese authorities for information regarding cases of avian flu.[139] Had the lessons of SARS been taken to heart, or were older values such as fear of losing face or hiding information from central officials at work? Policy-makers and security experts wrestled with an essential question: To what extent can history help us understand the international ramifications of disease control and prevention measures?[140]

And finally, to return to the experience of individuals and health care professionals, what can historians do to ensure that memories of these events are not silenced or ignored? Have colleagues studying the history of nursing undertaken interviews with hospital staff and public health nurses who worked throughout SARS? Who is providing the historical background for the court challenges that nurses' groups launched in 2005?[141] Who is collecting the memories and experiences of SARS patients?[142] Have any of these recollections appeared as autobiography, fiction, or blog entries? What artistic or cultural products have emerged to valorize the heroism of front-line workers or to condemn the laxity of officials during the SARS incident? And how will historians who lived through the event respond to the challenge of explaining its impact on Canadian society?

Canadian novelists, playwrights, and filmmakers have already begun to use the 1918 pandemic and SARS as plot devices or creative sources. How extensively were historians or their work consulted by writers such as Frances Itani, Daniel Kalla, and Jean Little when they wrote their fictional accounts of the 1918 epidemic or used SARS as a literary motif?[143] Did *Plague City*, the 2005 made-for-TV movie of the SARS episode, based on the experiences of clinical and nursing staff with occasional glimpses of the work of municipal public health staff and the World Health Organization, provide a balanced recounting?[144] And how do these cultural products affect popular understanding of disease and public policy? Do historians have an obligation to participate in their creation or to provide thoughtful critiques? And where should their concerns be voiced – in academic journals or the daily press?

Will SARS fade from public memory as quickly as influenza did in the 1920s?[145] In 2006, Dr. Danuta Skowronski, an epidemiologist with the BC Centre for Disease Control, launched a call for survivors of the 1918 flu pandemic to share their memories with her staff and other health care professionals because, as a result of reading various historians' accounts, she realized that personal stories would provide an excellent way to reassure the public that most people survive pandemics and to educate health professionals about the past. In recognition of the ninetieth anniversary of the influenza pandemic, Skowronski worked with Helen Branswell, a medical reporter for the Canadian Press, to create a set of interviews that led to news stories and video clips describing how Canadians survived the 1918 virus. The results of this collaboration appeared in newspapers across Canada in mid-September, and several are available online.[146] Ironically, there has been little reaction to these stories, though they will provide future historians with visual images and auditory proof of some survivors' conflicted and conflicting memories. But clearly, much investigation into collective memory and the choices that societies and individuals make about what will be remembered and what will be forgotten remains to be done.

Infectious diseases have never respected individuals or national boundaries, and analyzing the history of epidemics offers numerous ways for historians to contribute to a deeper understanding of both past and present. Their work must attempt to bridge the divide between theory and the lived experience by examining what happened and explaining why it occurred. Such studies must also be alert to both public rhetoric and the social silences that privilege some events, actions, and recollections but not others. Historians' work must be shared with policy-makers, politicians, bureaucrats, and health care professionals because science and society are no longer separate entities.[147] Determining how best to penetrate the policy-making process will require moving beyond the academy to make professional links with local health units, non-governmental organizations, interested scientific researchers, newspapers, digital media outlets, and the general public. Sharing the results of our research with the wider community will enhance public debate about future pandemic plans and ensure that social and cultural issues receive the same level of attention as legal, political, and economic concerns. For, as Virginia Berridge observes,

> historians as policy prescribers would only join the ranks of the "usual suspects" in policy making. But as analysts offering the classic function of "enlightenment" they have a perspective which no other discipline can offer. History as analysis offers great insight, interpretative richness and a sophisticated understanding of the past. For the lack of these, current policy is poorer.[148]

ACKNOWLEDGMENT

This chapter was originally published in the *Journal of the History of Medicine and Allied Sciences* 62,1 (January 2007): 56-89. The postscript is dedicated to the memory of Dr. Sheela Basrur (1956-2008), Toronto's medical officer of health during the SARS outbreak and Ontario's chief medical officer from 2004 to 2006.

NOTES

1 André Picard, "Mommy, Are You Going to Die?" *Toronto Globe and Mail,* 5 April 2003, F5. This news story revealed the name of the index case and noted that it was an alert Chinese-speaking nurse at Scarborough Grace Hospital who informed the emergency room physician (who had already called Toronto Health because he was concerned about infectious TB) that there was an atypical pneumonia outbreak in China, according to the Chinese-language press. Their combination of an alert medical and nursing care team meant that, although the index patient had infected nursing staff and other patients while initially waiting for attention in the ER, local health authorities in the hospital and in the community moved to quarantine and isolation procedures in both areas promptly. This story also exemplifies the way that reporters use individual cases to alert their readers of the dangers inherent in outbreaks. See also Chris Daniels, "The SARS Fighters: Agnes Wong, Ontario/Dr. Sheela Basrur, Ontario/Dr. Mona Loutfy, Ontario," *Time Canada,* 5 July 2004, 32.

2 Charles Rosenberg, *The Cholera Years: The United States in 1832, 1849 and 1866* (Chicago: University of Chicago Press, 1962); Geoffrey Bilson, *A Darkened House: Cholera in Nineteenth-Century Canada* (Toronto: University of Toronto Press, 1980); Judith W. Leavitt, "Politics and Public Health: Smallpox in Milwaukee, 1894-1895," in *Sickness and Health in America: Readings in the History of Medicine and Public Health,* ed. Judith W. Leavitt and Ronald L. Numbers (Madison: University of Wisconsin Press, 1985), 372-82; John Joseph Heagerty, *Four Centuries of Medical History in Canada* (Toronto: Macmillan, 1928), 17-211; Margaret Humphreys, "No Safe Place: Disease and Panic in American History," *Am. Lit. Hist.* 14 (2002): 845-57; Martin S. Pernick, "Contagion and Culture," *Am. Lit. Hist.* 14 (2002): 858-65; and Nayan Shah, *Contagious Divides: Epidemics and Race in San Francisco's Chinatown* (Berkeley: University of California Press, 2001).

3 The historical literature on epidemics both past and present is best understood through reading Charles Rosenberg, *Explaining Epidemics and Other Studies in the History of Medicine* (Cambridge: Cambridge University Press, 1992); Caroline Hannaway, Victoria A. Harden, and John Parascandola, eds., *AIDS and the Public Debate: Historical and Contemporary Perspectives* (Amsterdam: IOS Press, 1995); and Shah, *Contagious Divides.*

4 In her study *The Gospel of Germs: Men, Women, and the Microbe in American Life* (Cambridge, MA: Harvard University Press, 1998), Nancy Tomes presents a convincing argument about the impact of the "germ" theory on American attitudes to infectious disease and demonstrates how various groups adapted new behaviour patterns and beliefs as a result. More recently, in "Epidemic Entertainments: Disease and Popular Culture in Early-Twentieth-Century America," *Am. Lit. Hist.* 14 (2002): 625-52, she examines how contemporary problems such as the AIDS, Ebola, and West Nile viruses have been used by the media to create a climate of fear that prompts citizens to ignore significant public health threats by focusing on exotic and unlikely "risks." But her focus is on the way that advertising agencies used scientific discoveries in the mid-twentieth century to sell products by claiming to educate consumers in basic health principles. The use of radio and film for similar purposes is also analyzed to demonstrate the way that science becomes part of popular discourse and is, in turn, modified by popular perceptions.

5 The major North American studies of the 1918 flu epidemic include Alfred W. Crosby, *Epidemic and Peace, 1918* (Westport, CT: Greenwood Press, 1976); Alfred W. Crosby,

America's Forgotten Pandemic: The Influenza of 1918, 2nd ed. (New York: Cambridge University Press, 2003); Gina Kolata, *Flu: The Story of the Great Influenza Pandemic of 1918 and the Search for the Virus That Caused It* (New York: Farrar, Straus and Giroux, 1999); Eileen Pettigrew, *The Silent Enemy: Canada and the Deadly Flu of 1918* (Saskatoon: Western Producer Prairie Books, 1983); Kirsty Duncan, *Hunting the 1918 Flu: One Scientist's Search for a Killer Virus* (Toronto: University of Toronto Press, 2003); and Carol R. Byerly, *Fever of War: The Influenza Epidemic in the U.S. Army during World War I* (New York: New York University Press, 2005). An excellent historiographical overview is found in Howard Phillips, "The Re-Appearing Shadow: Trends in the Historiography of the 1918-19 Influenza Pandemic," *Canadian Bulletin of Medical History* 21,1 (2004): 121-34.

6 For a popular history of virology, see Peter Radetsky, *Invisible Invaders: The Story of the Emerging Age of Viruses* (Boston: Little, Brown, 1991), especially Chapter 12, which discusses the 1918 flu epidemic. See also Eugenia Tognotti, "Scientific Triumphalism and Learning from Facts: Bacteriology and the 'Spanish Flu' Challenge of 1918," *Social History of Medicine* 16 (2003): 97-110.

7 Anne McIlroy, "1918 Redux?" *Toronto Globe and Mail,* 5 April 2003, F9. In this article, the *Globe's* science reporter provided readers with specific parallels between 1918 and 2003 but argued that virologists would be able to sequence the genetic makeup of the corona virus thought to cause SARS.

8 J.M.S. Careless, *Toronto to 1918: An Illustrated History* (Toronto: James Lorimer and National Museums of Canada, 1984), 157-72, 183-202.

9 James Lemon, *Toronto since 1918: An Illustrated History* (Toronto: James Lorimer and National Museums of Canada, 1985), 11-23, 92-94, 113-87. See also Lila Sarick, "Visible Minorities Flock to City," *Toronto Globe and Mail,* 18 February 1998, A8. Sarick stated that 1996 census data indicated that 32 percent of the Greater Toronto Area's population was visible minorities. The story noted that Toronto's services and language classes were provided in many different languages and that these were under threat because of provincial plans to reorganize the education funding system.

10 Gay Abbate, "Toronto Board of Health Defies Order to Cut Budget," *Toronto Globe and Mail,* 30 July 1997, A5; and John Spears, "Budget Blueprint Holds Line on Taxes," *Toronto Star,* 10 March 1998, B1. According to a TPH *Budget Fact Sheet* dated 10 March 1998, the department received 1.6 percent of the $5.9 billion gross budget for the city. The $44.2 million allocated for TPH services in 1998 was 4.6 percent less than in 1997 and 9.4 percent less than in 1996.

11 In 1867, the British North America Act, now known as the Constitution Act, 1982, divided legislative powers between the federal and provincial governments. Health, education, and social services were allocated to the provinces, while the federal government was responsible for national economic policy, the military, criminal law, agriculture, immigration, and only minor health duties such as immigrant inspection, quarantine, and care of sick mariners and Aboriginals.

12 R.D. Defries, ed., *The Development of Public Health in Canada* (Toronto: Canadian Public Health Association, 1940); and R.D. Defries, ed., *The Federal and Provincial Health Services in Canada* (1959; repr., Toronto: Canadian Public Health Association, 1962).

13 Ian Hugh Maclean Miller, *Our Glory and Our Grief: Torontonians and the Great War* (Toronto: University of Toronto Press, 2002), 185. Miller notes that from August to mid-September 1918, Torontonians received news that 2,127 men were killed, wounded, or missing.

14 Heather MacDougall, *Activists and Advocates: Toronto's Health Department, 1883-1983* (Toronto: Dundurn Press, 1990), 26-32.

15 K.M. Yorke, "Saving Lives on the Wholesale Plan: How Toronto Has Been Made the Healthiest of Large Cities," *Maclean's*, July 1915, 20-22, 93-96.

16 Charles J. Hastings, "The Modern Conception of Public Health Administration," *Conservation of Life* 3 (July 1917): 49-54; Charles J. Hastings, "The Modern Conception of Public Health Administration," *Conservation of Life* 4 (October 1917): 86-90, both reprinted in *Saving the Canadian City: The First Phase, 1880-1920*, ed. Paul Rutherford (Toronto: University of Toronto Press, 1974), 123-36.

17 "A Pull All Together," *Public Health Journal* 9 (1918): 32-34; F.N. Stapleford, "Causes of Poverty," *Public Health Journal* 10 (1919): 157-61; and F.N. Stapleford, "The Policy, Spirit and Programme of the Neighborhood Worker's Association," *Public Health Journal* 10 (1919): 382-86.

18 MacDougall, *Activists and Advocates*, 60-64.

19 Crosby, *America's Forgotten Pandemic*, 17-41.

20 H.O. Howitt, "Some Observations on the Recent Epidemic," *Public Health Journal* 10 (1919): 508.

21 "The Present Epidemic," *Canadian Medical Association Journal* 8 (1918): 1028-29.

22 See Heather MacDougall, "'Enlightening the Public': The Views and Values of the Association of Executive Health Officers of Ontario, 1886-1903," in *Health, Disease and Medicine: Essays in Canadian History*, ed. Charles G. Roland (Toronto: Clarke Irwin, 1984), 436-64; Michael Bliss, *Plague: A Story of Smallpox in Montreal* (Scarborough, ON: HarperCollins Canada, 1991); and Barbara Craig, "A State Medicine in Transition: Battling Smallpox in Ontario, 1882-1885," *Ontario History* 75 (1983): 319-47.

23 Charles Hastings, "The Value of a Credit Balance in Public Health Administration," *American Journal of Public Health* 6 (1916): 115. See also MacDougall, *Activists and Advocates*, 140-41.

24 Provincial Board of Health of Ontario, "Spanish Influenza," *Public Health Journal* 9 (1918): 478. This item is followed on pages 482-85 by an article reprinted from Chicago papers of 3 October 1918. Chicago's health commissioner, John Dill Robertson, provided citizens with information from Surgeon-General Blue of the US Public Health Service that focused on the origin of the disease, its symptoms, and treatment. An editorial on page 495, entitled "Influenza," reminded *Public Health Journal* readers that there was ongoing controversy over Pfeiffer's bacillus as the cause of influenza and noted that the Connaught Laboratories of the University of Toronto was undertaking to study whether the causative agent was a filterable virus or *B. influenzae* and if a prophylactic vaccine were possible.

25 "The Provincial Board of Health of Ontario," *Public Health Journal* 19 (1919): 27-30.

26 "Mayor Clashes with Two MOH," *Toronto Globe*, 9 October 1918, 8; and "Can Keep Down the Mortality," *Toronto Globe*, 11 October 1918, 6. In the latter article, Mayor Church apologized for criticizing Hastings for failing to improve conditions in the military hospitals because the mayor now understood that the city's MOH did not have jurisdiction over such facilities. Judith Walzer Leavitt, *The Healthiest City: Milwaukee and the Politics of Health Reform* (Princeton: Princeton University Press, 1982), 227-39.

27 Hastings was also attending an emergency APHA Executive Committee meeting in New York City because it was clear that the annual meeting would have to be postponed due to the ravages of the epidemic in eastern and central North America. See "The Annual Meeting Postponed," *American Journal of Public Health* 8 (1918): 786-87.

28 Miller, *Our Glory*, 185-86.

29 Ibid., 186.

30 Pettigrew, *Silent Enemy*, 48.

31 J.T.H. Connor, *Doing Good: The Life of Toronto's General Hospital* (Toronto: University of Toronto Press, 2000), 203-4.

32 Irene McDonald, *For the Least of My Brethren: A Centenary History of St. Michael's Hospital* (Toronto: Dundurn Press, 1992), 79.

33 John W.S. McCullough, "The Control of Influenza in Ontario," *Canadian Medical Association Journal* 8 (1918): 1084-85.

34 "Hearty Response Made by Nurses," *Toronto World*, 17 October 1918, 5.

35 *Activities of Central Neighbourhood House*, City of Toronto Archives, Central Neighbourhood House fonds, formerly Sc 5, series D, box 1, Toronto. See finding aid number 1005 for current content records.

36 Ibid. The Health Department recognized the additional need in poorer districts and used Salvation Army cadets to assist the public health nurses in their home visits. See "S. Army Cadets Fighting 'Flu,'" *Toronto Globe*, 31 October 1918, 10.

37 "Sunshine Aid to Combat Flu," *Toronto Globe*, 10 October 1918, 6; and "Can Keep Down the Mortality," 6.

38 *History of Public Health Nursing*, November 1963, 10, City of Toronto Archives, file 34081, series 952, file 7.

39 Pettigrew, *Silent Enemy*, 53.

40 "Deaths from 'Flu' Are on Increase," *Toronto World*, 18 October 1918, 4. See also *Toronto Globe*, 18 October 1918, 4; and *Toronto Globe*, 29 October 1918, 10.

41 Ibid.

42 "University Classes Cancelled," *Toronto World*, 17 October 1918, 5. The news story stated, "All students in the faculty of medicine are asked to volunteer their services to fight the epidemic."

43 "Victorian Order of Nurses," *Public Health Journal* 10 (1919): 290. The VON usually cared for maternity cases but their small staff of eighteen volunteered to care for the sick during the flu epidemic. The St. Elizabeth Visiting Nurses performed similar duties for Catholic Torontonians.

44 Marion Royce, *Eunice Dyke: Health Care Pioneer* (Toronto: Dundurn Press, 1983), 69-70. The *Canadian Journal of Medicine and Surgery* 45 (1919): 212, states that Toronto suffered 1,408 deaths from influenza and 1,307 from pneumonia for a total of 2,715, which was 1,980 in excess of the normal October death rate of 735.

45 "The Provincial Board of Health of Ontario," *Public Health Journal* 9 (1918): 542, noted that since influenza was not a reportable disease, "the only means we have of getting anywhere near the deaths caused by the epidemic is from returns made by Undertakers." The result was an ongoing recalculation of the provincial morbidity and mortality rates as new information arrived. By 1919, McCullough had concluded that Ontario had experienced roughly forty to fifty thousand cases with ten thousand deaths.

46 "Get Busy with Masks," *Toronto World*, 18 October 1918, 4.

47 "Conditions in Industry," *Toronto Globe*, 29 October 1918, 13, estimated that production had declined 35-39 percent as a result of the epidemic. See also Miller, *Our Glory*, 188-89. Miller notes that "officials estimated the loss in [coal] production from the flu to be about 50,000 tons daily" (188).

48 "Want Follows 'Flu' Ravages," *Toronto Globe*, 31 October 1918, 10; and *History of Public Health Nursing*, 10.

49 Miller, *Our Glory,* 187-92.

50 Charles J.O. Hastings, "Democracy and Public Health," presidential address to the American Public Health Association, 9 December 1918, reprinted in *American Journal of Public Health* 9 (1919): 13.

51 "To Organize Dept. of Public Health – Federal Government Will Ask Parliament to Pass Bill," *Toronto Globe,* 25 October 1918, 2. See also Janice P. Dickin McGinnis, "The Impact of Epidemic Influenza: Canada, 1918-1919," *Historical Papers* 12,1 (1977): 120-40, reprinted in *Medicine in Canadian Society: Historical Perspectives,* ed. S.E.D. Shortt (Montreal and Kingston: McGill-Queen's University Press, 1981), 447-78.

52 McCullough, "Control of Influenza." This article was republished in the *Canadian Medical Association Journal* on 26 April 2005 accompanied by an article in "The Left Atrium" section by Dr. Gillian Arsenault called "Lessons from History," in which she reminds her readers that we still do not have an effective treatment for influenza and that we too should use early-twentieth-century techniques of providing information and immediate closure of all but essential services to ensure that "when our time comes, we will be able to match the intelligence, energy, co-ordination and co-operation of our forebears." Gillian Arsenault, "Lessons from History," Left Atrium, *Canadian Medical Association Journal* 172,9 (26 April 2005), http://www.cmaj.ca/.

53 P.A. Bator with A.J. Rhodes, *Within Reach of Everyone: A History of the University of Toronto School of Hygiene and the Connaught Laboratories,* vol. 1, *1927-1955* (Ottawa: Canadian Public Health Association, 1990), ix-24.

54 Tognotti, "Scientific Triumphalism," 102-8, n. 24.

55 Robert D. Defries, *The First Forty Years 1914-1955: Connaught Medical Research Laboratories University of Toronto* (Toronto: University of Toronto Press, 1968), 49-50; and Toronto, Local Board of Health, *Monthly Report,* November 1919, 4.

56 J.J. Heagerty, "Influenza and Vaccination," *Canadian Medical Association Journal* 9 (1919): 226-28; "Official Report on Influenza Epidemic, 1918," *Canadian Medical Association Journal* 9 (1919): 351-54; T.F. Cadham, "The Use of a Vaccine in the Recent Epidemic of Influenza," *Canadian Medical Association Journal* 9 (1919): 519-27; and F.H. Wetmore, "Treatment of Influenza," *Canadian Medical Association Journal* 9 (1919): 1,075-80. See also Tognotti, "Scientific Triumphalism," for an overview of the Italian response to the epidemic.

57 In the *Toronto Globe,* there were daily reports about the role of civilian volunteers, and the women's pages during and after the epidemic listed the work of local chapters of the Liberal Association, the IODE (Imperial Order Daughters of the Empire), the Samaritan Club, the Red Cross Society, and women's church groups. See *Toronto Globe,* 16 October 1918, 4; *Toronto Globe,* 25 October 1918, 4; *Toronto Globe,* 2 November 1918, 10; and *Toronto Globe,* 6 November 1918, 10. See also Esyllt Jones, "Contact across a Diseased Boundary: Urban Space and Social Interaction during Winnipeg's Influenza Epidemic, 1918-1919," *Journal of the Canadian Historical Association,* n.s., 13 (2002): 119-39.

58 *History of Public Health Nursing,* 10.

59 "The Provincial Board of Health of Ontario," *Public Health Journal* 10 (1919): 29-30.

60 "A Working Program against Influenza," *American Journal of Public Health* 9 (January 1919): 1-13.

61 T.H. Whitelaw, "The Practical Aspects of Quarantine for Influenza," *Canadian Medical Association Journal* 9 (1919): 1070-74. Edmonton had to enforce Alberta provincial board of health regulations requiring modified quarantine and found that many citizens objected because their neighbours were not subject to the same limitations, even though they too had mild cases of the disease.

62   S. Boucher, "The Epidemic of Influenza," *Canadian Medical Association Journal* 8,12 (December 1918): 1087-92.

63   *Public Health Journal* 11 (1920): 98; and "University Course in Public Health Nursing Established in Ontario," *Public Health Journal* 11 (1920): 430-31.

64   "Preliminary Programme," *Public Health Journal* 10 (1919): 189.

65   MacDougall, *Activists and Advocates,* 123-25; Paul Bator, "The Health Reformers versus the Common Canadian: The Controversy over Compulsory Vaccination against Smallpox in Toronto and Ontario, 1900-1920," *Ontario History* 75 (1983): 348-73; and Katherine Arnup, "Victims of Vaccination? Opposition to Compulsory Immunization in Ontario, 1900-90," *Canadian Bulletin of Medical History* 9 (1992): 159-76.

66   MacDougall, *Activists and Advocates,* 157-58.

67   Jane Gadd, "Tuberculosis Makes Comeback among Homeless and Poor," *Toronto Globe and Mail,* 7 March 1996, A1, A10; and Trish Crawford, "Return of White Plague," *Toronto Star,* 18 April 1997, B1-2.

68   Andrew Nikiforuk, *The Fourth Horseman: A Short History of Epidemics, Plagues, Famine and Other Scourges* (Harmondsworth: Viking, 1991); Laurie Garrett, *The Coming Plague: Newly Emerging Diseases in a World Out of Balance* (New York: Farrar, Strauss and Giroux, 1995); and Laurie Garrett, *Betrayal of Trust: The Collapse of Global Public Health* (New York: Hyperion, 2000). See also the Epilogue to Nancy Tomes's study *The Gospel of Germs* and her article "The Making of a Germ Panic, Then and Now," *American Journal of Public Health* 90 (2000): 191-98.

69   Frank O'Connor, *Report of the Walkerton Inquiry: The Events of May 2000 and Related Issues* (Toronto: Ministry of the Attorney General, 2002).

70   Abbate, "Toronto Board of Health," A5; and Colin Vaughan, "The Gap between Promise and Reality," *Toronto Globe and Mail,* 5 August 1997, A5. As Colin Vaughan noted, the province was arguing that amalgamation would save money, but previous cuts to Toronto's Health Department had already reduced staffing levels by 25 percent, and the Toronto region had been designated as underfunded in a 1996 provincial study called *Towards Equitable Funding for Public Health.*

71   "The Toronto Experiment," *Toronto Globe and Mail,* 6 September 2003, M10-11.

72   Ibid. The figures, which are derived from the 2001 Canadian census, do not include the 35.5 percent of the population who identified their origin as "Other European." The census also allowed citizens to indicate up to six different ethnic origins, with the result that the overall totals equal more than 100 percent.

73   Toronto Public Health, *Public Health Budget Fact Sheet,* 10 March 1998.

74   Archie Campbell, *The SARS Commission Interim Report – SARS and Public Health in Ontario* (Toronto: Queen's Printer, 2004), 46, http://www.health.gov.on.ca/.

75   Canada, National Advisory Committee on SARS and Public Health, *Learning from SARS: Renewal of Public Health in Canada: A Report of the National Advisory Committee on SARS and Public Health* (Ottawa: Health Canada, 2003), 2-3, http://www.hc-sc.gc.ca/.

76   Ibid., 3-7.

77   Sheela V. Basrur, Barbara Yaffe, and Bonnie Henry, "SARS: A Local Public Health Perspective," *Canadian Journal of Public Health* 95 (2004): 22.

78   Archie Campbell, *The SARS Commission Second Interim Report: SARS and Public Health Legislation* (Ottawa: Queen's Printer, 2005), 213-30, http://www.health.gov.on.ca.

79   Campbell, *The SARS Commission Interim Report,* 146.

80   Weizhen Dong, "Beyond SARS: Health Care in a Highly Diversified Society – A Case Study of Toronto," in University of Toronto Centre for Health Promotion, *14th Annual*

Report 2003-2004, 9-10, http://www.utoronto.ca/chp/download/AnnualReports/2003 -04.pdf.

81 Mark Hume, "In Search of a SARS Vaccine: 'It's Been a Heck of a Ride,'" *Toronto Globe and Mail,* 7 February 2004, F6.

82 Campbell, *The SARS Commission Interim Report.* See Inadequate Infectious Disease Information Systems, 100-10, and Lack of Surge Capacity: The Toronto Example, 146-52.

83 Campbell, *The SARS Commission Interim Report,* 147-49. Justice Campbell noted a variety of criticisms about the lack of sustained follow-up by TPH staff who were familiar with the individual or family's case and several instances where TPH staff called to inquire about the health status of patients, only to discover that they had died in hospital days earlier. See also Basrur, Yaffe, and Henry, "SARS: A Local Public Health Perspective," 22-23. In Chapter 8 of *The SARS Commission Second Interim Report,* Mr. Justice Campbell discussed the legal meaning of the term "quarantine." He also cited Clete DiGiovanni et al., "Factors Influencing Compliance with Quarantine in Toronto during the 2003 SARS Outbreak," *Biosecurity and Bioterrorism: Biodefense Strategy, Practice and Science* 2 (December 2004): 265-72, in which Torontonians and health care personnel who had been quarantined reported that they complied with quarantine requests "to reduce the risk of transmission to others," to protect community health, and because they saw it as their "civic duty." Fear of legal consequences had little influence in their decision to undergo the hardship that ten days in isolation imposed.

84 Caroline Alphonso, "Hospitals Scramble to Protect SARS Staff," *Toronto Globe and Mail,* 22 April 2003, A1, 4; and Carolyn Abraham, "Virus Can Live 24 Hours outside Host," *Toronto Globe and Mail,* 22 April 2003, A1, 4. The second story notes that a team from the Centers for Disease Control in Atlanta had arrived in Toronto to assist infection control experts at Mount Sinai and Sunnybrook and Women's College Health Sciences Centre in determining what measures to take to protect health care workers from infection. Torontonians seemed calm about the outbreak, and even those who regularly used the GO transit system to commute to work were not unduly worried about the possibility of having shared the train with a symptomatic nurse from Mount Sinai on 14 and 15 April. See Colin Freeze, "Commuters into Toronto Ride Out Scare," *Toronto Globe and Mail,* 22 April 2003, A5.

85 Chapter 2 of *Learning from SARS* describes the "quest for Containment" between 8 and 23 April, and notes that the media highlighted each story about possible community spread, leaving the impression that TPH and provincial authorities were not doing their jobs effectively. Canada, *Learning from SARS,* Chapter 2, sec. 2e: "The Quest for Containment (April 8, 2003-April 23, 2003)," 10-12.

86 Rhea Seymour, "Courage under Fire," *University of Toronto Magazine* 31,2 (Winter 2004): 30. The writer notes that medical and nursing students at the University of Toronto had their classes and clinical rotations cancelled as a result of the SARS outbreak. In contrast to 1918, they were not asked to volunteer their services.

87 André Picard, "Outbreak Is Easing, Expert Says," *Toronto Globe and Mail,* 24 April 2003, A1, A8.

88 Campbell, *The SARS Commission Interim Report,* 56-63.

89 Carolyn Abraham and Caroline Alphonso, "Crossed Wires Put Toronto on Hit List," *Toronto Globe and Mail,* 24 April 2003, A1, A7.

90 Seymour, "Courage," 32-33.

91   Danylo Hawaleshka, "SARS: Is This Your Best Defence?" *Maclean's*, 14 April 2003, 24;
     Murray Campbell, "Disease Is Damaging Ontario's Economy, Cabinet Officials Say,"
     Toronto Globe and Mail, 23 April 2003, A4; Jonathon Gatehouse, "SARS: Fear and Loathing
     of Toronto," *Maclean's*, 5 May 2003, 19-22; and Mary Janigan, "Room at the Table,"
     Maclean's, 5 May 2003, 24-25.
92   Kylie Taggart, "Independent SARS Commission Set Up in Ont.," *Medical Post* 25 (2003):
     5. In this story, Taggart notes that a ninety-six-year-old man who died at NYGH was thought
     to be the index case for the second SARS wave because a health care worker on the same
     floor may have contracted SARS from her mother, who had been a patient in the Scar-
     borough Grace Hospital.
93   Canada, *Learning from SARS*, 1, 4. According to Hume, "In Search of a SARS Vaccine,"
     China experienced 5,000 cases with 349 deaths and was leading in the race to produce a
     vaccine against SARS. Worldwide, the disease infected 8,500 people in thirty countries
     and killed 800 including the 44 in Toronto.
94   Terry Murray, "Health-Care Staff Have a 'Duty' to Treat," *Medical Post* 39,20 (2003): 6.
95   Seymour, "Courage," 26-29. See also Terry Murray, "MD's Illness Gave Her a Unique View
     of SARS," *Medical Post* 39,19 (2003): 5.
96   Jackie Smith, "First, Tell the Real Story," *Toronto Globe and Mail*, 28 April 2003, A13; Carolyn
     Abraham and Lisa Priest, "Cutbacks Fed SARS Calamity, Critics Say," *Toronto Globe and
     Mail*, 3 May 2003, A1, A6; and Richard Mackie and Murray Campbell, "Public-Health
     Spending Cuts Went Too Far, Critics Say," *Toronto Globe and Mail*, 6 May 2003, A9.
97   Campbell, *The SARS Commission Interim Report*, 132.
98   Ibid., 133.
99   Nick McCabe-Lokos, "Know What Is Known about SARS," *Toronto Star*, 28 March 2003,
     D5; and André Picard, "Fear Factor: So Just How Big a Risk Is SARS?" *Toronto Globe and
     Mail*, 5 April 2003, F8.
100 Gatehouse, "SARS: Fear and Loathing," 22. What made the statement more surprising is
     that Pat Green's husband was a Toronto firefighter, and her son, Derek, was a Toronto
     Transit Commission bus driver, indicating that all three of them were in occupations which
     would be at risk if SARS had been spreading in the community.
101 Campbell, *The SARS Commission Interim Report*, 60-61.
102 The *Learning from SARS* report estimated that SARS would cost Canada $2 billion, while
     the former Ontario auditor, Erik Peters, stated that SARS-related spending by the provincial
     government would cost $720 million, only $250 million of which would come from federal
     coffers. See Campbell, *The SARS Commission Interim Report*, Appendix E: "The Economic
     Impact of SARS."
103 "Voices from the Front," *Maclean's*, 5 May 2003, 23-24. Tess Malolos, a member of the
     Bukas-Loob sa Diyos congregation, explains the misinformation that was harming her
     family and the Filipino community.
104 Paul Farmer, "Pestilence and Restraint: Haitians, Guantánamo, and the Logic of Quaran-
     tine," in Hannaway, Harden, and Parascandola, *AIDS and the Public Debate*, 139-52.
105 Hawaleshka, "Is This Your Best Defence?" 21-23; and Picard, "Mommy, Are You Going
     to Die?"
106 *Learning from SARS* points out that "SARS has provoked welcome discussion of the oc-
     cupational culture in health care ... Countless health care workers faced a fundamental
     conflict between self-preservation, and a professional obligation to serve the greater good

... The Committee would like to salute each and every one of them for their courage and commitment." Canada, *Learning from SARS,* 16.

107 Judy Gerstel, "Doctor's Diary of Deadly Disease, Hong Kong M.D. Shares Experience, His Notes Help Toronto's Battle," *Toronto Star,* 28 March 2003, D1, D4.

108 *Learning from SARS* states that "nurses have long voiced concerns that their knowledge and experience are not taken seriously by senior decision makers. At North York General Hospital, nurses alleged that administrators ignored their warnings of an impending second SARS outbreak." Canada, *Learning from SARS,* 16. For the nurses' perspective, see "SARS War's Unsung Heroes – Nurses at Their Posts through Crisis Despite Stress, Danger," National Nursing Week Supplement, *Toronto Globe and Mail,* 12 May 2003, N1. In a more pointed critique of the system, thirty nurses who contracted SARS as a result of nursing patients decided to sue the provincial government. See "Nurses Sue over SARS," *Record,* 26 March 2004, A1, A2. The case is still pending.

109 Celia Milne, "SARS Will Strike Again – And Again," *Medical Post* 39,26 (2003): 5, quotes Dr. Mark Lipsitch of Harvard University, who stated that "TPH did a very good job under completely uncertain circumstances." See also City of Toronto, press release, 12 July 2004, http://wx.toronto.ca/.

110 Campbell, *The SARS Commission Second Interim Report,* 51.

111 Prithi Yelaja, "Fear Recalls Past Outbreaks," *Toronto Star,* 28 March 2003, D2; McIlroy, "1918 Redux?" F9; and Danylo Hawaleshka, "Killer Viruses," *Maclean's,* 2003, 50-51.

112 Hume, "In Search of a SARS Vaccine," F6; "SARS Vaccine Team Hits Serious Hurdle," *Record,* 29 November 2004, A3; small news item, *Toronto Star,* 20 June 2005, A13; and Sheryl Ubelacker, "SARS Link to Acute Lung Failure Discovered in Laboratory Mice," *Toronto Globe and Mail,* 12 July 2005, A11.

113 Carolyn Bennett, "Building a National Public Health System," *Canadian Medical Association Journal* 170 (2004): 9; and Richard Mackie, "Ontario to Put SARS Lessons into Practice," *Toronto Globe and Mail,* 23 June 2004, A9. As a result of experience during the SARS outbreak and growing concern about a future influenza pandemic, all three levels of Canadian government have created pandemic influenza plans. See http://www.health.gov. on.ca for information on the Ontario plan and its links to its federal counterpart. For the TPH plan, see "Pandemic Influenza," Toronto Public Health, http://www.toronto.ca/.

114 Jacalyn Duffin, "Introduction: Lessons and Disappointments," in *SARS in Context: Memory, History, Policy,* ed. Jacalyn Duffin and Arthur Sweetman (Montreal and Kingston: McGill-Queen's University Press, 2006), 3.

115 John Tosh, Introduction, in *Historians on History,* 2nd ed., ed. John Tosh (Harlow, UK: Longmans Pearson, 2008), 7.

116 As Tosh states, "In each generation the call for greater accessibility and greater account-ability on the part of historians has to be repeated." Tosh, *Historians on History,* 349. See also Virginia Berridge, "History Matters? History's Role in Health Policy Making," *Medical History* 53 (2008): 311-26.

117 Canada, National Advisory Committee on SARS and Public Health, *Learning from SARS: Renewal of Public Health in Canada: A Report of the National Advisory Committee on SARS and Public Health* (Ottawa: Health Canada, 2003), http://www.phac-aspc.gc.ca/.

118 He was also strongly supported by the editors of the *Canadian Medical Association Journal,* who argued that "this is not just another high-sounding recommendation (creating PHAC): the committee lays out a legislative roadmap to create such a body within the existing provincial-federal jurisdictional minefield ... But even with legislative amendments and a

real boost in funding, we still face the difficult and critical task of changing the culture of public health in this country. For too long public health professionals and medical officers of health, impeded by bureaucracy and political agendas, have struggled to make unencumbered decisions in the public interest. Like other physicians, medical officers of health diagnose and treat, but their patients are populations and their treatments – public health education and mass communication, quarantine, school and workplace closures, boil-water orders, travel advisories, bans on the sale of hazardous goods – readily become politicized by their social and economic consequences." Editorial, "A Canadian Agency for Public Health: If Not Now, When?" *Canadian Medical Association Journal* 169,8 (14 October 2003): 741.

119 Canadian Coalition for Public Health in the 21st Century, "Consultation on Strengthening the Pan-Canadian Public Health System and Meeting with the Minister of State (Public Health) March 10, 2004," *Canadian Journal of Public Health* 95 (July-August 2004): 1-15.

120 Michael Rachlis, "Moving Forward with Public Health in Canada," *Canadian Journal of Public Health* 95 (November-December 2004): 405-6. Butler-Jones had been a member of the Naylor committee and was a former medical officer of health from Saskatchewan.

121 Wayne Kondro, "Public Health on the Installment Plan," *Canadian Medical Association Journal* 170,9 (27 April 2004): 1378.

122 For the reappearance of SARS, see "China Reports First New SARS Cases in Months," *Waterloo Region Record,* 23 April 2004, A10; "SARS Deaths in China Spark Quarantines, Travel Precautions," *Waterloo Region Record,* 24 April 2004, A12; Mark Hume, "SARS Claims New Victim as Hong Kong, U.S. on Alert," *Toronto Globe and Mail,* 24 April 2004, A8; "China Probes New SARS Cases," *Waterloo Region Record,* 26 April 2006, A5; and "Medical Investigators Set Sights on SARS Cases," *Waterloo Region Record,* 29 April 2004, A8. For fears about the spread of pandemics, see Patricia Huston, "Thinking Locally about Pandemic Influenza," *Canadian Journal of Public Health* 95 (May-June 2004): 184-85.

123 "SARS Vaccine Team Hits Serious Hurdle," *Waterloo Region Record,* 29 November 2004, A3.

124 Eugenia Tognotti, "Scientific Triumphalism and Learning from Facts: Bacteriology and the 'Spanish Flu' Challenge of 1918," *Social History of Medicine* 16 (2003): 97-110.

125 Carolyn Abraham, "Scientists Create 'Cousin' of 1918 Killer Flu," *Toronto Globe and Mail,* 7 October 2004, A21.

126 J.K. Taubenberger et al., "Characterization of the 1918 Influenza Virus Polymerase Genes," *Nature* 437,7060 (6 October 2005): 889-93; "Deadly Virus Recreated, Linked to Avian Flu," *Waterloo Region Record,* 6 October 2005, A1-A2; and Carolyn Abraham, "Similarities between Avian Flu Mutations and 1918 Virus Fuel Fears of Next Pandemic," *Toronto Globe and Mail,* 6 October 2005, A1, A11.

127 Stéphane Barry, Luc Hessel, and Norbert Gualde, "La grippe, une menace éternelle," *Canadian Bulletin of Medical History* 24 (2007): 445-66.

128 "U.S. Warns of Bird Flu Pandemic," *Waterloo Region Record,* 11 October 2005, A7; and Erica Weir, "The Changing Ecology of Avian Flu," *Canadian Medical Association Journal* 173,8 (11 October 2005): 869-70. For summaries of the national plan and Toronto's and Waterloo Region's preparations and estimates, see Elaine Carey, "Bracing for the Pandemic," *Waterloo Region Record,* 26 February 2005, A1, A14; Jeff Gray, "City Gets Ready for a Global Flu," *Toronto Globe and Mail,* 10 May 2005, A12; and Anne Kelly, "Preparing for a Pandemic," *Waterloo Region Record,* 21 October 2005, D1. The provincial and regional plans are similar to those found in the rest of the country.

129 Esyllt W. Jones, *Influenza 1918: Disease, Death, and Struggle in Winnipeg* (Toronto: University of Toronto Press, 2007); and Eileen Pettigrew, *The Silent Enemy: Canada and the Deadly Flu of 1918* (Saskatoon: Western Producer Prairie Books, 1983).

130 Rodney Kort, Allison J. Stuart, and Erika Bontovics, "Ensuring a Broad and Inclusive Approach: A Provincial Perspective on Pandemic Preparedness," *Canadian Journal of Public Health* 96 (November-December 2005): 406-11.

131 See Kumanan Wilson and Harvey Lazar, "Planning for the Next Pandemic Threat: Defining the Federal Role in Public Health Emergencies," *Institute for Research in Public Policy Matters* 6 (November 2005): 1-36.

132 Heather MacDougall, "Reinventing Public Health: A New Perspective on the Health of Canadians and Its International Impact," *Journal of Epidemiology and Community Health* 61 (2007): 955-59. See also World Health Organization, *World Health Report 2008 – Primary Health Care: Now More than Ever* (Geneva: World Health Organization, 2008). The election of Stephen Harper's first minority government in January 2006 resulted in the elimination of the junior minister of state for public health and a shift in focus to the curative system. As André Picard observes in "We Need More than Mother Earth and Apple Pie Goals – Where's the Action?" *Toronto Globe and Mail,* 4 December 2008, L4, without specific targets, more funding for training public health professionals, stronger social welfare programs, and committed political leadership, these laudable aims will not be fulfilled. He could have strengthened his argument by pointing out that the Naylor, Walker, and Campbell reports as well as submissions from the Canadian Coalition for Public Health in the 21st century had presented the same recommendations years earlier.

133 Andrew Nikiforuk, *Pandemonium: Bird Flu, Mad Cow Disease, and Other Biological Plagues of the 21st Century* (Toronto: Viking Canada, 2006).

134 Vincent Lam and Colin Lee, *The Flu Pandemic and You: A Canadian Guide* (Toronto: Doubleday Canada, 2006).

135 Heather MacDougall, "Review of *The Flu Pandemic and You: A Canadian Guide,*" *Canadian Journal of Public Health* 99 (March-April 2008): 434.

136 Lam and Lee, *The Flu Pandemic,* 212-31. For an example of the way that health care professionals understand and use history, see ibid., Chapter 4, "Will History Repeat Itself? Influenza Pandemics over the Centuries" (42-67).

137 World Health Organization Western Pacific Region, *SARS: How a Global Epidemic Was Stopped* (Geneva: World Health Organization, 2006); Angela R. McLean et al., *SARS: A Case Study in Emerging Infections* (Oxford: Oxford University Press, 2005); Arthur Kleinman and James L. Watson, eds., *SARS in China: Prelude to Pandemic?* (Stanford: Stanford University Press, 2006); WHO News, "Health Is a Foreign Policy Concern," *Bulletin of the World Health Organization* 85 (March 2007): 167-68; and WHO News, "New Rules on International Public Health Security," *Bulletin of the World Health Organization* 85 (June 2007): 428-30.

138 "Stockpiling Flu Vaccines Questioned," *Waterloo Region Record,* 3 November 2006, A6.

139 Howard Markel et al., "Nonpharmaceutical Interventions Implemented by US Cities during the 1918-1919 Influenza Pandemic," *Journal of the American Medical Association* 298 (8 August 2007): 644-54; and "WHO Slams China on Bird Flu Info," *Waterloo Region Record,* 2 November 2006, C9.

140 Alexandra Minna Stern and Howard Markel, "International Efforts to Control Infectious Diseases, 1851 to the Present," *Journal of the American Medical Association* 292 (22-29 September 2004): 1474-79; and Theodore Brown, Marcus Cueto, and Elizabeth Fee, "The

World Health Organization and the Transition from 'International' to 'Global' Public Health," *American Journal of Public Health* 96 (January 2006): 62-72.

141 "SARS Lawsuits Allowed to Proceed," *Waterloo Region Record,* 24 August 2005, A4.

142 Maureen A. Cava et al., "The Experience of Quarantine for Individuals Affected by SARS in Toronto," *Public Health Nursing* 22 (2005): 398-406. See also Clete DiGiovanni et al., "Factors Influencing Compliance with Quarantine in Toronto during the 2003 SARS Outbreak," *Biosecurity and Bioterrorism: Biodefense Strategy, Practice and Science* 2 (2004): 265-72.

143 Frances Itani, *Deafening: A Novel* (Toronto: Harper Canada, 2003); Daniel Kalla, *Pandemic: A Novel* (New York: Tom Doherty, 2005); and Jean Little, *If I Should Die Before I Wake* (Toronto: Scholastic Press, 2005).

144 Jim Bawden, "*Plague City* Recreates SARS Scare of 2003," *Waterloo Region Record,* 4 January 2005, B5. See also Catherine Dawson March, "SARS Attacks," *Toronto Globe and Mail Television,* 28 May-3 June 2005, 6-7, who provides an interesting summary of current knowledge about the etiology of SARS and recollections of the outbreak as well as illuminating the choices that producers make when recreating historical events for television.

145 Howard Phillips, "The Re-Appearing Shadow of 1918: Trends in the Historiography of the 1918-19 Influenza Pandemic," *Canadian Bulletin of Medical History* 21,1 (2004): 121-34; and Helen Branswell, "90 Years after Spanish Flu We're More Vulnerable Now: Experts," *Toronto Star,* 16 September 2008, http://www.healthzone.ca/.

146 See Helen Branswell, "Spanish Flu Survivors Recount Fear, Nosebleeds, Makeshift Morgues," *Toronto Star,* 19 September 2008, http://www.healthzone.ca/; and "Surviving 'the Spanish Lady' (Spanish Flu)," CBC TV, 10 April 2003, http://archives.cbc.ca/.

147 See David M. Morens and Anthony S. Fauci, "The 1918 Influenza Pandemic: Insights for the 21st Century," *Journal of Infectious Diseases* 195 (1 April 2007): 1018-28; Donald E. Low, "Pandemic Planning: Non-Pharmaceutical Interventions," *Respirology* 13 (2008): Supplement 1, S44-S48; and Markel et al., "Nonpharmaceutical Interventions," 644-54, for examples of new topics for historical research and the application of existing historical knowledge to the second phase of pandemic planning.

148 Berridge, "History Matters?" 322.

Conclusion

ESYLLT JONES AND MAGDA FAHRNI

In May of 2010, just as the H1N1 scare was finally beginning to lose its front-page appeal, several contributors to this volume gathered for a roundtable discussion to explore the intersections between influenza's history and recent experience. We were especially interested in probing the question of the "usability" of influenza's past, given the degree to which the 1918-20 epidemic has become, as Ann Herring noted, the benchmark against which any current or future influenza pandemics are measured. It is the only one of the major twentieth-century influenza outbreaks for which we have good historical knowledge. A rather simplified and selective story of its devastation, presented by media outlets, has often been employed to highlight the potentially catastrophic impact of H1N1. The 1918-20 experience tends to serve as a narrative backdrop, setting the stage on which contemporary anxieties play out. Although attention to the history of influenza could allow for a rewarding engagement between past and present (helping us to understand the impact of social conditions, for example), there are also ways in which influenza's past is rather less than fruitfully engaged (present-day allusions to the 1918-20 pandemic tend to ignore the historical evidence of conflict during it), and much of the richness of historical knowledge is less apparent in public debate.

Since 2009, there has been considerable debate about what "lessons" might be learned from our experience with H1N1. Layered over the question of the usability of influenza's long history is now an attempt to evaluate our most recent experience. In a sense, H1N1 joins the list of twentieth-century influenza pandemics (actual or feared) and will become a subject of future research. At the same time, responses to H1N1 in Canada do allow us to draw some points of comparison and contrast with what we know about the 1918-20 outbreak. Despite the obvious and enormous differences in scale and the numbers of people who contracted the disease and died from it, the events associated with H1N1 resonated with Canadian historians of influenza in several ways.

One issue to which some media commentators and public health officials have paid attention is the impact of social inequality and poverty on flu morbidity and mortality. The history of influenza has demonstrated that socioeconomic factors contributed to significant differentials in mortality among Canadians, although much research remains to be done on this subject. Disease experience also goes beyond what statistics can tell us. Historians, trained in the use of sources and methodologies such as oral history, can illuminate the lived experience of influenza, from the point of view of patients and health care providers. We know that the illness historically poses particular challenges for the marginalized in our communities; we also know that mutual aid, kin, and community can be essential sources of support. Often, memories of the 1918-20 pandemic are centred on the supportive roles of family, friends, neighbours, and sometimes complete strangers; many, if not most, of these devoted family and community members were women. One of the key insights that this research brings to bear is the need to incorporate these supportive roles into pandemic preparation, even into health care planning more generally. Although there are definite limits to the capacity of voluntary care networks to respond to pandemics, and these limits must be recognized by the state, community and kin are never absent from the disease experience.

Scholarship on First Nations reveals that some Aboriginal communities were disproportionately at risk in 1918 through 1920 and beyond. Historical understanding of why that might be the case is becoming increasingly sophisticated. Karen Slonim's chapter in this collection is an example of such work. The need for a nuanced social awareness of the relationship between the disease and income, living conditions, and the availability of health care becomes evident when we look at the *differences between* First Nations, rather than focusing solely on their similarities. As Slonim demonstrates, not all experiences were the same. In 2009-10, H1N1 cases among First Nations received a great deal of media attention, but far less was paid to First Nations that were not suffering high rates of infection and death, or where material conditions on reserves were not obviously shocking. As is so often the case in Canadian history, First Nations' experiences are considered categorically.

This aspect of influenza's history becomes an important observation, considering the tension between a positive awareness of the impact of social conditions and victimization or stigmatization of flu victims. The influenza cases in communities such as Garden Hill and St. Theresa Point First Nations made national headlines in 2009 and attracted international attention from influenza experts. By 2010, as the virus became more widespread in Manitoba, many individuals requiring ventilators were from First Nations communities. However temporarily, this served to highlight both the inadequate living conditions in some reserves and the importance of disease interactions, where Aboriginal people also suffer disproportionately high rates of diabetes, tuberculosis, obesity, and other health challenges. Indeed, in Manitoba in 2009, the work of journalists such as Jen Skerritt underlined the risks posed by influenza in communities already dealing with high numbers of tuberculosis cases. TB, so rarely a threat to white middle-class Canadians that it has almost slipped outside of public awareness, serves to highlight the distinct realities of Aboriginal health in Canada and the lingering impact of colonial governance that has shaped the bodily experiences of Aboriginal people for several centuries.

As essential as it is for Canadians to comprehend the human face of disease, this awareness can serve to further deepen the stigmatization of Aboriginal people in Canada and to perpetuate an image of victimhood rather than agency. Recent responses to the presence of infectious disease in Canada and globally have demonstrated an increasing association of influenza with racialized others, be they Aboriginal, Asian, or Mexican. Consider the emptying of Asian restaurants in Toronto during the SARS epidemic or the association between Mexican workers and the flu. This is quite distinct from perceptions of influenza in Canada at the end of the Great War, when there was relatively little direct public scapegoating of the poor, non-Anglo immigrants, or First Nations people. Once the pandemic took hold in cities such as Winnipeg, residents of poor neighbourhoods were assumed to be not only highly at risk, but also passive victims incapable of staying healthy. Yet, though occasional racialized comments were voiced about the dissemination of influenza in Canada, evidence suggests that ethnic minorities were not generally blamed for either its spread or its initial appearance. During a time of war, the enemy was clearly identified, and rumours circulated that the flu had been brought to Canada by German U-boats. But this was not a prevalent notion.

Many public health officials also refrained from feeding any potential anti-immigrant feeling. Those most experienced with an ethnically diverse population, such as Winnipeg's A.J. Douglas, wanted to keep communication open and encourage non-English-speaking residents of the city to be aware of and follow health dictates. After decades attempting to limit the spread of diseases such as smallpox, diphtheria, scarlet fever, typhoid, measles, and tuberculosis, health officials drew on extensive practical experience and a changing ethos of public health, a movement away from direct coercion toward educational approaches. Organized opposition to compulsory smallpox vaccination, for example, had forced them to develop strategies for public health compliance that attempted to balance the dictates of disease control with the rights of the individual and the family unit. Although more research needs to be done in this area, many citizens sought influenza vaccination in 1918-19, which was offered for free and on a voluntary basis in some Canadian cities. But widespread public support for vaccination was by no means guaranteed in this era. The flu pandemic came at the end of a long period of agitation against compulsion in public health.

By the First World War, as the political franchise and a sense of working-class entitlement broadened, demand had grown for political accountability for health in general and for disease control measures more specifically. After all, provincial and local governments formally held extremely broad legislative powers to contain individuals and to destroy property in response to the presence of infectious disease in the community. Such legally permissive measures had been the target of popular opposition since the mid-nineteenth century in Canada and were on occasion framed as unjustifiable violations of bodily integrity and parental rights. In Britain, popular opposition had resulted in the introduction of a conscientious objector clause to compulsory vaccination laws.

From a historical perspective, then, it is not unexpected that vaccination would become an issue during H1N1. As in the late nineteenth and early twentieth centuries, we live in an era when opposition to vaccination circulates freely among dissenters. In addition, there exists a long-standing social critique of pharmaceutical companies on the grounds that they "push" unnecessary and in some cases unsafe drugs on doctors and patients, and in fact powerfully shape the very definition of disease. This, combined with older notions of bodily autonomy and the right to freedom from coercion (whether that coercion is direct or indirect), creates a heady mix. During the winter of 2009-10, many of us stood in university classrooms talking to our students about these issues, as young adults – a high-risk group in an influenza pandemic – were proving particularly uninterested in getting vaccinated. On social media, many expressed frank skepticism if not anxiety about the H1N1 vaccine. The history of vaccination tells us that popular opposition often becomes part of a broader critique of the state, as anti-vaccinators ally themselves with feminists, workers, and freethinkers in an impressive array of movements that challenge the right of the state to determine the fate of the disenfranchised body. Thus, the lessons of disease history are also lessons about the political relationship between citizen and state.

However, medical scientists and journalists, who purport to speak in the language of science, often resort to ad hominem and emotive attacks on those opposed to vaccination, referring to them as conspiracy theorists or at best as irrational. The challenges facing the vaccination campaign during H1N1 have been linked explicitly to the false claims of the MMR-autism controversy, which, it is argued, has damaged the public's trust in vaccination, with deleterious results. Yet, historical experience suggests that concern about the relationship between MMR vaccination and autism might be only the most obvious and visible element of a deeper anti-vaccination sentiment: the tip of the social movement iceberg. In fact, opposition to public health is a multifaceted and complex historical phenomenon, often moving considerably beyond any specified disease experience. It speaks more to issues of political disenfranchisement and a class and social justice critique of the social order: in today's case, the power of "big pharma." Many of its representatives have been women. It is an issue about power – who has it, who does not, and whether this balance is legitimate. Given this, it is difficult to address as a straightforward issue or with "good" science. Interestingly, low vaccination uptake is not mentioned in the government's 2010 report *Lessons Learned,* although it does offer some acknowledgment that the public is concerned about the availability, efficacy, and safety of H1N1 vaccines.

In 1918-20, at the height of the influenza pandemic and in the evaluations that followed, physicians and public health officials were not united in their views about how to respond to the disease. We know now, of course, that their understanding of the virus was extremely limited. And we know that the various branches of the Canadian state had a much more restricted capacity for effective intervention than they do today. But at the time, not unlike today, public health officials operated with the best knowledge that they had in hand. Controversies did arise, and practices varied even within Canada. Some practitioners and governments advocated the use of masks; others argued that masks would only worsen the chance of becoming ill. Some advocated strict quarantine; others asserted that quarantine was practically impossible to enforce and that any involuntary isolation would lead the public to conceal cases of influenza. Some believed in one or another vaccine serum; others doubted the efficacy of any available serum. Governments and health officials essentially had to make rapid decisions in a context of limited understanding of the disease they confronted. Their decisions were not perfect; sometimes, they were open to legitimate criticism. As Mark Humphries points out, public health took a back seat to the war effort, particularly during the fall 1918 wave. Geographic mobility played a role in the spread of disease in 1918-20, just as global migration does today. Health officials also faced economic pressures, as both business and government feared the financial consequences of an economy shut down by a pandemic. Indeed, public health policy never effectively dealt with the exigencies imposed by wage labour and poverty in an at-risk working-class population. History reminds us of the need to consider disease sufferers as people whose individual choices are proscribed by the material conditions of life.

Recent anxieties about avian and swine flu pandemics have created opportunities for an enhanced dialogue between historical and contemporary experience, both in terms of understanding the nature of the great influenza viruses and the nature of social and political responses to pandemic disease. Yet, this dialogue is never easy. Whereas historians set their examinations of events such as the 1918-20 epidemic in a rich historical context, seeking to complicate any single meta-narrative and to highlight national and local specificities, that context is often stripped away when their work is used to illustrate present-day situations. History cannot be employed to predict the future. But it provides ample matter for reflection.

Selected Bibliography

Books

Baer, Hans, Merrill Singer, and Ida Susser. *Medical Anthropology and the World System.* 2nd ed. Westport, CT: Praeger, 2003.

Baillargeon, Denyse. *Un Québec en mal d'enfants: la médicalisation de la maternité, 1910-1970.* Montreal: Éditions du remue-ménage, 2004.

Barry, John M. *The Great Influenza: The Epic Story of the Deadliest Plague in History.* New York: Viking, 2004.

Bernier, Jacques. *La médecine au Québec: naissance et évolution d'une profession.* Sainte-Foy: Presses de l'Université Laval, 1989.

Bilson, Geoffrey. *A Darkened House: Cholera in Nineteenth-Century Canada.* Toronto: University of Toronto Press, 1980.

Blakely, Debra. *Mass Mediated Disease: A Case Study Analysis of Three Flu Pandemics and Public Health Policy.* Lanham, MD: Lexington Books, 2006.

Bliss, Michael. *Plague: A Story of Smallpox in Montreal.* Toronto: HarperCollins, 1991.

Burnet, F.M., and E. Clark. *Influenza: A Survey of the Last 50 Years in the Light of Modern Work on the Virus of Epidemic Influenza.* London: Macmillan, 1942.

Byerly, Carol R. *Fever of War: The Influenza Epidemic in the U.S. Army during World War I.* New York: New York University Press, 2005.

Cliff, A.D., P. Haggett, and J.K. Ord. *Spatial Aspects of Influenza Epidemics.* London: Pion, 1986.

Cohen, Yolande. *Profession infirmière: une histoire des soins dans les hôpitaux du Québec.* Montreal: Presses de l'Université de Montréal, 2000.

Copp, Terry. *The Anatomy of Poverty: The Condition of the Working Class in Montreal, 1897-1929.* Toronto: McClelland and Stewart, 1974.

Côté, Louise. *"En garde!" Les représentations de la tuberculose au Québec dans la première moitié du XXe siècle.* Sainte-Foy: Presses de l'Université Laval, 2000.

Crosby, Alfred W. *America's Forgotten Pandemic: The Influenza of 1918.* Cambridge: Cambridge University Press, 1989.

–. *Epidemic and Peace, 1918.* Westport, CT: Greenwood Press, 1976.

Delaporte, François. *Disease and Civilization: The Cholera in Paris, 1832.* Cambridge, MA: MIT Press, 1986.

Duncan, Kirsty. *Hunting the 1918 Flu: One Scientist's Search for a Killer Virus.* Toronto: University of Toronto Press, 2003.

Evans, Richard J. *Death in Hamburg: Society and Politics in the Cholera Years, 1830-1910.* London: Penguin Books, 1987.

Farmer, Paul. *Infections and Inequalities: The Modern Plagues.* Rev. ed. Berkeley: University of California Press, 1999.

Fougères, Dany. *L'approvisionnement en eau à Montréal: du privé au public, 1796-1865.* Sillery: Septentrion, 2004.

Gagan, David Paul, and Rosemary R. Gagan. *For Patients of Moderate Means: A Social History of the Voluntary Public General Hospital in Canada, 1890-1950.* Montreal and Kingston: McGill-Queen's University Press, 2002.

Gagnon, Robert. *Questions d'égouts: santé publique, infrastructures et urbanisation à Montréal au XIXe siècle.* Montreal: Boréal, 2006.

Herring, D. Ann, ed. *Anatomy of a Pandemic: The 1918 Influenza in Hamilton.* Hamilton: Allegra Press, 2006.

Johnson, Niall. *Britain and the 1918-19 Influenza Pandemic: A Dark Epilogue.* London: Routledge, 2006.

Jones, Esyllt W. *Influenza 1918: Disease, Death, and Struggle in Winnipeg.* Toronto: University of Toronto Press, 2007.

Jordan, E.O. *Epidemic Influenza.* Chicago: American Medical Association, 1927.

Keating, Peter, and Othmar Keel, eds. *Santé et société au Québec XIXe-XXe siècle.* Montreal: Boréal, 1995.

Kelm, Mary-Ellen. *Colonizing Bodies: Aboriginal Health and Healing in British Columbia, 1900-1950.* Vancouver: UBC Press, 1998.

MacPhail, Andrew. *Official History of the Canadian Forces in the Great War, 1914-19: The Medical Services.* Ottawa: Department of National Defence, 1925.

McPherson, Kathryn. *Bedside Matters: The Transformation of Canadian Nursing, 1900-1990.* Toronto: Oxford University Press, 2003.

Morris, R.J. *Cholera 1832: The Social Response to an Epidemic.* London: Croom Helm, 1976.

Nicholson, G.W.L. *Canada's Nursing Sisters.* Toronto: Samuel Stevens, Hakkert, 1975.

–. *The White Cross in Canada: A History of St. John Ambulance.* Montreal: Harvest House, 1967.

Pettigrew, Eileen. *The Silent Enemy: Canada and the Deadly Flu of 1918.* Saskatoon: Western Producer Prairie Books, 1983.

Pettit, Dorothy A., and Janice Bailie. *A Cruel Wind: Pandemic Flu in America.* Murfreesboro, TN: Timberlane Books, 2008.

Phillips, Howard, and David Killingray, eds. *The Spanish Influenza Pandemic of 1918-19: New Perspectives.* London: Routledge, 2003.

Pyle, G.F. *The Diffusion of Influenza: Patterns and Paradigms.* Totowa, NJ: Rowman and Littlefield, 1986.

Ranger, Terence, and Paul Slack, eds. *Epidemics and Ideas: Essays on the Historical Perception of Pestilence.* Cambridge: Cambridge University Press, 1992.

Rice, Geoffrey. *Black November: The 1918 Influenza Pandemic in New Zealand.* 2nd ed. Christchurch, NZ: Canterbury University Press, 2005.

Rosenberg, Charles. *The Cholera Years: The United States in 1832, 1849 and 1866.* Chicago: University of Chicago Press, 1962.

–. *Explaining Epidemics and Other Studies in the History of Medicine.* Cambridge: Cambridge University Press, 1992.

Santé Canada. *Plan canadien de lutte contre la pandémie d'influenza dans le secteur de la santé.* Ottawa: Agence de santé publique du Canada, 2004.

Smith, Edward Arthur Warwick, and Ambrose McGhie Medical Museum. *Hamilton's Doctors 1932-1982.* Hamilton: Ambrose McGhie Medical Museum, 2004.

Summers, Anne. *Angels and Citizens: British Women as Military Nurses, 1854-1914.* London: Threshold Press, 2000.

Tomes, Nancy. *The Gospel of Germs: Men, Women, and the Microbe in American Life.* Cambridge, MA: Harvard University Press, 1998.

Waldram, James B., D. Ann Herring, and T. Kue Young. *Aboriginal Health in Canada: Historical, Cultural, and Epidemiological Perspectives.* Toronto: University of Toronto Press, 2006.

Articles and Book Chapters

Adams, Annmarie. "Borrowed Buildings: Canada's Temporary Hospitals during World War I." *Canadian Bulletin of Medical History* 16,1 (1999): 25-48.

Anctil, Hervé, and Marc-A. Bluteau. *La santé et l'assistance publique au Québec: 1886-1986.* Quebec City: Ministère de la santé et des services sociaux, Direction des communications, 1986.

Andrews, Margaret. "Epidemic and Public Health: Vancouver 1918-19." *BC Studies* 34 (Summer 1977): 21-44.

Baillargeon, Denyse. "Fréquenter les gouttes de lait: l'expérience des mères montréalaises, 1910-1965." *Revue d'histoire de l'Amérique française* 50,1 (1996): 29-68.

Beiner, Guy. "Out in the Cold and Back: New-Found Interest in the Great Flu." *Cultural and Social History* 3,4 (October 2006): 496-505.

Bilson, Geoffrey. "Dr. Frederick Montizambert (1843-1929): Canada's First Director General of Public Health." *Medical History* 29 (1985): 386-400.

Bristow, Nancy K. "'You Can't Do Anything for Influenza': Doctors, Nurses and the Power of Gender during the Influenza Pandemic in the United States." In Phillips and Killingray, *The Spanish Influenza Pandemic,* 58-69.

Chan, Andrea H.W., and Hagen F. Kluge. "The Epidemic Spreads through the City." In Herring, *Anatomy of a Pandemic,* 41-56.

Chen, Zheng W. "Immunology of AIDS Virus and Mycobacterial Co-Infection." *Current HIV Research* 2 (2004): 351-55.

Coburn, David. "The Development of Canadian Nursing: Professionalisation and Proletarianization." *International Journal of Health Services* 18,13 (1988): 437-56.

Dechêne, Louise, and Jean-Claude Robert. "Le choléra de 1832 dans le Bas-Canada: mesure des inégalités devant la mort." In *Santé et Société au Québec XIXe–XXe siècle,* ed. Peter Keating and Othmar Keel, 61-84. Montreal: Boréal, 1995.

Desrosiers, Georges, and Benoît Gaumer. "Les débuts de l'éducation sanitaire au Québec: 1880-1901." *Canadian Bulletin of Medical History* 23,1 (2006): 183-207.

Desrosiers, Georges, Benoît Gaumer, François Hudon, and Othmar Keel. "Le renforcement des interventions gouvernementales dans le domaine de la santé entre 1922 et 1936: le Service provincial d'hygiène de la province de Québec." *Canadian Bulletin of Medical History* 18 (2001): 205-40.

Dickin McGinnis, Janice P. "A City Faces an Epidemic." *Alberta History* 24,4 (Autumn 1976): 120-141.

–. "The Impact of Epidemic Influenza: Canada, 1918-19." In *Medicine in Canadian Society: Historical Perspectives,* ed. S.E.D. Shortt, 447-77. Montreal and Kingston: McGill-Queen's University Press, 1981.

Elliott, Jayne. "Blurring the Boundaries of Space: Shaping Nurses' Lives at the Red Cross Outposts in Ontario, 1922-1945." *Canadian Bulletin of Medical History* 2,12 (2004): 303-25.

Fahrni, Magda. "'Elles sont partout': les femmes et la ville en temps d'épidémie, Montréal, 1918-1920." *Revue d'histoire de l'Amérique française* 58,1 (2004): 67-85.

Farley, Michael, Othmar Keel, and Camille Limoges. "Les commencements de l'administration montréalaise de la santé publique (1865-1885)." In Keating and Keel, *Santé et société,* 85-114.

Gagan, Rosemary. "Disease, Mortality, and Public Health, Hamilton, Ontario, 1900-1914." *Urban History Review* 17,3 (1989): 161-75.

Guérard, François. "L'hygiène publique au Québec de 1887 à 1939: centralisation, normalisation et médicalisation." *Recherches sociographiques* 37,2 (1996): 203-27.

Herring, D. Ann. "The 1918 Influenza Epidemic in the Central Canadian Subarctic." In *Strength in Diversity: A Reader in Physical Anthropology,* ed. D. Ann Herring and Leslie Chan, 364-84. Toronto: Canadian Scholars Press, 1994.

–. "'There Were Young People and Old People and Babies Dying Every Week': The 1918-1919 Influenza Pandemic at Norway House." *Ethnohistory* 41,1 (1994): 73-105.

Herring, D. Ann, and L. Sattenspiel. "Death in Winter: The Spanish Flu in the Canadian Subarctic." In Phillips and Killingray, *The Spanish Influenza Pandemic,* 156-72.

–. "Social Contexts, Syndemics, and Infectious Disease in Northern Aboriginal Populations." *American Journal of Human Biology* 19,2 (2007): 190-202.

Humphries, Mark Osborne. "The Horror at Home: The Canadian Military and the 'Great' Influenza Pandemic of 1918." *Journal of the Canadian Historical Association,* n.s., 16,1 (2005): 235-60.

Johnson, N.P.A.S., and J. Mueller. "Updating the Accounts: Global Mortality of the 1918-1920 'Spanish' Influenza Pandemic." *Bulletin of the History of Medicine* 76,1 (2002): 105-15.

Jones, Esyllt W. "'Cooperation in All Human Endeavour': Quarantine and Immigrant Disease Vectors in the 1918-1919 Influenza Pandemic in Winnipeg." *Canadian Bulletin of Medical History* 22,1 (2005): 57-82.

Kash, John C., et al. "Genomic Analysis of Increased Host Immune and Cell Death Responses Induced by 1918 Influenza Virus." *Nature* 443,7111 (4 October 2006): 578-81.

Keene-Payne, Rhonda. "We Must Have Nurses: Spanish Influenza in America, 1918-1919." *Nursing History Review* 8 (2000): 143-56.

Kelm, Mary-Ellen. "British Columbia First Nations and the Influenza Pandemic of 1918-1919." *BC Studies* 122 (Summer 1999): 23-48.

–. "Diagnosing the Discursive Indian: Medicine, Gender, and the 'Dying Race.'" *Ethnohistory* 52 (Spring 2005): 371-406.

Kobasa, Darwyn, et al. "Aberrant Innate Immune Response in Lethal Infection of Macaques with the 1918 Influenza Virus." *Nature* 445,7125 (18 January 2007): 319-23.

Lisowska, Anna. "Healing and Treatment: Who Answered the Call of the Sick?" In Herring, *Anatomy of a Pandemic,* 89-104.

Loo, Y.-M., and M. Gale. "Fatal Immunity and the 1918 Virus." *Nature* 445,7125 (18 January 2007): 267-68.

Lux, Maureen. "'The Bitter Flats': The 1918 Influenza Epidemic in Saskatchewan." *Saskatchewan History* 49,1 (Spring 1997): 3-13.

MacDougall, Heather. "Public Health and the 'Sanitary Idea' in Toronto, 1866-1890." In *Essays in the History of Canadian Medicine,* ed. Wendy Mitchinson and Janice Dickin McGinnis, 62-87. Toronto: McClelland and Stewart, 1988.

Mamelund, Svenn-Erik. "A Socially Neutral Disease? Individual Social Class, Household Wealth and Mortality from Spanish Influenza in Two Socially Contrasting Parishes in Kristiania 1918-19." *Social Science and Medicine* 62 (2006): 923-40.

Minnett, Valerie, and Mary-Anne Poutanen. "Swatting Flies for Health: Children and Tuberculosis in Early Twentieth-Century Montreal." *Urban History Review* 37,1 (Fall 2007): 32-44.

Moffat, Tina, and D. Ann Herring. "Historical Roots of High Rates of Infant Death in Aboriginal Communities in Canada in the Early Twentieth Century: The Case of Fisher River, Manitoba." *Social Science and Medicine* 48 (1999): 1821-32.

Morens, David M., and Anthony S. Fauci. "The 1918 Influenza Pandemic: Insights for the 21st Century." *Journal of Infectious Diseases* 195 (1 April 2007): 1018-28.

Morton, Gladys. "The Pandemic Influenza of 1918." *Canadian Nurse* 72,12 (December 1976): 32-37.

Noymer, A. "Testing the Influenza-Tuberculosis Selective Mortality Hypothesis with Union Army Data." PAA Extended Abstract, 23 September 2005. http://paa2006.princeton.edu.

Noymer, A., and M. Garenne. "Long-Term Effects of the 1918 'Spanish' Influenza Epidemic on Sex Differentials of Mortality in the USA." In Phillips and Killingray, *The Spanish Influenza Pandemic,* 202-17.

–. "The 1918 Influenza Epidemic's Effects on Sex Differentials in Mortality in the United States." *Population and Development Review* 26,3 (2000): 565-81.

Olson, D.R., L. Simonsen, P.J. Edelson, and S.S. Morse. "Epidemiological Evidence of an Early Wave of the 1918 Influenza Pandemic in New York City." *Proceedings of the National Academy of Sciences of the United States of America* 102,31 (2005): 11059-63.

Osborne, John B. "Preparing for the Pandemic: City Boards of Health and the Arrival of Cholera in Montreal, New York, and Philadelphia in 1832." *Urban History Review* 36,2 (Spring 2008): 29-42.

Osterholm, M.T. "Preparing for the Next Pandemic." *Foreign Affairs* 84,4 (2005): 24-37.

Patterson, K.D., and G.F. Pyle. "The Geography and Mortality of the 1918 Influenza Pandemic." *Bulletin of the History of Medicine* 65 (1991): 4-21.

Phillips, Howard "The Re-Appearing Shadow of 1918: Trends in the Historiography of the 1918-19 Influenza Pandemic." *Canadian Bulletin of Medical History* 21,1 (2004): 121-34.

Pierre-Deschênes, Claudine. "Santé publique et organisation de la profession médicale au Québec, 1870-1918." *Revue d'histoire de l'Amérique française* 35,3 (December 1981): 335-75.

Pope, Mara. "The Essence of Altruism: The Spirit of Volunteerism in Hamilton during the 1918 Influenza Pandemic." In Herring, *Anatomy of a Pandemic*, 105-19.

Quiney, Linda J. "Borrowed Halos: Canadian Teachers as Voluntary Aid Detachment Nurses during the Great War." *Historical Studies in Education* 15,1 (Spring 2003): 78-99.

–. "'Filling the Gaps': Canadian Voluntary Nurses, the 1917 Halifax Explosion, and the Influenza Epidemic of 1918." *Canadian Bulletin of Medical History* 19,2 (2002): 351-74.

Ray, Arthur J. "Diffusion of Diseases in the Western Interior of Canada, 1830-1850." *Geographical Review* 66,2 (April 1976): 139-57.

Reid, A.H., and J.K. Taubenberger. "The Origin of the 1918 Pandemic Influenza Virus: A Continuing Enigma." *Journal of General Virology* 84 (2003): 2285-92.

Robert, Jean-Claude. "The City of Wealth and Death: Urban Mortality in Montreal, 1821-1871." In *Essays in the History of Canadian Medicine,* ed. Wendy Mitchinson and Janice Dickin McGinnis, 18-38. Toronto: McClelland and Stewart, 1988.

Sattenspiel, Lisa, and D. Ann Herring. "Simulating the Effect of Quarantine on the Spread of the 1918-19 Flu in Central Canada." *Bulletin of Mathematical Biology* 65,1 (2003): 1-26.

–. "Structured Epidemic Models and the Spread of Influenza in the Central Canadian Subarctic." *Human Biology* 70,1 (1998): 91-115.

Sattenspiel, Lisa, Ann Mobarry, and D. Ann Herring. "Modeling the Influence of Settlement Structure on the Spread of Influenza among Communities." *American Journal of Human Biology* 12 (2000): 736-48.

Stuart, Meryn. "War and Peace: Professional Identities and Nurses' Training, 1914-1930." In *Challenging Professions: Historical and Contemporary Perspectives on Women's Professional Work,* ed. Elizabeth Smyth, Sandra Acker, Paula Bourne, and Alison Prentice, 171-93. Toronto: University of Toronto Press, 1999.

Taubenberger, J.K., and D.M. Morens. "1918 Influenza: The Mother of All Pandemics." *Emerging Infectious Diseases* 12,1 (2006): 15-22.

Taubenberger, J.K., A.H. Reid, and T.G. Fanning. "Le virus retrouvé de la grippe espagnole." *Dossier pour la science* 50 (2006): 52-59.

Taubenberger, J.K., Ann H. Reid, Raina M. Lourens, Ruixwe Wang, Guozhong Jin, and Thomas G. Fanning. "Characterization of the 1918 Influenza Virus Polymerase Genes." *Nature* 437 (6 October 2005): 889-93.

Tétreault, Martin. "Les maladies de la misère: aspects de la santé publique à Montréal (1880-1914)." *Revue d'histoire de l'Amérique française* 36,4 (None 1983): 507-26.

Venus, Cheryl, and Kiran Persaud. "Hamilton's Epidemic Wave." In Herring, *Anatomy of a Pandemic*, 31-40.

THESES AND DISSERTATIONS

Farmer, Tracy. "Putting Health in Its Place: Women's Perceptions and Experiences of Health in Hamilton's North End." PhD diss., Department of Anthropology, McMaster University, 2004.

Moffat, Tina. "Infant Mortality in an Aboriginal Community: A Historical and Biocultural Analysis." Master's thesis, Department of Anthropology, McMaster University, 1992.

Quiney, Linda J. "'Assistant Angels': Canadian Women as Voluntary Aid Detachment Nurses during and after the Great War, 1914-1930." PhD thesis, Department of History, University of Ottawa, 2002.

Riegler, Natalie M. "The Work No and Networks of Jean I. Gunn, Superintendent of Nurses, Toronto General Hospital, 1913-1941: A Presentation of Some Issues in Nursing during Her Lifetime, 1882-1941." PhD thesis, Department of Education, University of Toronto, 1992.

Contributors

Francis Dubois (Master's in geography from the Université de Montréal) has been a researcher with the Office des personnes handicapées du Québec since 2008. He is currently implementing and evaluating a program titled Equals in Every Respect: Because Rights Are Meant to Be Exercised, as well as carrying out a study of secondary conditions experienced by disabled persons.

Magda Fahrni is an associate professor in the Department of History at the Université du Québec à Montréal, where she teaches women's history, family history, and the history of twentieth-century Quebec and Canada. She is the author of the prize-winning *Household Politics: Montreal Families and Postwar Reconstruction* (2005) and the co-author of the third edition of *Canadian Women: A History* (2011). With Robert Rutherdale, she co-edited *Creating Postwar Canada: Community, Diversity, and Dissent* (2008).

Denis Goulet, adjunct professor at the University of Sherbrooke's Faculté de médecine et des sciences de la santé, specializes in the history of health and medicine. He has published numerous books and articles on the history of medicine in Canada, notably *Histoire de la neurologie, Histoire de la dermatologie au Québec, Histoire de la néphrologie au Québec, Histoire de la gastro-entérologie au Québec,* and *La Faculté de médecine et des sciences de la santé de l'Université de Sherbrooke 1966-2006.* He also teaches the history of medicine and the sociology of health in various medical faculties.

Ann Herring is professor of anthropology at McMaster University, Hamilton, Ontario. Her research centres on the anthropology of infectious disease and on emerging infections and the social circumstances that encourage them to flourish. Her current research interests include the health of Aboriginal people in Canada, nineteenth- and twentieth-century epidemics, and the concept of syndemics. Recent publications include *Plagues and Epidemics: Infected Spaces Past and Present* (edited with A.C. Swedlund, 2010), "The Coming Plague of Avian Influenza" (with S. Lockerbie, 2010), and "Syndemics in Global Health" (with M. Singer, J. Littleton, and M. Rock, 2011).

Mark Humphries is an assistant professor in the Department of History at Memorial University of Newfoundland. He has published widely on the social and military history of the Great War and the history of medicine in Canada including a monograph titled *The Last Plague: Spanish Influenza and the Development of Public Health in Canada* (2012). His article "War's Long Shadow: Masculinity, Medicine, and the Gendered Politics of Trauma, 1914-1939" won the 2010 Canadian Historical Review Prize.

Esyllt W. Jones is the author of *Influenza 1918: Disease, Death and Struggle in Winnipeg* (2007), which was awarded the Canadian Historical Association Clio Prize for Prairie History. Her work on influenza focuses on the relationship between the pandemic, family life, and social inequality, as well as questions of embodiment and mourning. She is currently researching the emergence of medicare in Saskatchewan from a transnational perspective. She is an associate professor in the Department of History at the University of Manitoba, where she teaches the history of health and disease, local history, and the history of social movements.

Mary-Ellen Kelm is the Canada Research Chair in history, medicine and society in the History Department at Simon Fraser University. Her most recent book, *A Wilder West: Rodeo in Western Canada,* was published by UBC Press in 2011. She is currently writing about the history of Aboriginal health research in North America.

Heather MacDougall is an associate professor at the University of Waterloo, specializing in Canadian history of medicine and health care. Her most recent publication, *Making Canadian Medicare: Healthcare in Canada, 1914-2007,* can be viewed at www.civilization.ca/medicare. She is

currently researching the history of anti-vaccination discourse and rhetoric, and its impact on contemporary public policy.

Linda Quiney teaches Canadian and medical history with the Department
of History at the University of British Columbia. Her research interests
focus on women's voluntary efforts in the area of nursing and medical
services during the First World War. She has published on the work of
Canadian volunteer nursing in the Great War, as well as the role of women's
wartime voluntary efforts as a contribution to the peacetime mandate of
the Canadian Red Cross.

Karen Slonim recently completed her PhD in anthropology at the
University of Missouri-Columbia. She currently teaches at McMaster
University and works as a consultant in issues relating to health at DPRA
Canada. Her work on the determinants of health, evolutionary medicine,
political economy, syndemics, and informal networks of care research helps
us to understand the ways in which humans are transformed by and
transform the parasitic pathogens with which they interact.

Jean-Pierre Thouez was a professor at the Université de Montréal and a
research fellow in various hospitals until his retirement in 2005. A pioneer
in the study of medical geography in Canada, he has published numerous
papers and books that explore the relationships between human health
and the environment as well as the influence of territory on aging.

Index

Printed and bound in Canada by Friesens
Set in Garamond by Artegraphica Design Co. Ltd.
Copy editor: Deborah Kerr
Proofreader: Jean Wilson
Indexer: Dianne Tiefensee